THE
STREETMEDIC'S
HANDBOOK

THE STREETMEDIC'S HANDBOOK

Owen T. Traynor, MD
Emergency Medicine Services Fellow
University of Pittsburgh
Associate Medical Director for
    Paramedic Education
Center for Emergency Medicine of
    Western Pennsylvania
Pittsburgh, PA

Patrick R. Coonan, RN, EdD, CEN, EMT-CC
Assistant Dean, Advanced Practice
Director, Critical Care Program
Columbia University School of Nursing
New York, NY

Thomas J. Rahilly, MS, EMT-CC
Chief Instructor
Nassau County Emergency Medical Service
    Academy
Plainview, NY

Jonathan S. Rubens, MD, FACEP
Attending Physician, Emergency Center
Medical Director
St. Mary's Hospital
Athens, GA

 F. A. DAVIS COMPANY • Philadelphia

F. A. Davis Company
1915 Arch Street
Philadelphia, PA 19103

Printed in Canada

Last digit indicates print number: 10 9 8

Publisher: Jean-François Vilain
Editor: Lynn Borders Caldwell
Production Editor: Marianne Fithian
Cover Designer: Louis J. Forgione

As new scientific information becomes available through basic and clinical research, recommended treatments and drug therapies undergo changes. The authors and publisher have done everything possible to make this book accurate, up to date, and in accord with accepted standards at the time of publication. The authors, editors, and publisher are not responsible for errors or omissions or for consequences from application of the book, and make no warranty, expressed or implied, in regard to the contents of the book. Any practice described in this book should be applied by the reader in accordance with professional standards of care used in regard to the unique circumstances that may apply in each situation. The reader is advised always to check product information (package inserts) for changes and new information regarding dose and contraindications before administering any drug. Caution is especially urged when using new or infrequently ordered drugs.

Library of Congress Cataloging-in-Publication Data
The streetmedic's handbook / Owen T. Traynor . . . [et al.].
    p.   cm.
  Includes bibliographical references and index.
  ISBN 0-8036-0012-7 (alk. paper)
  1. Medical emergencies—Handbooks, manuals. etc. 2. Emergency medical technicians—Handbooks, manuals, etc. I. Traynor, Owen T. II. Title: Street medic's handbook.
  [DNLM: 1. Emergencies—handbooks. 2. Emergency Medical Technicians—handbooks. WB 39 S915 1995]
RC86.8.S77 1996
616.02'5—dc20
DNLM/DLC   95-13932
for Library of Congress   CIP

This book is dedicated to the providers of prehospital emergency medical services everywhere who must be at their best when conditions and circumstances are at their worst.

FOREWORD

The advances in emergency medical services systems in the past 25 years have been extraordinarily dramatic. We have gone from patients withering and dying, while waiting excessive amounts of time for help to arrive or simply being whisked away in the back of police cruisers without even basic care, to timely response by well-trained paramedics. These healthcare professionals arrive at the scene of a medical crisis with the skills, drugs, and equipment to initially treat medical emergencies that are beyond the expertise of many physicians.

Advanced level Emergency Medical Technicians (EMTs) are expected to know more now than ever before to properly carry out their more sophisticated responsibilities. They must quickly assess and treat almost any medical, surgical, or behavioral emergency that can occur to a human being—from the first days of life in the womb over a lifetime that can span more than 100 years. It is difficult to maintain this immense knowledge base, particularly for those ailments that the EMT does not treat on a daily basis.

The Streetmedic's Handbook serves many roles—peripheral brain, review text, continuing education tool, and so on. Most importantly, however, you will find it has lasting value as a quick, reliable reference. This text deserves to be an essential part of the equipment of every advanced level EMT. What differentiates this text from others is its practical streetwise approach to the common problems facing prehospital providers. Two medics carrying this text are almost as effective as a three-person crew.

As the list of prehospital drugs and allowed interventions continues to grow, reference manuals become essential. This text will make a positive contribution in providing just the mechanism necessary for medics to learn and relearn the important job of caring for another individual during a medical emergency. Take the time to make use of the material in this book. You will find it an indispensable supplement to the skills that make you an essential component of the emergency health system.

Paul Paris, MD, FACEP
Professor and Chief, Division of Emergency Medicine
University of Pittsburgh School of Medicine Medical Director
Bureau of Emergency Medical Services, Chief Medical Officer
Center for Emergency Medicine
Pittsburgh, Pennsylvania

INTRODUCTION

Welcome to *The Streetmedic's Handbook!*

This book is designed to be a concise, pocket-size reference for advanced level Emergency Medical Technicians (EMTs). Its approach is unlike any other book because it identifies the 45 most important and common prehospital emergencies, then tells you how to manage each emergency. It is written the way patients present to you—in a problem-oriented format.

No other book organizes as much practical information as *The Streetmedic's Handbook*. Its problem-oriented approach helps you to evaluate and treat a patient quickly. Most other EMT books review anatomy and physiology first, then tell you what problems may be present. Although this is an excellent method for understanding emergencies, it is not the best way to evaluate and treat quickly, especially because emergency medical problems do not typically present themselves in a system-related manner.

This book can be used by the experienced, "streetwise" medic, especially during recertification and in-service training. It is also excellent for first-time students, because it allows them to match patient assessment to clinical management and helps them take what they are learning in the classroom directly to the field.

Each of the 45 prehospital emergencies in the book contains the following components:
- Statement of the problem
- Thought-provoking questions (with answers) that start the paramedic thinking while en route to the emergency.
- Differential diagnosis for the problem
- Summary of key historical information to obtain
- Key physical examination findings
- Suggested therapy
- References for further study
- Space for personal notes

Only the essential information is given for each emergency so that you can learn or review quickly—either during "down time" or en route. Use the blank space at the end of each emergency to jot down any additional information that you already know or have learned so that it is easy to find the next time you need it.

In addition, the following special sections help you review other important, related topics:

- Special situations such as multiple casualty incidents, infectious disease exposure, and the pediatric patient
- Important procedures such as medication administration and airway management interventions
- Medicolegal documentation, including oral and written case presentation
- Emergency medications commonly used by paramedics
- Commonly prescribed medications, likely to be used by patients
- An appendix, containing useful charts and tables such as the Glasgow Coma Scale and the Trauma Score

A detailed index appears at the end of the book, allowing you to find specfic information as quickly as possible.

One of the greatest challenges in writing this book was the difficulty in making it appropriate for EMTs, both nationally and internationally, because each Emergency Medical Service (EMS) system has different needs, resources, and approaches to prehospital emergency care. We state the therapy we recommend, even if controversial, as well as other currently used options. Although we may be criticized for not taking a firm stand on certain issues, we have provided one place where EMS providers can easily find out about other patient care options. Please keep in mind, however, that this information must only be used when authorized by medical control or to change existing protocols through the appropriate medical advisory committee or board in a particular EMS system. It does not constitute authority to deviate from the off- or on-line medical direction of an Advanced Life Support system.

Not every medic has the discipline to become a true learner, but for those who possess the traits of a streetmedic, this book was written for you. We wish you continued success in your profession and encourage you to improve your knowledge and patient care skills. It is also important to make sure you share this knowledge with those around you. All streetmedics bear the responsibility of ensuring that the system we work in continually improves its quality of care.

We would appreciate hearing your thoughts on this book. Please tell us what you like or what can be improved. Write to us in care of Lynn Borders Caldwell, F. A. Davis Company, 1915 Arch Street, Philadelphia, PA 19103 or e-mail us at strt medic@aol.com.

Owen T. Traynor
Patrick R. Coonan
Thomas J. Rahilly
Jonathan S. Rubens

ACKNOWLEDGMENTS

The authors would like to express their sincere appreciation to
- The many contributors who provided a wealth of practical information that will make this book a valuable tool for the streetmedic
- The staff of the F. A. Davis Company, particularly Lynn Borders Caldwell, Ona Kosmos, Herb Powell, Peter Faber, and Marianne Fithian
- The following manuscript reviewers who provided many thoughtful comments and criticisms

Jane E. June, RN, MSN
Program Coordinator
EMT—Intermediate/Paramedic Programs
Quinsigamond Community College
Worcester, Massachusetts

Kay Lewis, RN, PhD
Chair
Emergency Medical Technology Program
Phoenix College
Phoenix, Arizona

Gregg Margolis, BS, EMT-P
Associate Director of Education
Center for Emergency Medicine of Western Pennsylvania
Pittsburgh, Pennsylvania

James L. Paturas, EMT-P
Director
Emergency Medical Services
Bridgeport Hospital
Bridgeport, Connecticut

Erika Reich, RN
Program Director
Paramedic Institute
Torrance, California

Donnie S. Sides, NREMT-P
ALS Instructor
North Carolina Office of Emergency Medical Services
Raleigh, North Carolina

Amy M. Tremel, BS, EMT-P
Emergency Medical Service Education Specialist
Center for Emergency Medicine of Western Pennsylvania
Pittsburgh, Pennsylvania

- Our family members and friends who gave us the encouragement and support that was needed to complete the book

CONTRIBUTORS

David R. Adamovich, EdD, FACSM, EMT-P
Vice President
EMS Consultants, Inc.
Farmingdale, NY

Deborah Barclay, NREMT-P
Coordinator of Medical Education
Center for Emergency Medicine of Western Pennsylvania
Pittsburgh, PA

Douglas Barnaby, EMT-P
Emergency Department Technician
North Shore University Hospital
Manhasset, NY

Michael Baumann, MD
Emergency Medicine Resident Physician
University of Pittsburgh
Affiliated Residency in Emergency Medicine
Pittsburgh, PA

Bernard Beckerman, MD, FACEP
Emergency Medicine Attending Physician
North Shore University Hospital
Manhasset, NY

Russell Bradley, MD
Emergency Medicine Resident Physician
Allegheny General Hospital
Combined Emergency Medicine/Internal Medicine Residency
Pittsburgh, PA

Clifton W. Callaway, MD
Emergency Medicine Resident Physician
University of Pittsburgh
Affiliated Residency in Emergency Medicine
Pittsburgh, PA

Bruce M. Cohn, JD, EMT-CC
Instructor
Nassau County Emergency Medical Service Academy
Plainview, NY

Elizabeth Cohn, RN, EMT-CC
Emergency Nurse
Department of Emergency Medicine
North Shore University Hospital
Manhasset, NY

Patrick R. Coonan, RN, EdD, CEN, EMT-CC
Assistant Dean, Advanced Practice
Director, Critical Care Program
Columbia University School of Nursing
New York, NY

Alan Cooper, MA, EMT-P
Director
Center for Emergency Training and Development
Manhasset, NY

Roy E. Cox Jr., BS, EMT-P
Patient Care Coordinator
Department of Public Safety
Bureau of Emergency Medical Services
City of Pittsburgh, PA

Gary T. Ferrucci, EMT-CC
Instructor Coordinator
Nassau County Emergency Medical Service Academy
Plainview, NY

John Fitzwilliam, BS, BA, EMT-CC
Ex-Chief
Bethpage New York Fire Department
Lieutenant
Emergency Ambulance Bureau
Police Department
Nassau County, NY

Deepi Goyal, MD
Emergency Medicine Resident Physician
University of Pittsburgh
Affiliated Residency in Emergency Medicine
Pittsburgh, PA

Myles Greenberg, MD
Emergency Medicine Resident Physician
University of Pittsburgh
Affiliated Residency in Emergency Medicine
Pittsburgh, PA

Donna M. Harrison, MD
Emergency Medicine Resident Physician
University of Pittsburgh
Affiliated Residency in Emergency Medicine
Pittsburgh, PA

Lorraine Hartnet, MD, FACEP
Emergency Department Attending Physician
North Shore University Hospital
Manhasset, NY

Micelle Haydel, MD
Emergency Medicine Resident Physician
University of Pittsburgh
Affiliated Residency in Emergency Medicine
Pittsburgh, PA

Rebecca Humes, MD
Emergency Medicine Resident Physician
University of Pittsburgh
Affiliated Residency in Emergency Medicine
Pittsburgh, PA

Carol Johnson, RN, MSN
Emergency Nurse
Department of Emergency Medicine
The Mercy Hospital of Pittsburgh
Pittsburgh, PA

Dean Johnson, MD
Emergency Medicine Resident Physician
University of Pittsburgh
Affiliated Residency in Emergency Medicine
Pittsburgh, PA

Scott Jolley, MD
Emergency Medicine Resident Physician
University of Pittsburgh
Affiliated Residency in Emergency Medicine
Pittsburgh, PA

Donall E. Kenny, EMT-P
Paramedic
Oakland Veterans Administration Medical Center
Pittsburgh, PA

Robert L. Kerner, Jr., RN, CEN, EMT-CC
Instructor Coordinator
Nassau County Emergency Medical Service Academy
Plainview, NY

R. Todd Kiskaddon, MD
Emergency Medicine Attending Physician
Yale University School of Medicine
New Haven, CT

Gregg Margolis, MS, NREMT-P
Associate Director of Education
Center for Emergency Medicine of Western Pennsylvania
Pittsburgh, PA

Kemedy K. McQuillen, MD
Pediatric Resident Physician
Childrens Hospital of Pittsburgh Pediatric Residency
Pittsburgh, PA

Thomas Pangburn, MD
Emergency Medicine Resident Physician
University of Pittsburgh
Affiliated Residency in Emergency Medicine
Pittsburgh, PA

Thomas Platt, NREMT-P
Coordinator of Emergency Medical Service Education
Center for Emergency Medicine of Western Pennsylvania
Pittsburgh, PA

Thomas J. Rahilly, MS, EMT-CC
Chief Instructor
Nassau County Emergency Medical Service Academy
Plainview, NY

Jonathan S. Rubens, MD, FACEP
Attending Physician, Emergency Center
Medical Director
St. Mary's Hospital
Athens, GA

Ritu Sahni, MD
Emergency Medicine Resident Physician
University of Pittsburgh
Affiliated Residency in Emergency Medicine
Pittsburgh, PA

Mark Scheatzle, MD
Emergency Medicine Resident Physician
University of Pittsburgh
Affiliated Residency in Emergency Medicine
Pittsburgh, PA

Andrew W. Stern, MPA, MA(PS), NREMT-P
Senior Paramedic
Town of Colonie
Emergency Medical Services
Albany, NY

Walt Stoy, PhD, NREMT-P
Director of Education
Center for Emergency Medicine of Western Pennsylvania
Pittsburgh, PA

Owen T. Traynor, MD
Emergency Medicine Resident Physician
University of Pittsburgh
Affiliated Residency in Emergency Medicine
Pittsburgh, PA

John Wilkinson, MD
Emergency Medicine Resident Physician
Henry Ford Residency in Emergency Medicine
Detroit, MI

Mike Yee, BS, EMT-P
Paramedic
Department of Public Safety
Bureau of Emergency Medical Services
City of Pittsburgh, PA

CONTENTS

SECTION I

Commonly Encountered Problems

CHAPTER 1

Abdominal Pain
Jonathan S. Rubens, MD, FACEP

Presentation

The multiple etiologies of abdominal pain range from the life-threatening to the trivial. The pain is very subjective, and the neuroanatomy of the systems involved makes abdominal pain one of the most difficult entities to diagnose. Visceral pain (from the walls of hollow organs and the capsules of solid organs) tends to be vague, poorly localized, and is often described as "crampy," "gaslike," or "dull." Frequently associated symptoms of visceral pain are autonomic responses that produce nausea, vomiting, pallor, and diaphoresis. By contrast, somatic pain (from the peritoneum and diaphragm) is better localized and described as sharper.

Immediate Concerns

- **What is the status of the patient's airway?** If a patient is vomiting, is he alert enough to protect his airway?
- **What is the patient's hemodynamic status?** Are signs or symptoms of shock present? If so, immediate resuscitative measures should be instituted.

  NOTE: Patients with aortic dissections or rupture are often initially hypertensive. Once the aorta has ruptured, they rapidly become hypotensive.

Important History

- **What is the onset and duration of the pain?** Abdominal pain that begins abruptly and is severe can indicate serious disorders, such as a vascular catastrophe, perforation of a hollow organ, or a kidney stone. Abdominal pain that has a slower onset and is less severe usually suggests inflammatory causes, such as cholecystitis, appendicitis, and diverticulitis.

- **Where is the pain and does it move?** The location of pain and its pattern of radiation or migration, or both, can give clues to the underlying etiology. For instance, the pain of appendicitis classically begins as central abdominal pain that moves to the right lower quadrant (RLQ). Similarly, the pain of acute cholecystitis often starts in the midepigastrium and moves to the right upper quadrant (RUQ).
- **What are the quality and severity of the pain?** Pain that comes in waves, like cramps, is known as colicky pain. Colicky pain results from the intermittent contraction of smooth-muscled hollow organs like the gallbladder, intestines, and uterus.
- **Are there any symptoms associated with the pain?** Does the patient give a recent history of nausea, vomiting, or diarrhea? Hematemesis, melena, or hematochezia may suggest bleeding in the gastrointestinal (GI) tract. Dysuria, hematuria, and urinary frequency may implicate a urologic source of pain. Cardiopulmonary symptoms must always be elicited because pulmonary embolism, pneumonia, and acute myocardial infarction manifest abdominal pain as the primary symptom.
- **Current and past medical history?** This may significantly influence the assessment of the patient with abdominal pain. Patients often have experienced a similar pain. Prior abdominal surgery can be important in offering specific evidence for or against a specific cause of pain. Menstrual and gynecologic histories are especially important.

Differential Diagnosis

To narrow the diagnoses responsible for a patient's complaint of acute abdominal pain, a regional approach may be employed. Such an approach recognizes that many entities may cause pain in more than one area; for example, the location and length of the appendix is highly variable, and therefore may cause pain in any abdominal quadrant.

RIGHT UPPER QUADRANT

- **Pneumonia** can be a cause of abdominal pain. Pain is usually referred from irritation of the diaphragm from pleural fluid or inflammation. In particular, children with pneumonia often present with abdominal pain as the chief complaint. Pneumonia should be suspected in the patient with upper respiratory complaints in addition to the complaint of abdominal pain, particularly if there is a history of recent upper respiratory infection (URI), respiratory disease, or sputum production. The appreciation of a fever, auscultation of rhonchi or rales, and even the detection of wheezing may help in establishing this as a potential cause of the patient's discomfort.

- The pain from **pulmonary embolism** likewise can cause abdominal complaints because of pleura irritation from the infarcted area of lung. Patients often have pleuritic pain but this can be referred to the diaphragm if the lower segments of the lung are involved. Complaints of shortness of breath, hemoptysis, and concurrent chest pain should be elicited to help make this diagnosis.

- *Liver.* **Hepatitis** usually occurs after an incubation period of 1 to several weeks. Patients may or may not have a history of exposure to the viruses that cause it or may have a history of risks of such exposure. In acute viral hepatitis, the early symptoms or prodrome (signs and symptoms that preceded an illness) can be quite variable and include anorexia, nausea and vomiting, fatigue, generalized malaise, and alterations in olfaction and taste sensations. Low-grade fevers are common. Patients may complain of dark "Coca-Cola"-colored urine and "clay-colored" stools before onset of jaundice. It is usually with the onset of jaundice that the liver becomes enlarged and tender and may cause RUQ pain and discomfort.

- Right upper quadrant pain due to **heart failure** is actually caused by a similar mechanism: venous system pressures behind the failing right ventricle rise, causing congestion of the hepatic vessels and occasionally RUQ pain. Look for signs and symptoms of congestive heart failure as a clue to this diagnosis. Other primary hepatic diseases, including infection or abscess and cirrhosis, can cause RUQ pain.

- *Duodenum.* The most common symptom of **peptic ulcers** is pain. The pain is usually sharp or burning and gnawing in character. Generally the pain is epigastric, but approximately 10% of patients have RUQ pain, some with radiation to the back. There is a history of pain that occurs from 90 minutes to 3 hours after eating and awakens the patient at night. It may be relieved by eating or taking antacids, and this can be helpful in making the diagnosis. Abrupt, severe pain with a rigid, quiet abdomen is characteristic of ulcer perforation. In addition, ulcer disease can be a source of GI bleeding, as indicated by hematemesis, hematochezia (blood in the stool), or melena.

- *Gallbladder.* Symptoms of gallbladder disease are usually due to inflammation, obstruction, or infection. Biliary colic is the most characteristic symptom of gallbladder disease. The pain, due to increased bile duct pressure and distention of the gallbladder, is often severe. It is an aching steady RUQ pain with frequent radiation to the shoulder, back, and scapular areas. Pain usually begins suddenly and may persist for hours. A positive Murphy sign (pain produced by deep inspiration or cough during subcostal palpation of the RUQ on examination) is highly specific for this disease. Patients are usually anorectic and nauseated. Vomiting is common. Biliary colic may be associated with eating a large or particularly fatty meal. If there is a fever or chills, cholecystitis (inflammation or infection) should be suspected.

- *Heart.* **Acute myocardial infarction** pain, particularly that of inferior wall myocardial infarctions, can be referred to the epigastrium and upper abdomen. This diagnosis should always be suspected in any patient with any cardiac risk factor, including, some say, all patients older than 35 years of age. Always elicit a cardiac history and signs and symptoms in any patient with upper abdominal pain.

- *Pancreas.* **Pancreatitis** pain can vary from mild and vague to severe and intolerable. The pain is usually steady and boring and located anywhere from the epigastric area to the RUQ and peribilical areas. Pain may be worse when the patient is supine. Nausea and vomiting are common. Patients will usually appear distressed and have a low-grade fever and marked abdominal tenderness. In severe cases, the abdomen may appear rigid, and the patient may present with tachycardia and hypotension. Ten percent of patients also have pulmonary findings (rales, effusions). Pain often seems out of proportion to the physical examination. Bowel sounds may be diminished or absent, and a bluish discoloration around the umbilicus (Cullen's sign) may occur as a result of hemoperitoneum. Similarly, a bruising discoloration may be appreciated at the flanks (Turner's sign). If either of the latter signs are present they are indicative of severe necrotizing pancreatitis, a condition from which many patients will not recover.

- *Kidney.* Pain from a **kidney stone**, due to distention of the proximal collecting system or the renal capsule, may be referred to the RUQ. The pain is usually steady but may be colicky in nature. The pain of a kidney stone often radiates to the lower abdomen, flank, or the testes or labia. A history of frequent urination, hematuria, or oliguria and acute onset of pain are associated with renal colic. Patients with a prior history of this disease will usually know what is wrong. These patients characteristically "cannot get comfortable" and writhe or pace owing to pain.

In contrast, the symptoms of pylonephritis (kidney infection) develop over several hours to days. These patients will usually be febrile, have rigors (shaking chills), and nausea and vomiting. Urinary complaints include dysuria, frequent urination, hematuria, and urgency. Patients may have upper quadrant pain and generally have marked tenderness on deep palpation in these areas and over the costovertebral angles (where the vertebrae and ribs connect).

- Another potential cause of RUQ pain includes: retrocecal appendicitis (see following discussion).

RIGHT LOWER QUADRANT PAIN

- **Aneurysm** and **dissection of the aorta** and other large arteries in the abdomen can cause pain primarily by compression of adjacent structures. Acute dissection usually presents as sudden onset of severe, sharp, or "tearing" pain. The pain may be anywhere along the route the aorta travels, including the mid to lower abdomen, and may radiate to the back. As the dissection progresses so might the pain. These patients may have a history of syncope, diaphoresis, or extremity weakness. Initially, these patients are generally hypertensive; however, hypotension, loss of distal pulses, and mottling of the lower extremities may soon ensue. An enlarging, tender, pulsatile mass in the abdomen is the most ominous physical finding of an impending aneurysmal rupture.

- *Appendix.* **Acute appendicitis** is an ailment most patients with abdominal pain fear and is likely to be the reason for an emergency medical call. Appendicitis is classically a diagnosis made by history and examination. The typical sequence of symptoms includes diffuse periumbilical pain, anorexia, and nausea and vomiting, followed by more well-defined RLQ pain. Given the variability of the location and size of the appendix, the pain of appendicitis can be felt in any quadrant, making the diagnosis of this disease more challenging. Thus, this diagnosis should always be suspected in anyone with abdominal pain and an appendix. Diagnostic clues include a history of anorexia, localized tenderness, rebound tenderness, rigidity, and guarding.
- *Bladder and Prostate.* Disorders of the lower urinary tract, in particular **cystitis** and **prostatitis**, are relatively common and can all produce lower abdominal pain. Patients with cystitis usually have symptoms of urinary frequency, urgency and dysuria with occasional hematuria. Suprapubic or back pain, or pain in both locations, may also be present. Patients may give a history of change in the color or odor of their urine. In contrast, patients with prostatitis may have all of the above urinary symptoms but usually have chills, fever, varying degrees of obstruction to urination and usually appear acutely ill.
- *Pelvic Organs.* Pelvic inflammatory disease (PID), ectopic pregnancy, ovarian cyst, Mittleschmertz, tubo-ovarian abscess (see Chapter 35, Pelvic Pain).
- *Ureter.* Ureteral stone (see Kidney Stone).
- **Other less common causes** of RLQ pain include:
    External genitalia — testicular torsion and trauma
    Small bowel — enteritis, Meckel's diverticulum
    Large bowel — cecal diverticulitis, perforation

LEFT UPPER QUADRANT PAIN

- *Pancreas.* **Pancreatitis** usually causes severe abdominal pain, usually epigastric, but pain may radiate to the left or right upper quadrants. This condition was previously mentioned under RUQ pain.
- *Spleen.* Traumatic injury of the spleen is a diagnosis suggested by a mechanism of injury or trauma, localized tenderness in the LUQ or rigidity of the abdomen and absent

or diminished bowel sounds. Splenic rupture can cause massive intra-abdominal hemorrhage and therefore hypotension and shock. It should be suspected in anyone with an appropriate mechanism of injury and abdominal symptoms. It is a surgical emergency.

Patients with acute mononucleosis may have splenomegaly as a complication of this illness, usually several weeks into the illness. These patients are at an increased risk of traumatic, generally not spontaneous, rupture.

- **Gastritis** or inflammation of the gastric mucosa can be a result of erosion (ie, chronic aspirin or nonsteroidal anti-inflammatory drug [such as Motrin] use) or inflammation or infection (bacterial, drug related, or radiation related). In the intensive care setting it may be caused by severe systemic trauma or stress (ie, burns, multisystem trauma, hemorrhage). Patients generally complain of nausea, burning or sharp pain, and vomiting and occasionally have hematemesis.
- **Gastric ulcer** pain can vary depending on the location— LUQ to epigastric for gastric ulcers and RUQ for duodenal ulcers. A history of relief with antacids or prior history of ulcer may be helpful in the diagnosis.
- Also consider:
    Large bowel—splenic flexure syndrome or crampy pain caused by trapped gas diverticulitis (see Left Lower Quadrant section)
    See Right Upper Quadrant pain section for discussion of the following:
    Lung—pneumonia, pulmonary embolism
    Heart—acute myocardial infarction
    Kidney—renal stone, pyelonephritis

LEFT LOWER QUADRANT PAIN

- *Descending Colon.* **Diverticular disease**, an "outpouching" of the colon, is a common disease. In **diverticulitis**, there is an inflammation of the outpouching producing LLQ pain and fever. **Diverticulosis** is often asymptomatic and the patient's primary complaint may be only GI bleeding.
- **Bowel obstruction** is an important cause of lower abdominal pain. The abdomen is usually distended and tender

and loud hyperactive bowel sounds can be heard. This condition may be a surgical emergency.

The following causes have all been discussed previously under Right Lower Quadrant pain or elsewhere in this text:

    Aortoiliac vessels—aneurysm
    Bladder and prostate—cystitis, prostatitis
    Pelvic organs—PID, ectopic pregnancy, ovarian cyst,
       Mittleschmertz, tubo-ovarian abscess
    Ureter—ureteral stone

DIFFUSE, POORLY LOCALIZED PAIN

- **Acute Gastroenteritis** is characterized by a constellation of symptoms that may include nausea, vomiting, diarrhea, abdominal cramping, and anorexia. Likewise, the character and severity of symptoms varies with the patient. Onset is usually sudden. Generally, vomiting and diarrhea are more severe than pain is. Fever, chills, and muscle aches may all be present. Occasionally the abdomen may be distended and tender with guarding. Hyperactive bowel sounds may be present.

- **Obstruction** of the small or large intestine can be caused by adhesions (from prior insults to the peritoneum, including surgeries), hernias, tumors, feces, or foreign bodies. Vomiting may appear early and obstipation, or inability to pass flatus, is frequently encountered. If the blood supply to the obstructed area of bowel becomes compromised, patients will progress from the above to steady, severe pain and may exhibit signs and symptoms of shock.

- Other diagnoses to consider include:
  - Sickle cell crisis (see Chapter 39, Sickle Cell Crisis)
  - Early appendicitis (see previous discussion)

Key Physical Examination Findings

- ABCs
- *General Appearance.* Observe for pallor and or diaphoresis. Little or no patient movement may indicate an inflamed peritoneum (patient sitting with knees to chest). Classically patients with kidney stones are very restless and unaffected by movement. A similar presentation occurs with ruptured diverticula.
- *Chest.* Listen for adventitial breath sounds, rales, or

rhonchi, which may give clues to thoracic causes of abdominal pain.

- *Abdomen.* Inspect for distention and scars. Auscultate for bowel sounds, their presence or absence; pitch, and activity. Peritoneal irritation and ileus (paralyzed intestine) generally result in decreased or absent bowel sounds versus the high-pitched, hyperactive bowel sounds associated with approximately 50% of small bowel obstructions. Palpation generally yields the most information. Localizing the area of maximal tenderness helps to narrow the diagnostic possibilities. Palpation also allows the prehospital care provider to determine the presence or absence of involuntary guarding and rebound tenderness, signs of peritoneal irritation.

Treatment Plan

- **Assess patient continually.** Vital signs should be monitored for changes or signs of shock. Consider cardiac monitoring in all patients with upper abdominal pain and be **liberal with the use of supplemental oxygen** in all patients. **Remember to protect the airway** in vomiting patients.
- **Treat shock** as appropriate (see Chapter 38, Shock).
- *Transport.* Expedite the transport of critical patients, and attempt to ensure the comfort of all patients.

Bibliography

Tintinalli JE, Krome LR, and Ruiz E (eds): Emergency Medicine: A Comprehensive Study Guide, ed 3. McGraw-Hill, New York, 1992, pp 303–336.

Trott AT: Acute Abdominal Pain. In Rosen P and Barkin RM (eds): Emergency Medicine: Concepts and Clinical Practice, ed 2. CV Mosby, St. Louis, 1988, pp 1389–1525.

Notes

CHAPTER 2

Altered Mental Status
Jonathan S. Rubens, MD, FACEP

Presentation

Altered mental status (AMS) represents not an entity unto itself but a continuum of disorders of consciousness, ranging from
mild alterations to coma. A patient may present anywhere along
this continuum.

Immediate Concerns

- **ABCs.** Airway management with cervical spine immobilization should always be the first priority. A good rule of
  thumb is to assume that any comatose patient has a cervical spine injury until proven otherwise. Assessment of
  breathing and circulatory or cardiac status complete the
  initial evaluation. Patients without an active gag reflex will
  require positive airway control to prevent aspiration. All
  patients with an AMS should receive supplemental oxygen, and any evidence of hemodynamic compromise should
  be treated aggressively. Establish intravenous access and
  administer naloxone hydrochloride (Narcan), thiamine, and
  dextrose per protocol.

Important History

- There is no unimportant source of history. The patient may
  be unreliable or unable to give the history, so other sources
  must be sought.
- All persons present should be interviewed and encouraged
  to follow the patient to the hospital in a safe manner.
- The scene should be searched for toxins (ie, food, alcohol,
  drugs, chemicals, medications, etc).
- The patient should be checked for a medic alert bracelet or
  identification cards.

Differential Diagnosis

Two mnemonics (AEIOU and TIPS) are useful in ensuring that important causes of altered mental status are not over-looked:

A — **alcohol/acidosis.** Alcohol, ethanol being the most common, also methanol, ethylene glycol (found in antifreeze), and paraldehyde, results in altered mental status from direct central nervous system depression or from the metabolic acidosis with which they are associated.

E — **epilepsy.** Epileptics are prone to seizures that would not ordinarily induce them in most individuals. The aura that precedes the seizure is character-ized by such altered mental states as olfactory, visual, auditory, or taste hallucinations.

I — **infection.** Infectious processes, meningitis, encephalitis, brain abscess, both from direct effects on the brain and from resultant fever and toxin production can cause altered mental status.

O — **overdose.** Almost all substance abuse, especially when substances are abused in large quantities, can greatly alter the patient's mental status.

U — **uremia.** Uremic patients have shifts of intracellu-lar free water that, if rapidly changed in brain cells, may precipitate changes in mental status.

T — **trauma/tumors.** Trauma resultant in subdural or acute epidural hematomas, or concussion. Space occupying lesions, neoplasms, and blood (hemor-rhages and hematomas) affect mental status by exerting increased intracranial pressure.

I — **insulin.** Hypoglycemia, hyperglycemia, and associated metabolic acidosis are common causes of a depressed sensorium that are too often misdiag-nosed as substance abuse.

P — **psychosis.** Psychiatric disorders can result in an altered mental status ranging from states of depres-sion to agitation and hostility.

S — **stroke.** Sudden blockages of cerebral blood flow can depress the mental status of the stroke victim. Space occupying lesions, neoplasms, blood (hemor-rhages and hematomas) affect mental status by exerting increased intracranial pressure.

Key Physical Examination Findings

- *Initial Assessment.* Look for signs of shock
- *Vital Signs.* Be alert for signs of hypertension and hypotension, bradycardia, and abnormal body temperature. Respiratory rates and patterns may be helpful in identifying the cause of the AMS.
- *HEENT.* Look for signs of trauma — Battle's sign (late sign), hematomas, lacerations, raccoon eyes. Check for pupillary reaction and eye movements. Check breath for odors: alcohol and the acetone (fruity) smell of diabetic ketoacidosis.
- *Skin.* Inspect for needle marks, cyanosis, bites, stings, or rashes. Relative hypothermia is especially significant in the elderly and the very young.
- *Neurologic Examination.* Observe for abnormal respiratory pattern, AVPU mental status (Alert, responsive to Verbal or Painful stimuli, Unresponsive), facial asymmetry, pupil size and reaction, extra ocular movements and nystagmus, motor abnormalities, and abnormal posturing.

Treatment Plan

Treatment of the patient with altered mental status is one of the few situations where the prehospital care provider may be called upon to begin treatment of the patient before completion of a full examination.

- **Immobilize the cervical spine** if a mechanism of injury indicates a need.
- **Assure airway control** and **treat respiratory compromise.** Administer **oxygen** and **provide ventilatory support** as needed. Monitor O_2 saturation with pulse oximetry if available. Intubate and hyperventilate the patient if appropriate.
- **Treat shock** as appropriate (see Chapter 38, Shock).

  NOTE: The use of the MAST is controversial in patients with isolated or known head injury.
- **Establish IV access** with **0.9% NaCl or lactated Ringer's solution** KVO.
- Monitor ECG.
- **Draw blood** (red-top tube) and determine blood glucose level if possible. **Administer 50 ml of 50% dextrose IV** and 100 mg of Thiamine (IM or IV).

- Administer 1 to 2 mg of Narcan IV if a narcotic overdose is suspected.
- Transport to the appropriate ED.

Bibliography

Plum F and Posner JB: The Diagnosis of Stupor and Coma, ed 3. FA Davis, Philadelphia, 1980.
Tintinalli JE, Krome LR, and Ruiz E (eds): Emergency Medicine: A Comprehensive Study Guide, ed 3. McGraw-Hill, New York, 1992, pp 150–158.

Notes

CHAPTER 3

Anaphylaxis

Donna M. Harrison, MD

Presentation

Anaphylaxis (from the Greek "removal of protection") describes the clinical syndrome of severe hypersensitivity reaction that occurs after exposure to certain foreign substances. A wide variety of substances are known to produce anaphylactic reactions; common examples include foods, radiographic contrast material, insect stings, and medications (especially the penicillins, aspirin, and sulfa drugs). The patient with anaphylaxis may present in several different ways: with dyspnea, total airway obstruction, pruritus (itching), urticaria (hives), or dysrhythmias.

Immediate Concerns

- **What is the patient's respiratory status?** Upper airway obstruction, as a consequence of laryngeal spasm and edema, may manifest as a tightening sensation in the throat and chest, hoarseness, and stridor. Obstruction may progress to severe respiratory distress and suffocation. Urgent intervention includes high-flow oxygen administration, possibly endotracheal intubation and the administration of epinephrine and inhaled bronchodilators. In extreme cases, surgical interventions (ie, needle cricothyrotomy) may be needed to sustain life.
- **What is the patient's hemodynamic status?** Cardiovascular collapse and hypotensive shock can occur because of peripheral vasodilation and enhanced vascular permeability. Immediate resuscitation includes large-bore IV access and possibly PASG.

Important History

- **Has there been itching, hives or both, or airway problems?** Pruritus and urticaria suggest exposure by injection, inhalation, or ingestion of a substance tha﹗ ﹍ hypersensitivity reaction. This reaction is mild b﹍ progress to a more serious state rapidly. The patient's ﹍ ity to communicate implies adequate cerebral oxygenatic﹍. Inability to speak or stridor could indicate upper airway obstruction from laryngospasm or laryngeal edema.

- **Was there any witnessed exposure to an allergen?** The patient, family members, or witnesses may be able to tell you whether the patient is taking new medications or was stung by an insect, or what foods the patient was eating before the event.
- **Is there a history of allergies?** If the history is positive for allergies, determine the nature of past problems. The incidence and severity of allergic reactions are variable, depending on the antigen involved and the patient's sensitivity. Allergic manifestations may be subtle, and severity can range from mild to life-threatening. Because there is frequently no history of prior allergic reactions, symptoms may be unpredictable A high index of suspicion is necessary for early recognition and early treatment. A history of asthma may be suggestive of the person at higher risk for developing anaphylaxis. The respiratory, cardiovascular, and cutaneous systems demonstrate the major clinical manifestations of anaphylaxis.
- **Does the patient have a history of asthma?** Patients with a history of reactive airway disease often have more severe bronchospasm in anaphylaxis, and this may interfere with resuscitation.
- **What medications is the patient taking?** Anaphylaxis can occur from a variety of agents, including medications, foods, venoms, pollens, and serum. The most common medications causing anaphylaxis are penicillins, cephalosporins, tetracycline, amphotericin, and local anesthetics. Aspirin and other nonsteroidal anti-inflammatory drugs can also cause anaphylactic reactions. In addition to identifying possible allergens, obtaining a list of the patient's medications is important because ongoing treatment with beta-adrenergic blocking agents (beta blockers) may predispose patients to more severe reactions; also, these medications may make patients refractory to standard epinephrine doses.

Differential Diagnosis

The recognition of systemic anaphylaxis rests almost entirely on observation of the typical clinical features in association with temporal exposure to a foreign substance. Essential to the diagnosis of anaphylaxis is the presence of airway obstruction, hypotension, gastrointestinal symptoms, and generalized cutaneous reactions, alone or in combination.

Other conditions that share certain signs and symptoms with the anaphylactic syndrome must be excluded. These include:

- *Chronic Obstructive Pulmonary Disease.* Emphysema and chronic bronchitis account for a large percentage of paramedic calls for shortness of breath. These patients almost universally have a significant smoking history. In addition, these patients often have a history of chronic cough, sputum production, and dyspnea on exertion.
- *Asthma.* Asthma is characterized by a hypersensitivity of the tracheobronchial tree to a variety of stimuli, leading to bronchoconstriction, inflammation, and increased airway secretions.
- *Congestive Heart Failure.* This is often overlooked as a cause of wheezing, but wheezing may be the only sign of congestive heart failure. This diagnosis should be suspected in every middle-aged or older person who complains of wheezing, especially if there is also a history of heart disease.
- *Aspiration and Airway Obstruction.* Persistent localized wheezing can suggest the diagnosis of foreign body aspiration, especially in individuals who may not protect their airways well, such as young children and older debilitated patients. Foreign body aspiration, however, usually produces an obstruction of the upper airway and therefore is more likely to produce stridor (a continuous sound more prominent during inspiration than expiration) than frank wheezing.
- *Other Causes.* Pneumonia, pulmonary embolism, thoracic cage deformities, tuberculosis, and lung cancer are among the other causes of wheezing. Wheezing, however, is a less common manifestation of these disorders than those just mentioned.

- *Vasovagal Reaction.* This can also cause acute hy↳ from cardiovascular collapse, but is usually associat▵ bradycardia and resolves quickly when lying down.
- *Shock.* Various types of shock will have a presentation similar to that of anaphylaxis without airway compromise.

Key Physical Examination Findings

- *Initial Assessment.* Be alert for upper airway compromise—stridor or hoarseness may be present. Respirations may be ineffective. Look for signs of inadequate perfusion.
- *Vital Signs.* Assess for tachycardia, tachypnea, and hypotension.
- *Cutaneous Manifestations.* Observe for signs of generalized erythema (redness), urticaria (hives), and angioedema (swelling of the hands, face, neck, and upper airway). Flushing, chills, and diaphoresis may occur.
- *Lungs.* Check breath sounds for bronchoconstriction—wheezing and a prolonged expiratory phase.
- *Mental Status.* Assess for impaired mentation, altered mental status, or loss of consciousness as any of these conditions may indicate significant respiratory compromise and the need for immediate respiratory support.

Treatment Plan

- *Patient Assessment.* Perform a rapid and systematic primary survey initially and institute therapy as life-threatening problems are discovered. Prompt transport to the appropriate ED is a key intervention. A secondary survey should be performed once the primary survey and all primary survey interventions have been accomplished. Frequent reassessment of the patient in anaphylactic shock is necessary owing to the potential for worsening of the respiratory and hemodynamic status. Be prepared—potential for cardiac arrest exists.
- *Communications.* Consult with a medical control physician for guidance and institution of appropriate orders. Such consultation may prove valuable in the care of the patient in shock.
- *Airway.* Provide a high flow of oxygen via face mask. Im-

mediate **endotracheal intubation may be required** but may be extremely difficult if angioedema or severe laryngospasm is present.

- Administer **epinephrine 0.3 to 0.5 mg of a 1:1000 solution SC** (pediatric dose: 0.01 mg/kg SC, not to exceed 0.5 mg) if the patient is hemodynamically stable, or
- Administer **epinephrine 0.3 to 0.5 mg of 1:10,000 solution IV** (pediatric dose: 0.1 mg/kg IV, not to exceed 0.5 mg) if the patient is hemodynamically unstable. This dosage may be repeated every 5 minutes.
- If the patient is hemodynamically unstable, place in the **shock position** (supine with legs elevated) or use **PASG** if indicated. The use of PASG remains controversial; follow local protocol.
- Establish **large-bore IV access** with 0.9% NaCl or LR.
- Administer **diphenhydramine (Benadryl) 10 to 50 mg slow IV bolus** or deep IM injection (pediatric dose: 2 to 5 mg/kg IV or deep IM; usual dose is 10 to 30 mg).
- Administer **hydrocortisone 100 to 500 mg IV or IM** (pediatric dose: 0.16 to 1.0 mg/kg IV/IM), or
- Administer **methylprednisolone 100 to 200 mg IV/IM** (not recommended for prehospital use in pediatric patients).
- Provide **aerosolized albuterol (0.5 ml in 3 ml saline)** to manage bronchospasm. Other beta agonists such as terbutelene, metaproterenol, and (Bronchosol) may also be considered.
- **Transport expeditiously to appropriate ED**. Do not needlessly delay patient transport—expedite transport.

Bibliography

Bochner BS and Lichtenstein LM: Anaphylaxis. *N Engl J Med*, 324: 1785–1790.

Caroline NL: Anaphylaxis. In Emergency Care in the Streets, ed 4. Little, Brown & Co, Boston, 1991, pp 595–602.

Haist SA, Robbins JB, and Gomella LG (eds): Anaphylactic Reaction. In Internal Medicine on Call. Appleton & Lange, Norwalk CT, 1991, pp 22–24.

Salome JA: Anaphylaxis. In Tintinalli JE, Krome LR, and Ruiz E (eds): Emergency Medicine: A Comprehensive Study Guide, ed 3. McGraw-Hill, New York, 1992, pp 901–903.

Notes

CHAPTER 4

Bites And Envenomation

Scott Jolley, MD

Presentation

Patients who have been bitten or stung present with a wide spectrum of reactions, depending on the source and site of the injury. The vast majority of patients present with a local reaction—pain, burning, redness or other discoloration, itching, swelling, and discoloration at, or surrounding, the site of injury. Mild to moderate systemic signs and symptoms may include headache, flushing, weakness, dizziness, nausea, vomiting, fever, and sweating. There may be enlarged lymph nodes; tingling in the skin, scalp, face, and extremities; muscle twitches, arthritis, or photophobia. Others may present with more severe systemic complaints of hypotension, hypertension, tachycardia, difficulty breathing, airway obstruction, convulsions, paralysis, or massive bleeding. Other more severe conditions are hemolytic anemia, coagulation defects, renal failure, anaphylaxis, coma, and death.

Immediate Concerns

- **Is the scene safe?** Make sure that the patient and all rescue personnel are out of striking distance from the trouble-causing creature. Be sure to call the appropriate agency for help in securing the scene (ASPCA, Game Warden, etc.). If possible, have the authorities capture the insect or animal for identification and testing.
- **What is the status of the patient's airway?** Some bites can cause an acute anaphylactic reaction with severe airway compromise. Prompt recognition and intervention is required. Positive pressure ventilation, endotracheal intubation, and administration of medications may be required to maintain a patent airway and oxygenation.
- **What is the patient's hemodynamic status?** Certain tox-

ins can cause significant hypotension. Others can result in severe coagulopathy, causing uncontrollable bleeding. Hemodynamic instability, regardless of its cause, requires aggressive management. In the case of envenomation, expeditious transport to a medical facility should be considered a high priority with treatment en route.

Important History

- **Has the patient been bitten?** Has there truly been an insult? Where is it located? If the patient provides a poor or incomplete history and is in an environment where a bite or sting is possible, visually inspect the patient for the classic signs of such an injury.
- **What type of creature bit or stung the patient?** Identify unique situations such as a bite by an exotic snake or creature endemic to the specific geographic location. In many cases, emergency medical service (EMS) personnel will be the only source of vital information needed for effective treatment. Details such as whether the animal exhibited strange behavior or showed symptoms of rabies will help determine specific therapeutic interventions at the medical facility.
- **Is there a history of a previous bite or envenomation?** Occasionally, the patient may have a history of being bitten before. Previous exposure, particularly if there was a severe systemic reaction (ie, anaphylaxis or shock), may indicate that the patient is at risk for another severe reaction. Find out if the patient has had a previous reaction to the antivenom or antidote. This patient may lose consciousness or suffer an altered mental status, causing the patient to become incapable of communicating with the providers in the ED.

SYMPTOMS

Bites and envenomation have predictable symptoms that coincide with the amount and potency of the venom, site of injection, allergy to venom, progression of the ill effects of the injury, and elapsed time from the initial insult. Venom does not necessarily come from snakes or other animals. Envenomation should be considered from bees and other insects as well.

OTHER IMPORTANT CONSIDERATIONS

- *Site.* Identify the site of the bite or sting. Then, establish that the bite or sting has been accompanied by the injection of venom, follow the progression of clinical signs and symptoms. Is there streaking, redness, hives, or excessive swelling moving away from the site? These signs are particularly important as they may highlight an underlying more serious condition.
- *Time.* Identify the time of the bite or sting. This establishes a framework for expected symptoms to occur and allows you to follow progression of symptoms.
- *Bystander Interventions.* Determine the type of interventions that may have been initiated by bystanders to identify complications that may occur from harmful or non-standard therapy, or both (ie, incisions, ice, suction, wrapping).
- *Allergies.* Obtain information regarding known allergies. This information can prevent further complications resulting from treatment and can direct possible alternate therapeutic interventions.
- *Medications.* Obtain information about medications currently being taken by the patient. These may interfere with therapy or treatment medications.
- *Tetanus Status.* Question all patients about their current immunization status.

Differential Diagnosis

SNAKES

Dangerous snakes are classified as belonging to one of two families: Crotalidae (pit vipers) are commonly known as rattlesnakes, cottonmouths, and copperheads. Elapidae (coral snakes) are of the Eastern, Texan, and Arizonan varieties. The majority of bites occur between April and October and involve the upper or lower extremities. The victims tend to be males between 10 and 19 years of age.

- **Pit viper** bites have one or two fang marks and manifest local and systemic signs and symptoms. Local symptoms include pain, numbness, edema, bruising, hemorrhagic blisters, and lymphangitis (inflammation of lymphatic vessels, characterized by a red streak). Patients may experience systemic symptoms including a metallic taste; numbness (most notably around the mouth, scalp, fingers, and toes); weakness; nausea and vomiting; hypotension and bleeding from the skin, nose, or gastrointestinal tract.

- **Coral snakes** must be identified by their stripe pattern. An effective mnemonic developed for this purpose is: "red on black venom lack; red or white on yellow kill a fellow." These snakes tend to bite and chew, leaving small pinpoint bite marks. Because they have small mouths, they tend to bite fingers and toes. Their venom primarily attacks the nervous system. Patients may present early with euphoria, drowsiness, difficulty swallowing, blurry vision, slurred speech, salivation, nausea, vomiting, or weakness. Later they may present with complete motor or respiratory paralysis.

SPIDERS

The black widow (Lactrodectus) and the brown recluse (Loxosceles) are the most worrisome spider bites encountered by medical personnel. Spiders will generally leave only one set of bite marks.

- **Widow spiders** are oval shaped and dark black with red, orange, or yellow bellies. The bite of the female widow is said to secrete one of the most potent venoms harmful to humans. The bite is typically unnoticed, followed by salivation, dizziness, numbness (particularly in the soles of the feet), nausea and vomiting, diffuse muscle spasm, particularly in the back and abdomen, progressing to a rigid abdomen and pain. Symptoms come in waves and may induce hypertension or hypertensive crisis.
- **Brown spiders,** of the violin or fiddle back types, are known to have local and systemic symptoms from their bites. The bite leaves a "bullseye" type mark. Locally, the skin becomes hard, swollen, and painful. Within 1 to 2 hours local pain and erythema develops followed by a blister or vesicle over the bite that will burst in a few days, leaving a necrotic ulcer. Systemic symptoms may include fever, chills, and a scarlatini form of rash.

SCORPIONS

Centruroides exilicauda is the most dangerous species of scorpion found in the United States. They are found in Arizona, New Mexico, and parts of California, and Colorado.

Envenomation is followed by intense local pain, sensitivity to touch, pressure, or temperature and may culminate in extremity weakness. Systemic symptoms include hyperexcitability, salivation, convulsions, paralysis, and respiratory failure.

BEES, ANTS, AND WASPS

Stings most often occur on the head and neck and less commonly on hands, legs, and feet. Immediate pain followed by redness, swelling, and itching are common. Systemic signs and symptoms include shortness of breath, flushing, nausea, vomiting, hives, and fever. Anaphylaxis may occur within minutes to 2 hours and is associated with hives, shortness of breath, airway edema and increased secretions, weakness, vomiting, and hypotension. Patients often report chest tightness and the feeling of impending doom.

ANIMAL AND HUMAN BITES

These injuries commonly occur on the upper extremity and hand, especially the fingers. Other areas that may be involved include the head and neck, trunk, lower extremities, and genitalia. The majority of animal bites tend to come from dogs. Bites come in many forms from punctures to avulsions, and the common result is a crush injury with an abundance of devitalized tissue. Human bites tend to be more serious because of the virulent bacteria in the mouth. Signs and symptoms include initial evidence of a laceration and progress to redness, swelling, clear or pussy discharge, and later enlarged lymph nodes and a reduced range of motion in the joints.

OTHER OFFENDING CREATURES

Ticks, gila, caterpillars, sucking bugs, beetles, mosquitoes, biting flies, lice, fleas, mites, parasites, centipedes, millipedes, and aquatic organisms and animals are potentially anaphylactic. Whereas most of these are not as serious as those mentioned previously, all bites and stings should receive careful evaluation by EMS and other medical personnel.

Key Physical Examination Findings

- *Initial Assessment.* Assess ABCs. Look for signs of airway compromise, breathing difficulty, hemodynamic instability, or external bleeding.

- **Vitals Signs.** Assess resuscitation needs, signs and symptoms of decompensation, or progression of symptoms.
- **Site of Insult(s).** Identify the site for fang marks, stingers, swelling, redness, bleeding, bruising, or laceration. If swelling or bruising are present, measure and document the circumference or margins to permit the tracking of their progression. Remove stingers with a knife, tweezers, or razor.
- **Signs and Symptoms.** Evaluate the patient for signs and symptoms of severe envenomation or resultant anaphylaxis. These can include shortness of breath, flushing, nausea, vomiting, hives, and fever. Anaphylaxis, may occur within minutes to 2 hours and is associated with hives, shortness of breath, airway edema and increased secretions, weakness, vomiting, and hemodynamic collapse. Patients often report chest tightness and the feeling of impending doom.

Treatment Plan

GENERAL TREATMENT GUIDELINES: HEMODYNAMICALLY STABLE PATIENT

- Administer O_2 and provide **ventilatory support** as needed. Monitor O_2 saturation with pulse oximetry if available.
- Remove all constricting items, including rings and jewelry. This intervention will prevent any neurovascular constrictive compromise secondary to massive swelling.
- Loosen constrictive clothing.
- Place patient in the **shock position** (supine with legs elevated), protecting the cervical spine as indicated.
- **Treat non-life-threatening injuries** as appropriate (ie, control minor bleeding, splint fractures, etc).
- Establish **large-bore IV access** with 0.9% NaCl or LR.
- **Transport to appropriate ED**. Ensure patient comfort en route.

GENERAL TREATMENT GUIDELINES: HEMODYNAMICALLY UNSTABLE PATIENT

- Administer O_2 and provide **ventilatory support** as needed. Monitor O_2 saturation with pulse oximetry if available.
- Remove all constricting items, including rings and jewelry. This intervention will prevent any neurovascular constrictive compromise secondary to massive swelling.

- Loosen constrictive clothing.
- Place patient in the **shock position** (supine with legs elevated) or use PASG if indicated. The use of **PASG** is controversial; follow local protocol.
- Establish **large-bore IV access** and begin **fluid resuscitation with 0.9% NaCl or LR** if hypotension develops. If transportation is delayed, or if there is inadequate response to 2 to 3 liters of crystalloid infusion, consider infusing colloid solutions, such as plasmanate or hespan. If there has been inadequate response to ongoing fluid resuscitation, consider using vasopressors, such as dopamine 2 to 20 μg/kg per minute. IV infusion (pediatric dosing: start at 1.0 μg/kg per minute) titrated to systolic BP greater than 90 mm Hg. Vasopressors are a temporary "last-ditch" effort to be used only after the patient does not respond to fluid resuscitation.
- Immobilize any affected extremity and keep the patient calm.
- **Transport expeditiously to the appropriate ED.** Do not needlessly delay patient transport—treat the patient en route.

ANAPHYLAXIS

- The patient who has been bitten or stung should be treated using the previous guidelines, with the addition of the following therapeutic modalities:
- Protect airway: A high flow of O_2 via non-rebreathing face mask is indicated. Do not delay endotracheal intubation if the patient exhibits respiratory compromise. Immediate **endotracheal intubation may be required** but may be extremely difficult if angioedema or severe laryngospasm is present. Use caution to prevent trauma during the attempted intubation. If local protocol allows, intubation should be performed while the airway is uncompromised.
- Administer **epinephrine, 0.3 to 0.5 mg of a 1:1000 solution SC** (pediatric dose: 0.01 mg/kg SC, not to exceed 0.5 mg) if the patient is hemodynamically stable, or
- Administer **epinephrine 0.3 to 0.5 mg of 1:10,000 solution IV** (pediatric dose: 0.1 mg/kg IV, not to exceed 0.5 mg) if the patient is hemodynamically unstable. Dosage can be repeated every 5 minutes.
- Administer **diphenhydramine (Benadryl), 10 to 50 mg**

slow IV bolus or deep IM injection (pediatric dose: 2 to 5 mg/kg IV or deep IM; usual dose is 10 to 30 mg).
- Administer **hydrocortisone 100 to 500 mg IV or IM** (pediatric dose: 0.16 to 1.0 mg/kg IV or IM), or
- Administer **methylprednisolone (Solumedrol) 100 to 200 mg IV or IM** (not recommended for prehospital use in pediatric patients).
- Provide **aerosolized albuterol (0.5 ml in 3 ml saline)** to manage bronchospasm.
- Transport expeditiously to an appropriate ED.

SPECIFIC TREATMENTS

Human and Animal Bites

- Apply direct pressure to control bleeding.
- Cover the wound—do not attempt to close the wound with suture or tape.

Snake Bites

- Apply constrictive bandage (one that occludes venous blood flow but not arterial) in cases of coral snake bites. Although controversial, it has proven beneficial in such cases if applied within 30 minutes.
- Consult your EMS guidelines for treatment of bites from snakes indigenous to the region.

    NOTE: Do not apply ice or cold packs, make any incisions, or attempt to suck out venom. A suction device alone may be beneficial if applied within 30 minutes of envenomation.

Spider Bites

- If muscle spasms are present administer 10 ml of 10% calcium gluconate or diazepam, 2 mg IV.
- Apply a cold pack to attack site.

Scorpion Bites

- Apply a cold pack to the sting site.

Stings

- Scrape away the stinger with a knife or sharp edge.
- Apply a cold pack to the site of the sting.

Bibliography

Animal Attacks. In Auerbach PS (ed): Medicine for the Outdoors. Little, Brown & Co, Boston/Toronto, 1986, pp 254–256.

Bites and Stings. In Stewart CE, et al. (eds:) Environmental Emergencies. Williams & Wilkins, Baltimore, 1990, pp 160–258.

Envenomation. In Rippe JM, et al.: Critical Care Medicine, ed 2. Little, Brown & Co, Boston/Virgules/Toronto/London, 1991, pp 1266–1278.

Insect Bites. In Auerbach PS (ed): Medicine for the Outdoors. Little, Brown & Co, Boston/Toronto, 1986, pp 235–244.

Snake Bites. In Auerbach PS (ed): Medicine for the Outdoors. Little, Brown & Co, Boston/Toronto, 1986, pp 210–218.

Notes

CHAPTER 5

Bradycardia
Owen T. Traynor, MD

Presentation

The adult patient with a pulse rate of less than 60 bpm may be considered bradycardic. Bradycardia may be a normal physiologic finding, as in the well-conditioned athlete, or pathologic, causing syncope, hypotension, or heart failure.

Immediate Concerns

- **What is the patient's hemodynamic status?** If the patient is hemodynamically unstable, immediate resuscitation is warranted, including oxygen administration, IV access, IV medications, and possibly pacing. Patients with bradycardia caused by central nervous system (CNS) injury and increased intracranial pressure (ICP) may need to be hyperventilated.

Important History

- **Is the patient symptomatic?** Bradycardia may lead to inadequate cardiac output, resulting in the following common complaints: chest pain, dyspnea, fatigue, syncope, dizziness, or neurologic deficits. Chest pain may either be the result of a myocardial infarction (MI), which may be causing the bradycardia, or the consequence of poor coronary perfusion due to the bradycardia. Asymptomatic patients require less aggressive immediate therapy.
- **Is the patient taking any medication?** Many medications, particularly beta-adrenergic blockers, calcium channel blockers, clonidine, and antiarrhythmic agents, such as digitalis, can cause bradycardia.
- **Is there a history of hypothyroidism?** The thyroid hormones must be present in sufficient amounts for the hormones of the sympathetic nervous system to function

properly. Therefore, hypothyroidism may lead to brady-cardia.

- **Is the patient hypothermic?** Hypothermia can cause conduction abnormalities and myocardial irritability (see Chapter 26, Hypothermia).
- **Does the patient have a pacemaker?** Pacemakers are often implanted to treat bradycardias and heart blocks. Pacemaker failure may lead to the return of the rhythm disturbance.

Differential Diagnosis

- **Sinus bradycardia** can result from increased vagal tone, decreased sympathetic tone, and pathologic changes to the sinus node. It may occur in the well trained athlete also. Increased ICP, cervical tumors, mediastinal tumors, hypothyroidism, hypothermia, severe hypoxia, and certain medications (see previous discussion) can cause sinus bradycardia as well. Sinus bradycardia occurs in 10% to 15% of patients with acute MI and more commonly in inferior wall MIs than in anterior wall MIs. It is usually transient. Sinus bradycardia has been noted during reperfusion with thrombolytics.
- **Sinus pause or arrest** is recognized by a pause in the sinus rhythm. The PP interval of the pause is not a multiple of the PP interval of the underlying sinus rhythm. It may result in episodes of ventricular asystole if no latent pacemakers initiate an escape rhythm. These are usually of little significance unless there are no escape beats.
- **Sinoatrial exit block pause** occurs secondary to the absence of the normally expected P wave. The duration of the pause is a multiple of the PP interval of the underlying sinus rhythm. It is usually transient and of little significance.
- **Wandering atrial pacemaker** results in the transfer of the dominant pacemaker focus from the SA node to other supraventricular pacemaker sites with the next highest level of automaticity. Characterized by more than two P wave morphologies it can be normal in young healthy athletes. Persistence of atrioventricular (AV) junctional rhythms for extended periods may indicate underlying heart disease. Treatment is usually not necessary.
- **Hypersensitive carotid sinus syndrome** develops as a re-

sult of direct pressure or extension on the carotid sinus from head turning, neck tension, or tight collars and can cause syncope by stimulation of a hypersensitive carotid sinus. Most frequently characterized by asystole secondary to cessation of atrial activity from sinus exit block or sinus arrest. AV blocks may also occur. There are two types:

- **Cardioinhibitory carotid sinus hypersensitivity**, characterized by periods of asystole, and
- **Vasodepressor carotid sinus hypersensitivity**, characterized by a decrease in the systolic BP of 50 mm Hg or more without associated cardiac slowing, or a decrease in the systolic BP of 30 mm Hg or with cardiac slowing.
- **Sick sinus syndrome** is a sinoatrial (SA) node abnormality that includes persistent spontaneous inappropriate sinus bradycardia, episodes of sinus arrest or sinus exit block, a combination of SA or AV node conduction anomalies, or an alternation of periods of paroxysmal atrial tachycardias with slow atrial and ventricular rhythms. This is also known as the bradycardia tachycardia syndrome.
- *AV Blocks*
  - **First degree AV block**—Each P wave is conducted. The PR interval is greater than 0.20 seconds. Increased vagal tone or an acceleration of the atrial rate may convert first degree AV block into second degree AV block type I.
  - **Second degree AV block type I**—PR intervals increase until a P wave is not conducted. Second degree AV block type I with normal QRS complexes is not likely to progress to complete heart block.
  - **Second degree AV block type II**—P waves are not consistently conducted; however, PR intervals are constant. Second degree AV block type II may progress to complete heart block. In the context of an anterior wall MI, second degree AV block type II may require either temporary or permanent pacing. It is associated with an increased mortality, generally due to pump failure.
  - **Third degree AV block**—No atrial activity is conducted to the ventricles. The most common causes in adults are drug toxicity and coronary artery disease.

Key Physical Examination Findings

- *Initial Assessment*. Look for signs of shock.
- *Vital Signs.* Assess for hypotension. The presence of hy-

pertension and bradycardia in a patient with an altered mental state may indicate increasing ICP and CNS injury.
- *Lungs.* Listen for rales, which if present, indicate CHF.
- *Heart.* Listen for gallop rhythm.
- *Mental Status.* Monitor mental status; inadequate perfusion can cause an altered mental status.

ECG

An important diagnostic tool that will help determine therapy. See discussion on Treatment Plan that follows.

Treatment Plan

- *Patient Assessment.* Frequently reassess patient owing to the potential for a worsening of hemodynamic status and CHF. Cardiac monitoring is necessary. Be prepared—potential for cardiac arrest exists. Treat for an MI if the bradycardia is occurring in the context of a myocardial infarction.

HEMODYNAMICALLY STABLE PATIENT

- Administer O_2 and **provide ventilatory support** as needed.
- Have an external pacemaker standing by.
- **Transport to appropriate ED**. Continue to reassess the patient's ECG and hemodynamic status.
- Ensure patient comfort en route.

HEMODYNAMICALLY UNSTABLE PATIENT

- Administer O_2 and **provide ventilatory support** as needed. Monitor O_2 saturation with pulse oximetry if available.
- Place patient in the **supine position with legs elevated** unless pulmonary edema is present.
- Establish **IV access** with 0.9% NaCL or LR.
- Administer **0.5 to 1.0 mg atropine IV bolus**. Dosage may be repeated every 3 to 5 minutes as needed to a maximum total dose of 0.04 mg/kg.
- Begin **external pacing if the atropine fails** to improve the patient's condition.
- Consider the following options when atropine has failed and external pacing is unavailable or the patient remains hypotensive:

- **Dopamine, 5 to 20 μg/kg** per minute infusion or
- **Epinephrine, 2 to 10 μg** per minute infusion.
- **Isoproterenol 2 to 10 μg/min** infusion when atropine has failed and external pacing in unavailable.

  NOTE: The use of isoproterenol results in increased myocardial oxygen demand increasing the size of the infarct.
- **Transport to appropriate ED.** Continue to reassess the patient's ECG and hemodynamic status.

PATIENTS WITH BRADYCARDIA SECONDARY TO CNS INJURY

- Hyperventilate to decrease ICP (see Chapter 8, Central Nervous System Injury: Traumatic).

HYPOTHERMIC PATIENTS WITH BRADYCARDIA.

- Treat as a hypothermic patient (see Chapter 26, Hypothermia).

  NOTE: Use extreme caution when using lidocaine in the presence of bradycardia. Use of lidocaine in the presence of a ventricular escape rhythm will lead to asystole.

Bibliography

Braunwald E, (ed): Heart Disease: A Textbook of Cardiovascular Medicine, ed 4. WB Saunders, Philadelphia, 1992, pp 674–686.

Essentials of ACLS. In Textbook of Advanced Cardiac Life Support, ed 3. American Heart Association, Dallas TX, 1994, pp 1-28 to 1-32.

Guidelines for Cardiopulmonary Resuscitation and Emergency Cardiac Care. JAMA, 268: 2220–2222, 1992.

Notes

CHAPTER 6

Burns

Michael Bauman, MD

Presentation

The patient with burns may present in many different ways, depending on the type of burn severity and complexity of the burn injury. Burns may be chemical or thermal in nature and range from a superficial burn (ie, first degree such as sunburn), resulting only in mild discomfort, to a full-thickness burn (third degree), resulting in large amounts of charred and destroyed tissue. Initial attention should be directed to the systemic care of the burn patient.

Immediate Concerns

- **Is the scene safe?** Do not become a patient yourself. Watch for unsafe situations at the scene of chemical accidents and fires. Be sure to contact support agencies, such as the fire department, police department, or utility companies if their services are required.
- **Stop the burning process!** The patient with thermal burns is best cooled in the first minutes after injury. After several minutes the burn is not advancing, and excessively cooling the burn patient may cause profound hypothermia. Hypothermia is dangerous in the burn patient because it shifts the patient's metabolism to a catabolic metabolism, one where tissues are being broken down to create heat to warm the patient, leading to an increased mortality.
- **What is the patient's airway or respiratory status?** If the patient has been exposed to fire and smoke, ensure adequate ventilation and oxygenation. The most immediate threat to life is inhalation injury. These injuries are secondary to superheated gas, steam, smoke, or other toxic fumes. The diagnosis is made on clinical criteria. Airway management is the first priority with any patient. Carbon

monoxide and other products of combustion can impair oxygenation; high-flow oxygen is indicated.
- **Is the patient hemodynamically stable?** Large burns can cause significant loss of blood volume. In addition, severely burned patients may have other serious injuries that may cause hypovolemic shock. A large-bore IV fluid infusion can help prevent hemodynamic compromise.

Important History

- **Did the patient lose consciousness?** This finding along with the physical findings of circumoral burns; intraoral burns; singed facial hair; singed nasal hair; and the development of hoarseness, wheezing, dyspnea, a rasping cough, or hemoptysis leads to a diagnosis of a probable pulmonary injury. Other indicators of significant pulmonary injury include history of burning in an enclosed space. Early recognition is important, as postburn pulmonary injury may lead to a significant oxygenation-perfusion defect and complete respiratory failure. In general, 95% of patients with inhalation injuries have associated burns of the neck and face. However, the simple presence of these injuries alone does not mean that the patient has an inhalation injury.
- **What is the history of the event?** Burns caused by a wide variety of agents have the same effect on the layers of the skin but are approached differently in treatment. The extent and ultimate depth of burn depends on both the nature and the length of exposure. This is especially true for chemical burns.
- **What is the patient's chief complaint?** It may not be the burn. Do not let a surface burn distract from a thorough search for other injuries. Obtain a complete medical history and perform a thorough physical examination.
- **Were there other hazardous conditions?** Fire, steam, and many chemicals or vapors can cause inhalation injury in addition to a surface burn. In addition, there may be substantial risk of exposure to hazardous materials, placing healthcare workers at risk. Electrical injury can cause minor damage to the body surface, but extensive tissue destruction occurs below the surface, including fractures.
- **Does the patient have any underlying medical prob-**

lems? Chronic illnesses, specifically heart, kidney disease, diabetes mellitus, and pulmonary problems, can complicate the course of the patient's recuperation. Other pertinent data should be gathered including age, weight, height, previous state of health, and medication history.

Differential Diagnosis

DEPTH OF BURNS

- *Superficial* (first degree). Reddened, painful skin.
- *Partial Thickness* (second degree). Partial thickness, blisters present, destruction of the epidermis and dermal layers. Skin is moist and mottled.
- *Full Thickness* (third degree). Burn destruction of all layers down to subcutaneous layer. Skin may be leathery, charred, and anesthetic (loss of pain).

ETIOLOGY OF BURNS

- *Chemical.* Many chemicals cause tissue destruction. Make an attempt to bring the name of the causative agent to the hospital.
- *Thermal.* Thermal burns can be caused by any heat source: sun, stove, open flame, steam, or scald injuries from hot liquids.
- *Electrical.* Many sources exist for electrical burns, including household current to lightning. There is often severe muscle damage, causing rhabdomyolysis. The kidneys are at high risk of renal failure secondary to the presence of muscle breakdown products in the blood. Aggressive IV hydration may help limit or prevent renal failure.
- *Radiation.* Radiation burns may not show as an external injury. These patients may present with a myriad of complaints and are very difficult to diagnose unless the patients tells of a radiation accident.

SEVERITY OF BURNS

- *Critical Burns*
  ○ Covering more than 25% of the body surface area (BSA)
  ○ Third degree burns covering more than 10% BSA
  ○ Respiratory burns

- ○ Burns of face, hands, feet, genitalia
- ○ Electric burns, deep chemical burns
- ○ In patients with underlying chronic disease
- ○ Complicated by major injury

NOTE: The extent of of a burn may be determined by using the "Rule of Nines." Lund and Browder charts may be found in Appendix H.

Key Physical Examination Findings

- *Initial Assessment.* Ensure adequate airway and ventilatory support. Look for signs of shock. If the patient is in shock, look for another injury as the source of shock. Do not let a surface burn distract from a thorough search for other injuries.
- *Vital Signs.* Check for orthostatic vital signs owing to fluid loss. Watch for hypothermia.
- *HEENT.* Look for signs of inhalation injury: soot, burns, swelling, discoloration around or in the nares or mouth. Chemical burns to the eyes.
- *Neck.* Check for circumferential burns.
- *Cardiac Status.* Monitor victims of electrical injury. These patients can have abnormal cardiac rhythms that often respond readily to intervention.
- *Lungs.* Assess breath sounds for pulmonary edema, or pneumothorax.
- *Skin.* Assess skin for depth, extent, and presence of critical burns. Use the rule of nines to estimate the extent of the burn.
- *Extremities.* Check for circumferential burns, fractures, soft tissue injuries, and distal pulses.

Treatment Plan

- *Patient Assessment.* Frequently reassess the patient due to the potential for airway compromise and massive fluid loss. Life-threatening conditions often coexist with a large burn: arrhythmias; long bone fractures, particularly in electrical injury; and hypovolemia in patients with extensive thermal injury. Consequently, every burn patient warrants a complete examination and frequent reassessment. Although minor burns are usually considered a low-priority

injury, burns in the young and elderly patient carry increased morbidity and mortality.
- General management of burn wounds:
  - **Put out the fire.**
  - **Safeguard the airway**, and watch for clues to airway compromise.
  - Give high-flow O_2 and **provide ventilatory support**. Monitor O_2 saturation with pulse oximetry if available.
  - Ensure circulation. Establish **large-bore IV** with **0.9% NaCl or lactated Ringer's solution.** Burns patients suffer increased loss of body fluids; therefore, they require large volumes of IV rehydration. For example, the Parkland formula specifies that 4 cc/kg/% BSA burned of either LR or 0.9% NaCl be infused during the first 24 hours. Usually half of this amount is given during the first 8 hours, while the second half is given during the remaining 16 hours.

NOTE: Avoid insertion of the IV catheter through the burn site. Fluid resuscitation, however, is an essential component of burn care, and insertion of an IV catheter may, of necessity, be through burned tissue.

  - Treat the burns: cover the burns with clean or sterile dressings. Excessive use of moist dressings may cause hypothermia. It is, therefore, recommended that their use be limited. The use of wet versus dry dressings is currently a controversial topic and is usually guided by local or regional protocols.
  - Remove jewelry and elevate the patient's extremities.
  - Splint fractures.
  - Keep patient warm.
  - Administer morphine sulfate, 2 to 4 mg IV, for pain control.
- Add for electrical burns:
  - Monitor cardiac rhythm.
  - Run 0.9% NaCl or LR wide open.
- Add for chemical burns:
  - Remove clothes. Promptly remove chemical from contact with skin. Dry chemicals should be brushed away and then copiously irrigated with water. Irrigation should be continued during transport.
- Special cases:
  - Dry lime: brush off first, then irrigate with water.

 ° Hydrofluoric acid: may need an injection of calcium gluconate into the wound; therefore, expedite transport.

Bibliography

Braen GR: Thermal Injury. In Rosen P (ed): Emergency Medicine: Concepts in Clinical Practice, ed 3. Mosby-Year Book, St. Louis, 1992, pp 894–904.

Burns and Electrical Injuries. In Tintinalli JE (ed): Emergency Medicine, ed 2. McGraw-Hill, New York, 1988, pp 796–799.

Caroline NL: Wounds and Burns. In Emergency Care in the Streets, ed 4. Little, Brown & Co, Boston, 1991, pp 284–293.

Dressler DP, Hozid JL, and Nathan P: Thermal Injury. CV Mosby, St. Louis, 1988, pp 29–36.

Richard RL and Staley MJ. Burn Care and Rehabilitation: Principles and Practice. FA Davis, Philadelphia, 1994, pp 29–46.

Treat RC: Burns. In Campbell JE, Alabama ACEP: Basic Trauma Life Support, ed 2. Prentice-Hall, Englewood Cliffs, NJ, 1988, pp 210–226.

Notes

CHAPTER 7

Cardiac Arrest

Thomas Platt, NREMT-P

Presentation

By definition, cardiac arrest patients are unresponsive, apneic, and pulseless. There are several etiologies that may cause this event including lack of oxygenation, loss of oxygen-carrying capacity, failure of the heart as an adequate pump, and failure of the central nervous system.

Immediate Concerns

- **Is CPR indicated?** CPR is indicated for all apneic and pulseless patients who present without contraindications. Contraindications include obvious mortal injury, the presence of rigor mortis or extreme areas of dependent lividity, and a legal living will or DNR order, which expresses the patient's wishes that CPR not be performed.
- **Is the patient in ventricular fibrillation (VF) or ventricular tachycardia (VT) without a pulse?** After determining responsiveness and opening the airway, a rapid assessment for the presence of VF or pulseless VT is critical. The sooner that the patient is defibrillated, the more likely that defibrillation will be successful. The "quick-look" survey is performed by applying the defibrillator paddles to the patient's chest immediately. If a defibrillator is not available, chest compressions and ventilation should be initiated until the defibrillator is available. The precordial thump has been listed as acceptable, probably helpful, by the American Heart Association and may be attempted if the arrest was witnessed and a defibrillator is not immediately available. In the pulseless patient, however, VT and VF require immediate defibrillation, making a strong case for defibrillators being in close proximity to all monitored patients. (Other rhythms will be discussed in the treatment

plan.) Following the diagnosis of the rhythm and defibrillation (when indicated), the next concerns are to intubate the patient and to obtain vascular access. Remember to confirm placement of your endotracheal tube immediately after placement by auscultating breath sounds, by observing the rise and fall of the chest and by using devices such as end-tidal CO_2 detectors.

- **Has the cardiac arrest been caused by trauma or blood loss?** It is important to determine if this event is primarily cardiac or if it is the result of traumatic injuries. The management of traumatic arrest differs from a primary cardiac event. Arrests caused by blood loss or secondary to trauma generally require fluid resuscitation and surgical intervention. An additional concern is hypothermia. The management of a hypothermic patient also differs (see Chapter 26, Hypothermia).

Important History

- **Is CPR being performed adequately?** The importance of all healthcare providers having adequate knowledge and practice in the skills of basic life support (BLS) cannot be overemphasized. Without adequate ventilation and artificial circulation, the patient has no chance of survival.

Differential Diagnosis

Once the initial treatment priorities have been accomplished, it is important to determine the patient's rhythm and perfusion status. While evaluating the ECG, assess for a carotid pulse. Remember, treat the patient not the monitor. If there is a change in the patient's rhythm, assess for the return of a carotid pulse.

A variety of rhythms may be present. It is important that you have the ability to interpret ECGs rapidly. This ability combined with your knowledge of the American Heart Association (AHA) algorithms will allow you to make a diagnosis and to follow the correct treatment plan.

Key Physical Examination Findings

- *Initial Assessment.* Assess the apneic and pulseless patient according to the criteria presented in the Universal Algorithm for Adults.

Treatment Plan

- *Patient Assessment.* It is important to remember to frequently reassess the patient. Any change in the patient's perfusion status or rhythm will require you to change algorithms. Always treat the patient not the monitor.
- *The Team Leader.* If there is more than one EMS crew (ie, BLS and ALS) on the scene or multiple rescuers are present, identify a team leader early during the resuscitation effort. This person will facilitate the interventions to be followed. The team leader is responsible for interpreting the rhythms and assigning tasks to other members of the team.
- *Communications.* Along with the following standing orders, consultation with the medical control physician for guidance and institution of appropriate orders, including transportation or termination of resuscitation orders, may prove valuable in the care of the patient in cardiac arrest.
- *The Algorithmic Approach.* When using the AHA algorithms a number of assumptions are made: the condition in the algorithm persists, the patient remains apneic and pulseless, and that compressions and ventilations are continued throughout the resuscitation effort. The use of algorithms is to aid in treating the patient; they cannot replace clinical judgment.

THE UNIVERSAL ALGORITHM FOR ADULTS

This algorithm provides the recommended initial approach to the adult patient who may require ACLS interventions. In this chapter only those patients in cardiac arrest are considered. Please refer to the appropriate chapters for treatment of patients with arrhythmias, pulmonary edema, myocardial infarction, hypotension, or shock.

- Assess responsiveness—the responsive patient requires observation and treatment as indicated by their condition.
- Assess ABCs and perform CPR, if indicated, until a defibrillator is available. Be sure to protect the cervical spine, if indicated.
- Perform "quick-look" with the defibrillator paddles and assess rhythm. If VF or pulseless VT is present, perform the interventions listed in the following ventricular fibrillation and pulseless ventricular tachycardia algorithm. If there is electrical activity on the monitor and no pulse is

present, perform the interventions listed in the pulseless electrical activity (PEA) algorithm. If asystole is found, perform the interventions listed in the asystole algorithm.

VENTRICULAR FIBRILLATION AND PULSELESS VENTRICULAR TACHYCARDIA

The majority of cardiac arrest patients present in VF or VT. This, coupled with the fact that most of the survivors of sudden death will be the patients that respond to interventions in this sequence, makes it imperative that the paramedic understand the algorithm presented here.

- **Assess ABCs** and perform CPR until a defibrillator is available.
- **Perform "Quick-look"** with the defibrillator paddles and assess rhythm.
- **Defibrillate at 200 Joules** if VF or VT.
- Assess rhythm.

    NOTE: If defibrillation is effective and patient reverts to VF or VT, subsequent defibrillation should be performed, starting at the dose that was previously effective.

- If VF or VT persists, **defibrillate at 200 to 300 Joules**.
- Assess rhythm.
- If VF or VT persists, **defibrillate at 360 Joules**.
- Assess pulse and rhythm, keeping in mind that a change in pulse or rhythm will change the algorithm.
- Continue CPR.
- **Intubate** at once; remember to confirm tube placement.
- **Obtain vascular access** by the IV route.
- As soon as the patient is intubated or vascular access is obtained, administer **epinephrine** (1:10,000), **1 mg IV bolus**; repeat every 3 to 5 minutes. Epinephrine may be administered via the endotracheal route at 2 to 2.5 times the usual dose using appropriate dosage of epinephrine (1:1000) in sterile water or 0.9% NaCl to limit the fluid down the tube to no more than 10 ml at a time. When epinephrine is repeated, it may be given at the initial dose or at higher doses (up to 1.0 mg/kg) in a drug-shock, drug-shock pattern.
- **Defibrillate at 360 Joules**.
- Assess pulse and rhythm, keeping in mind that a change in pulse or rhythm will change the algorithm. If there has been no change in VF or VT, the patient is considered to be

in refractory VF or VT. The following antifibrillatory agents should be employed in a drug-shock, drug-shock pattern and the patient should be defibrillated at 360 Joules 30 to 60 seconds following each medication.

- Administer **lidocaine, 1.5 mg/kg IV bolus**. Dosage may be repeated in 3 to 5 minutes up to a maximum of 3.0 mg/kg. Follow the IV bolus instructions previously noted.
- Administer **bretylium, 5 mg/kg IV bolus**. Dosage may be repeated at 10 mg/kg every 5 minutes to a maximum of 35 mg/kg. Follow the IV bolus instructions previously indicated.
- Administer **procainamide, 30 mg per minute IV**, up to a maximum of 17 mg/kg. Follow the IV bolus instructions previously indicated.
- Should the patient's rhythm convert to a supraventricular rhythm after a defibrillation, an antifibrillatory agent should be employed to prevent recurrence. If no antifibrillatory agent has been given previously, give lidocaine, 1.0 to 1.5 mg/kg, followed by 2 to 4 mg per minute lidocaine infusion. The infusion dosage should be cut in half in patients in shock with hepatic dysfunction or in patients older than 70 years of age. If antifibrillatory agents have already been given, the patient should receive a maintenance infusion of whatever drug was helpful during defibrillation—lidocaine, 2 to 4 mg per minute, bretylium, 1 to 2 mg per minute, or procainamide, 1 to 4 mg per minute.

PULSELESS ELECTRICAL ACTIVITY (PEA)

Pulseless electrical activity includes electromechanical dissociation (EMD), pseudo-EMD, idioventricular rhythms, bradyasystolic rhythms, and postdefibrillation idioventricular rhythms.

- Continue **CPR** as initiated in the AHA universal algorithm.
- Intubate at once; remember to confirm correct tube placement.
- Consider possible causes and therapy:
  - **Hypovolemia**—begin volume infusion
  - **Cardiac tamponade**—transport expeditiously for pericardiocentesis
  - **Hypothermia**—see Chapter 26, Hypothermia
  - **Overdoses of drugs** such as tricyclics, digitalis, beta blockers, calcium channel blockers—transport

- ○ **Massive acute myocardial infarction**—see MI treatment in Chapter 10, Chest Pain.
- ○ **Hypoxia**—ensure adequate ventilations with high-concentration O_2
- ○ **Tension pneumothorax**—perform needle thoracentesis
- ○ **Massive pulmonary embolus**—transport expeditiously for surgery or thrombolytics
- ○ **Acidosis**—ensure adequate ventilations; consider sodium bicarbonate; transport
- ○ **Hyperkalemia** (patients in renal failure, tall peaked T waves)—consider calcium chloride and sodium bicarbonate; transport
- **Administer epinephrine** (1:10,000), **1 mg IV**; repeat every 3 to 5 minutes. Epinephrine may be given via the endotracheal route at 2 to 2.5 times the usual dose, diluted in 10 ml of either 0.9% Na CL or sterile water. When epinephrine is repeated, it may be given at the initial dose or at higher doses (up to 1.0 mg/kg or 5 mg). Remember to administer 20 to 30 ml of fluid and to perform effective CPR for 30 to 60 seconds after each medication bolus.
- **If patient is experiencing bradycardia, administer atropine, 1 mg IV push**. Dosage may be repeated every 3 to 5 minutes (maximum total dose: 0.04 mg/kg or 3 mg), remember to follow the IV bolus recommendations previously mentioned. Atropine may be given via the endotracheal route at 2 to 2.5 times the usual dose, diluted in 10 ml of either 0.9% NaCL or sterile water.

ASYSTOLE ALGORITHM

- Continue **CPR** as initiated in the AHA universal algorithm.
- **Intubate at once**; remember to confirm correct tube placement.
- Consider possible causes and therapy:
  - ○ **Hypoxia**—ensure adequate ventilations with high-concentration O_2
  - ○ **Hypokalemia**—transport
  - ○ **Drug overdose**—transport
  - ○ **Hyperkalemia** (patients in renal failure, tall peaked T waves)—consider calcium chloride and sodium bicarbonate; transport
  - ○ **Acidosis**—ensure adequate ventilations; consider sodium bicarbonate

○ **Hypothermia**—see Chapter 26, Hypothermia
• **Consider the immediate use of transcutaneous pacing.** Remember that the earlier the pacemaker is applied, the greater the chance of obtaining capture.
• **Administer epinephrine** (1:10,000), **1 mg IV**; repeat every 3 to 5 minutes. Epinephrine may be given via the endotracheal route at 2 to 2.5 times the usual dose, diluted in 10 ml of either 0.9% NaCL or sterile water. When epinephrine is repeated, it may be given at the initial dose or at higher doses (up to 1.0 mg/kg or 5 mg). Remember to administer 20 to 30 ml of fluid and to perform effective CPR for 30 to 60 seconds after each medication bolus.
• **Administer atropine, 1 mg IV push.** Dosage may be repeated every 3 to 5 minutes (maximum total dose: 0.04 mg/kg or 4 mg); remember to follow the IV bolus recommendations previously mentioned. Atropine may be given via the endotracheal route at 2 to 2.5 times the usual dose, diluted in 10 ml of either 0.9% NaCL or sterile water.
• If patient remains asystolic, after successful intubation and adequate ventilations and initial medications, and if reversible causes cannot be found, consider termination of efforts in consultation with the medical control physician.

Bibliography

Essentials of ACLS. In Textbook of Advanced Cardiac Life Support, ed 3. American Heart Association, Dallas TX, 1994, pp 1-10 to 1-28.

Grauer K and Cavallaro D: ACLS Certification Preparation, ed 3. Mosby-Year Book, St. Louis, 1992.

Guidelines for Cardiopulmonary Resuscitation and Emergency Cardiac Care. JAMA, 268:2222–2226, 1992.

Notes

CHAPTER 8

Central Nervous System Injury: Traumatic

Russell Bradley, MD

Presentation

The patient with a traumatic central nervous system (CNS) injury can vary in presentation from nearly asymptomatic with a cervical spine fracture and potential spinal cord injury, to mild and transient headache after a concussion, to coma and death after a major head injury. The presentation of CNS injury is generally related to the level along the CNS at which the injury takes place. With trauma, however, there are often multiple sites of injury, and one must take this into account when assessing the patient. Key in assessing multiple presentations of CNS injury is to identify a cause and mechanism of injury. This can include a direct blow to the head or body by some object; a penetrating injury such as from bullets, knives, or other sharp objects; or an indirect cause of injury, such as a transmitted force from a blow to the body, as in an motor vehicle accident (MVA), explosion, or a fall. This information will prove vital in the subsequent treatment and care of the patient. Because a CNS injury can have significant morbidity and mortality, the prehospital EMS provider must have a high index of suspicion and treat suspected cases of CNS injury based on mechanism of injury, history, and physical findings.

Immediate Concerns

- **Is there a mechanism of injury that could cause CNS injury?** Direct trauma to the head, spine, and back can obviously injure the CNS. The mechanism of injury is often apparent. However, there are times when a history of trauma must be actively sought. For example, alcoholic patients with subacute subdural hematomas may have fallen

49

and hit their head several days before becoming unconscious. Family members may not have taken notice of the
fall because the patient falls frequently. Have a high index
of suspicion. Although it usually may require significant
force to cause CNS injury, consider the elderly to be at
higher risk owing to the more brittle nature of their bones.
A cervical fracture may result from a fall to the ground
while standing. The paramedic should use spinal immobilization liberally. Be aware that there might not be signs
or symptoms of spinal cord damage. Vertebral spine injury
can remain silent until something causes a change in the
status of the injured area; that is, a fracture becomes displaced upon movement of the patient. Once again, the as-
sumption that there might be injury if there are any signs,
symptoms, or an appropriate mechanism of injury warrants appropriate cervical and spinal column immobilization.

- **Is the patient's airway patent and stable?** Patients with
  a CNS injury may be unable to protect their airway. Often
  there are associated facial injuries that cause both bleeding
  and swelling, leading to airway compromise. All airway
  interventions must be performed without endangering the
  cervical spine. Endotracheal intubation may be required.

- **Is the patient hemodynamically stable?** Hemodynamic
  instability in the context of a CNS injury usually means
  that there are other "hidden" injuries—look for evidence
  of internal trauma—intrathoracic, intra-abdominal,
  intrapelvic, and so forth. Treat the patient for shock while
  protecting the spine. Expedite transport to the closest appropriate ED.

- **Does the patient have an altered mental status?** The
  patient's mental status is the most sensitive indicator of brain
  function. The range of alteration of consciousness extends
  from the transient and mild, such as seeing stars, momentary amnesia, restlessness, vomiting, and headache, to the
  profound, such as focal neurologic deficits, stroke, paralysis, seizures, coma, shock, respiratory arrest, and death. It
  is prudent to assume that any patient with altered consciousness has also suffered damage to the cervical spine
  and spinal cord, and subsequent immobilization of the neck
  and spine must be used.

- **Did you inspect or gain information at the scene?** This is information that, if not recorded by the paramedic, will not be available at the ED. For example: in an MVA, telltale signs such as a cracked or "spidered" windshield, deformed steering column, the presence or absence of seatbelt use, and the location of automobile damage (ie, front, back, or side) can all help in determining the mechanism of injury. If the patient has fallen, it is important to note from how high and onto what type of surface. A fall that produces obvious gluteal, feet, or ankle injury might also cause compressive spinal fractures. Note the position in which the patient was found: extremity flexion and extension (known as decorticate and decerebrate posturing, respectively) can indicate a certain level of brain injury.

- **Are there distracting injuries, or is the patient's ability to feel pain impaired?** Often, the patient's self-reporting of symptoms is relied on to discover injury. If there are other significant painful injuries, the patient may not accurately report the pain of a skull or vertebral fracture. A patient who has been drinking alcohol or using pain medications or substances of abuse may be impaired and not report pain. These patients need to be considered as if they have an injury and be immobilized.

Important History

- **Is the patient's neurological injury improving or worsening?** The treatment on arrival at the ED may depend on the severity and progression of the injury. This requires sequential neurologic assessment. The Glasgow Coma Scale (GCS) should be noted initially and monitored during transport. A loss in the GCS of two or more points is an alarming sign: expedite transport. Know the signs of increasing intracranial pressure (ICP) that might indicate impending herniation: hypertension associated with bradycardia and an altered mental state. The development of a fixed and dilated pupil, implying third cranial nerve compression and possible herniation, should also spur quickened transportation. A simple way to look at CNS injuries is that they are of three types: those that are improving, those that are stable, and those that are worsening. Those that are worsening may require a more aggressive neurosurgical approach.
- **Has there been a loss of consciousness (LOC)?** If so,

for how long? Loss of consciousness requires significant force transmitted to the brain. Patients may not be reliable historians regarding LOC. A change in mental status for the better might have already occurred, and this information will be important in terms of future management in hospital. The patient might have lost consciousness before the event, thus precipitating the accident. Causes might include myocardial infarction (MI), seizure, cerebrovascular accident (CVA), syncope, or intoxication. A lucid interval may precede deterioration in an acute epidural hemorrhage. All trauma patients who have suffered an LOC require immobilization of the spine and transport to the hospital.

- **Is there any history of vomiting?** Children frequently vomit with any degree of head injury, but in the adult this can be a sign of deterioration. A history of vomiting might make one think of a cause for a blocked airway or possible aspiration.

- **Are there any comorbid medical problems or injuries?** The patient's LOC may have actually been caused by hypoglycemia, cardiac arrhythmia, an MI, alcohol or drug abuse, hypoxia, blood loss, or a seizure. There is no substitute for an accurate medical history—even in the face of an "obvious" injury. Often treatment and history may be obtained simultaneously.

Differential Diagnosis

SKULL FRACTURES

Skull fractures may be divided into two major groups: open fractures and closed fractures. In open fracture, a communication exists between the brain substance through the fracture to the outside of the skull. The dura, a layer of tissue around the brain that contains the cerebrospinal fluid (CSF), is disrupted in an open fracture. The dura is not disrupted in a closed fracture. Skull fractures may also be classified as depressed or nondepressed. A depressed skull fracture means that there is a step-off between the fractured piece of bone and the surrounding skull. Although skull fractures do not always cause brain injury; when present, there is a greater risk of underlying brain injury. The mechanism of injury can be secondary to penetration or crushing of the brain substance by a piece of bone. It can also be caused by the fracture disrupting cerebral vessels, leading to bleeding into or around the brain parenchyma (tissue). A basal skull fracture is another type of fracture where the fracture occurs through the bones at the base of the skull. Physical examination findings that suggest a basal skull fracture include Battle's sign, an ecchymosis found over the mastoid process that develops several hours after the trauma; raccoon eyes, a bilateral periorbital ecchymosis found without trauma to the eyes; and CSF leak from the nose or ears.

DIFFUSE BRAIN INJURIES

- *Concussion.* This may be defined as a temporary loss of neurologic function. It usually takes the form of a LOC. The duration of unconsciousness can range from seconds or minutes to several hours. It typically occurs as a result of a blow to the head. The movement of the brain within the skull may cause a transient impairment of the reticular activating system (RAS), which regulates consciousness. Although recovery is normally complete, some patients will experience headache, anxiety, memory difficulties, insomnia, and dizziness for weeks to months after the injury. More often than not, by the time the patient has been brought to the ED, return of consciousness has occurred. Concussion can be mild, moderate, or severe and potentially accompanies more critical brain injury.
- *Diffuse Axonal Injury.* This entity can be described as a very severe concussion. It is characterized by prolonged coma, often requiring long-term care. The pathology is described as microscopic injury scattered throughout the brain. This entity is often termed closed head injury (CHI) or brainstem injury, and its overall mortality is 33%.

FOCAL BRAIN INJURIES

- *Contusion.* This can be thought of as a bruise to the brain. Contusions can be small, large, single, or multiple. They usually occur directly under the site of impact, or on the opposite side of the head from the injury due to rebound of the brain and are known as coup and contrecoup injuries. A contusion might not exhibit any neurologic findings, but if sensory or motor cortex is injured, there will be focal deficits. Edema and hemorrhage can cause swelling, leading to increased ICP, and possible herniation or brainstem compression, both of which can cause immediate death.

INTRACRANIAL HEMORRHAGE

- *Acute Epidural Hematoma.* In the majority of cases, this results from an arterial injury in the dural covering of the brain causing bleeding between the skull and the dura. Bleeding can also occur from a disruption of venous vessels. Epidural hematomas are usually associated with a fracture over the middle meningeal artery, that is a fracture of the temporal or parietal bones of the skull. This can be a rapidly fatal process. As the skull is a confined space, an increase in the quantity of material, in this case blood where it should not be, compresses the brain and can cause herniation. In the classic description of an epidural hematoma, there is an initial LOC, followed by a lucid (but not necessarily symptom-free) interval, progressing to LOC. Although this is the classic description, it is not the most common presentation. There might be either no LOC or prolonged unconsciousness with this injury. A fixed dilated pupil on the side of the head injury is a hallmark of this injury. Immediate surgical intervention is the cure.
- *Acute Subdural Hematoma.* In this type of hematoma, the blood comes from bridging veins that span the gap between the brain tissue and the dura. The accumulation of blood is, therefore, between the dura and the brain. This is a much more common injury than an epidural hematoma; in fact, 30% of severe head injuries are subdural hematomas. Acceleration-deceleration forces are frequently the causative mechanism of injury. There is often quite extensive contusion, as well as injury caused by the increasing volume of blood compressing brain tissue. Acute subdural hematomas usually become symptomatic within 24 hours of injury, but subacute and chronic forms of this hemorrhage do exist. These forms take longer to show up after injury. Acute subdural hematomas require surgical intervention and, even with surgery, the mortality is 30%. The elderly and alcoholics are particularly susceptible to this type of injury because these patients' brains have undergone some atrophy and, therefore, the bridging veins must span a wider gap.

- ***Subarachnoid Hemorrhage***. Subarachnoid hemorrhage (SAH) occurs from bleeding vessels in the arachnoid space. Patients usually present with a severe headache, stiff neck photophobia, or some combination of these features. Patients may report that this is the worst headache of their life. SAH may occur in the absence of trauma secondary to a rupture of a cerebral aneurysm.
- ***Brain Hemorrhages and Lacerations***. These can be due to penetrating injuries and depressed skull fractures. If a major artery or venous sinus within the brain tissue is injured, the hemorrhage can be significant and life-threatening. If an object is impaled in the head or spine, it must be left in place until removal is performed by a neurosurgeon. Bullet wounds inflict injury greater than suggested by the bullet tract, secondary to the large amount of force dissipated into surrounding tissue. A bullet does not have to penetrate the skull to cause intracranial injury because of these transmitted forces.

SPINE INJURIES

Cervical Spine Injuries. These injuries can exist without spinal cord injury, and the potential for worsening always exists; immobilization is of paramount importance for a positive outcome. Always have a high index of suspicion for this type of injury, as missing it could be life-threatening. The mechanism of injury is often the best indicator that such an injury might have taken place. An unremarkable neurologic examination does not rule out cervical spine injury. The conscious patient will often be able to identify pain at the site of injury. If the patient is unconscious, various findings will lead one to suspect cervical cord injury, including diaphragmatic breathing, hypotension with bradycardia, especially without hypovolemia; flaccid motor tone; loss of bowel or bladder control, and grimacing to pain above but not below the clavicle. If the patient is unconscious and has been injured in a motor vehicle accident (MVA) or fall, the chance of a cervical spine injury is 5% to 10%. Remember that other injuries might be masked because of interrupted pain sensation.

Spinal Cord Injuries. These injuries can occur without vertebral injury, for example, where there is a hematoma or vascular compromise. Conversely, vertebral injury, such as fractures or herniated intervertebral discs, can exist without signs of cord injury. Once again, the cause and mechanism of injury will be crucial to the assessment of whether spinal cord injury is present. Complete spinal cord lesions create a total loss of motor and sensation distal to the site of injury.

Spinal cord injuries can cause neurogenic shock. Common findings include quadriplegia, absence of spinal reflexes, and absence of autonomic nervous system reflexes, all leading to poor vasomotor tone. Typical systolic blood pressure is between 80 and 100 mm Hg. The hypotension is accompanied by bradycardia and warm, pink, and dry skin. Thermoregulation is usually impaired secondary to loss of the ability to vasoconstrict or vasodilate appropriately, impaired sweating, and impaired ability to shiver. "Spinal" shock is usually a transient phenomena, lasting from hours to weeks. Not all spinal cord injuries, however, are complete cord injuries. It is possible to injure a part of the cord. Three common partial spinal cord lesions exist.

- In the **central cord syndrome**, the most common type of partial cord lesion, a ligament adjacent to the spine buckles into the cord during hyperflexion, causing a contusion of the central portion of the cord. The findings are usually characterized by weakness in the arms greater than in the legs, with the hands being affected more than the upper arms. This is due to the more central location of the nerves innervating the upper extremities and hands.

- The **anterior cord syndrome**, another partial syndrome, is caused by either compression of the anterior spinal cord or compression of the anterior spinal artery that supplies the anterior spinal cord. One finds paralysis and loss of pain and temperature sensation distal to the injury, but because the posterior aspect of the spinal cord is spared, the ability to sense light, touch, vibration, motion, and position is retained.

- The **Brown-Sequard syndrome**, or lateral cord syndrome, develops when a lateral half of the spinal cord is transected or injured, often due to a knife wound or gunshot wound. Here one finds loss of motor function distal to the injury on the same side of the body and loss of pain and temperature sensation distal to the injury on the other side of the body.

Key Physical Examination Findings

- *Initial Assessment.* Look for compromised airway, difficult breathing, signs of shock or acute hemorrhage. Consider the mechanism of injury and institute spinal precautions when indicated. If the patient is in shock, look for a hidden injury. Closed head injuries should not cause hypovolemia in adults.

- *Vital Signs.* Be alert for signs of increased ICP: hypertension, bradycardia, and altered mental status.
- *HEENT.* Look for raccoon eyes; Battle's sign; and clear fluid (CSF) or blood drainage from the nose or ears, a sign of basal skull fracture. Palpate skull for depression. Check facial bone instability. Check pupil size, symmetry, and reactivity to light. A specific measurement of size can provide precise information. Check for facial symmetry, and document deviation. Look for ecchymosis that might imply underlying fracture. Facial fracture might be associated with airway compromise and cervical spine injury. Palpate cervical spine.
- *Extremities.* Assess for any gross motor or sensory deficits.
- *Neurologic Examination.* Assess the level of consciousness, record GCS, perform assessment of motor and sensory status.

Treatment Plan

- *Patient Assessment.* Perform a rapid and systematic primary survey initially and institute treatment as life-threatening problems are discovered. Prompt transport to the appropriate ED is a key intervention. A secondary survey should be performed once the primary survey and all primary survey interventions have been accomplished. Frequent reassessment of the patient with a CNS injury is necessary owing to the potential for a rapidly worsening neurologic status. Be prepared—potential for cardiac arrest exists.
- *Communications.* Consult with the medical control physician for guidance and institution of appropriate orders. Such consultation may prove valuable in the care of the patient with a CNS injury.
- Administer O_2 and **provide ventilatory support**, including endotracheal intubation, as indicated. Protect the cervical spine if indicated. **If GCS is less than 9, the patient should be intubated** using the appropriate method (ie, oropharyngeal or nasopharyngeal) and hyperventilated.

- If there is no mechanism of injury to suggest cervical spine injury, place patient in the **Semi-Fowler or Fowler position**. The **coma position** is also useful to **reduce the aspiration risk** in patients with a compromised gag reflex or depressed consciousness.
- If there is a mechanism of injury that suggests the possibility of cervical spine injury, the patient requires spinal immobilization.
- Establish **large-bore IV access** with 0.9% NaCl or LR.
- Consider use of **methylprednisolone, 30 mg/kg IV**, followed by an IV infusion of 5.4 mg/kg per hour (doses less than 30 mg/kg are considered ineffective) to reduce cerebral edema in patients with GCS less than 10.
- **Treat for shock.** See Chapter 38, Shock.
- If the patient has an altered mental status, consider the administration of the following agents:
  - **Naloxone** (Narcan), 0.4 to 2.0mg IV bolus. Dose may be repeated in 2 to 3 minutes.
  - **Thiamine, 100 mg IM.**
  - **Dextrose 50%, 25 g IV if the patient is hypoglycemic** or if hypoglycemia is suspected in a diabetic patient.
- Treat symptomatic arrhythmias. See Chapters 5 and 43, Bradycardia and Tachycardia, respectively for specific options.
- Treat non–life-threatening injuries as appropriate (ie, control bleeding, splint fractures, etc).
- Transport to appropriate ED. Ensure patient comfort en route. Do not needlessly delay patient transport—expedite transport.

Bibliography

Caroline NL: Emergency Care in the Streets, ed 4. Little, Brown & Co, Boston, 1991, pp 297–328.

Committee on Trauma, American College of Surgeons: Head Trauma. In Advanced Trauma Life Support Student Manual, ed 5. American College of Surgeons, Chicago, 1993, pp 159–183.

Committee on Trauma, American College of Surgeons: Spine and Spinal Cord Trauma. In Advanced Trauma Life Support Student Manual, ed 5. American College of Surgeons, Chicago, 1993, pp 191–203.

Hockberger RS, Kirshenbaum K, and Doris PE: Spinal Trauma. In Rosen P (chief ed): Emergency Medicine: Concepts and Clinical Practice, ed 3. Mosby-Year Book, St. Louis, 1992, pp 371–412.

Mahoney BD: Spinal Injuries. In Tintinalli JE, Krome LR, and Ruiz E
(eds): Emergency Medicine: A Comprehensive Study Guide, ed 3.
McGraw-Hill , New York, 1992, pp 922–927.
Pons PT: Head Trauma. In Rosen P (chief ed): Emergency Medicine
Concepts and Clinical Practice, ed 3. Mosby-Year Book, St. Louis,
1992, pp 338–354.
Rockswold GL: Head Injury. In Tintinalli JE, Krome LR, and Ruiz E
(eds): Emergency Medicine: A Comprehensive Study Guide, ed 3.
McGraw-Hill , New York, 1992, pp 913–921.

Notes

CHAPTER 9

Cerebrovascular Accidents and Transient Ischemic Attacks

Russell Bradley, MD

Presentation

A stroke, or cerebral vascular accident (CVA), is a sudden neurologic injury related to impaired cerebral blood flow. In essence, it is a closed head injury. A transient ischemic attack (TIA) is like a stroke in presentation, but the symptoms last less than 24 hours. For all intents and purposes, a TIA must be treated in the prehospital arena like a stroke.

It is useful to divide strokes into two major categories: ischemic and hemorrhagic. Although there is no way to distinguish between hemorrhagic and ischemic strokes on the street, a hemorrhagic stroke is more likely to involve an altered level of consciousness or a severe headache that may rapidly progress to stupor or unconsciousness. A hemorrhagic stroke can occur secondary to trauma, either to the head or the body. Ischemic strokes are usually a result of either local clotting (thrombosis) of a blood vessel, or blockage caused by the blood vessel becoming plugged by material (an embolus) that comes from elsewhere in the body. Hemorrhagic strokes result from bleeding either directly into the brain tissue, or outside of the brain into the cerebrospinal fluid.

Strokes present according to which area of the brain is inadequately perfused. Symptoms can include:

- Paralysis or weakness of a lower limb, upper limb, one whole side of the body, or one or both sides of the face
- Altered mental state, including impaired judgment, insight, and memory
- Sensory deficits of the body or the face: numbness, pain, pins and needles, loss of pain, or temperature sensation

- Clumsiness and impaired gait
- Blindness in half of the visual field or in just one eye
- Pinpoint, dilated, or unequal pupils
- Aphasia: inappropriate use of language, poor understanding of language, difficulty finding words
- Dysarthria: slurred speech, difficulty with pronunciation
- Vertigo: the feeling of spinning or dizziness
- Syncope, loss of consciousness, coma
- Vomiting
- Headache
- Bowel and bladder incontinence
- Seizures
- Impaired or absent gag reflex
- Abnormal respiratory patterns, including respiratory arrest

Be aware that strokes may occur either suddenly or with a slow, insidious onset. If the patient is found at some point hours to days after the stroke, the presenting picture might also include dehydration and hypothermia.

Immediate Concerns

- **What is the status of the patient's airway?** A depressed mental status with or without an intact gag reflex can increase the risk of aspiration. If the airway is not patent or the patient is unconscious, intubation may be warranted. Placing the patient in the coma position can help decrease the aspiration risk.
- **Are the patient's respirations effective?** Injury to the respiratory centers of the brain can cause an altered respiratory pattern and ineffective ventilations. At the very least, supplemental oxygen should be administered. Intubation may be required.
- **Is the patient hemodynamically stable?** Circulatory collapse might occur secondary to disruption of the autonomic nervous system. Oxygen should be administered, a large bore IV placed, and 0.9% NaCl fluid started at KVO rate unless the patient exhibits signs of shock.
- **Is the patient hypoglycemic?** Blood glucose should be evaluated, and dextrose given if the blood glucose level is low. If glucose evaluation is not possible, glucose should only be given to diabetic patients in whom hypoglycemia is clinically suspected. By increasing the blood sugar level,

we increase the metabolism of the brain, thus increasing its oxygen requirements and increasing the size of the stroke. This can be disastrous in the already inadequately perfused brain.

- **What is the patient's neurologic status?** It is imperative that the paramedic assess the patient's level of consciousness, Glasgow Coma Scale, pupillary reaction, gross motor and sensory status, facial asymmetry, and the ability to speak and walk on the scene, as the examination might markedly change. If the patient presents with seizures, management should follow the guidelines discussed in Chapter 37, Seizure.

Important History

- **Does the patient have any risk factors for cerebrovascular disease?** These risk factors are the same as for cardiovascular disease and include a history of smoking, elevated cholesterol levels, hypertension, diabetes mellitus, and a family history. Both diabetes and hypertension predispose one to stroke through their deleterious effects on the small blood vessels of the brain.
- **Has the patient ever had a CVA or TIA before?** People who have a previous history of CVA or TIA are at increased risk for further episodes.
- **Is there any history of cardiac disease or cardiac arrhythmias?** Patients with heart disease are at higher risk for the development of a thrombus (clot) in the heart that may become dislodged, enter the blood circulation as an embolus, and travel to the brain to cause a stroke. Patients with chronic atrial fibrillation and those with prosthetic heart valves are often anticoagulated with warfarin (Coumadin) to decrease the risk of embolization. In the first 2 months after an acute myocardial infarction, the risk of stroke is 13 times greater than in people without recent AMIs. Patients with strokes are often found to have underlying "silent" MI. A stroke may result from the low flow state in the peri-MI period.
- **Is there any history of alcohol or drug abuse?** Intravenous drug usage can cause bacterial colonization of the heart valves, and the bacteria have the potential to break off in clumps and form emboli. Cocaine can cause marked

elevation in blood pressure, bursting cerebral blood vessels and causing hemorrhagic stroke. Alcohol lowers the seizure threshold, making seizures more likely, and withdrawal from alcohol can cause seizures.

- **What medications is the patient taking?** Oral anticoagulants, such as warfarin, can increase the risk of intracranial hemorrhage. Oral contraceptives also increase the risk of stroke due to the increased risk of clot formation. Nonsteroidal anti-inflammatory agents, through their antiplatelet properties, can make a hemorrhagic stroke bleed more actively.

Differential Diagnosis

ISCHEMIC STROKE

- **Local thrombosis** of cerebral or neck vasculature causes approximately 50% of all strokes. Diseases that predispose people to this type of stroke include hypertension, diabetes, polycythemia vera, sickle cell anemia, collagen vascular diseases, arteritis, and migraine headaches. Trauma can cause ascending aortic dissection and cerebral artery dissection, both of which lead to thrombus formation. Pregnancy can lead to a hypercoagulable state and therefore predispose to thrombus formation.
- **Embolic obstruction** accounts for another 33% of all ischemic strokes. The majority of emboli arise from a source in the heart. One quarter of all brain infarcts in patients younger than 40 years of age are secondary to cardiogenic emboli. The following diseases predispose the patient to development of an intracardiac clot and subsequent potential embolization: MI, atrial fibrillation, alcoholic cardiomyopathy, congestive heart failure, bacterial endocarditis, and any valvular disease or valvular prostheses. IV drug abuse can lead to bacterial endocarditis.

HEMORRHAGIC STROKE

- **Spontaneous intracerebral hemorrhage** is responsible for 8% to 11% of all acute strokes. The bleeding forms a hematoma that causes local tissue injury, decreased tissue perfusion, and an increase in intracerebral pressure. Predisposing conditions include hypertension, arteriovenous malformations (AVMs), and tumors. Other factors that can lead to hemorrhage include cocaine use, oral contraceptives, and anticoagulant and antiplatelet agents.

- **Arteriovenous malformations** (AVM) are tangles of connections between arteries and veins, usually present from birth. The walls of these connections are abnormally thin, and with advancing age grow thinner. They are often the cause of intracerebral hemorrhages in patients between the ages of 10 and 30 years. There is usually a familial inheritance with this disease entity; therefore, ask whether other family members might have had the same symptoms.
- *Brain Tumors.* A stroke can often be the first indication of a brain tumor, where the tumor has eroded into a blood vessel, causing bleeding. Find out if any other area of the body has had tumors, because this could indicate a metastatic tumor.
- **Subarachnoid hemorrhage** is caused by a leakage of blood into the subarachnoid space (between the brain and the first layer of surrounding membrane). These are most commonly caused by the rupture of an aneurysm. An aneurysm is a localized ballooning of a blood vessel, where the wall is weakened for some reason. Five percent of the general population have these aneurysms.

TRANSIENT ISCHEMIC ATTACKS

Transient ischemic attacks by definition are neurologic deficits that resolve within 24 hours. They are usually short-lived events, and can occur many times within 24 hours in a waxing and waning fashion. They are caused by a momentary lack of blood flow to some area of the brain, followed by the return of blood to that area. They are serious events and often indicate impending stroke.

There are many other disease states that may mimic CVAs, including the postictal state of a seizure disorder, hypoglycemia or hyperglycemia in diabetes mellitus, migraine headaches, multiple sclerosis, and toxic ingestions.

ECG

All patients who have experienced a CVA or TIA should receive cardiac monitoring. Cardiac monitoring may suggest evidence of possible MI, as well as reveal dysrhythmias that may be causing inadequate cardiac output and, therefore, inadequate cerebral blood flow.

Key Physical Examination Findings

- *Initial Assessment.* Look for compromised airway, ineffective breathing, and signs of shock.
- *Vital Signs.* Note the presence of hypertension, bradycardia, and an altered mental state, as these conditions may indicate rising intracranial pressure.
- *Neurologic Examination.* Assess mental status, pupillary responses, facial asymmetry, motor and sensory status.
- *HEENT.* Look for head or neck trauma, pupil asymmetry, and facial asymmetry. Check for blindness. Listen for carotid bruits.
- *Lungs.* Listen for rales that may suggest CHF and, therefore, a cardiac-related cause of the stroke.
- *Extremities.* Look for any gross motor and sensory deficits. Check for a Babinski reflex. This is done by rubbing a firm, but not sharp, object along the lateral edge of the sole of the foot from the heel to the ball of the foot and then across the ball to the medial edge of the foot. The reflex is positive when the initial movement of the great toe is upward, thus indicating a neurologic injury in either the spinal cord or brain. A Babinski reflex may be normal in children.

Treatment Plan

- *Patient Assessment.* Perform rapid and systematic primary survey initially and institute therapy as life-threatening problems are discovered. Prompt transport to the appropriate ED is a key intervention. Frequent reassessment of the patient with a CVA or TIA is necessary due to the potential for worsening of the neurologic status.
- Administer O_2 and **provide ventilatory support,** including endotracheal intubation as indicated.
- Place patient in the **Semi-Fowler or Fowler position**. The coma position is also useful to reduce the aspiration risk in patients with a compromised gag reflex or depressed consciousness.

- **Establish large-bore IV access** with 0.9% NaCl or LR as needed.
- If the patient has an altered mental status, consider the administration of the following agents:
  - **Naloxone** (Narcan) **0.4 to 2.0 mg IV bolus.** Dosage may be repeated in 2 to 3 minutes.
  - **Thiamine, 50 mg slow IV bolus and 50 mg IM.** If unable to establish IV access, 100 mg IM.

  NOTE: Rapid administration of thiamine may cause hypotension.

  - **Dextrose 50%, 25 g IV** if the patient is hypoglycemic or if hypoglycemia is suspected in a patient with diabetes.
- **Treat symptomatic arrhythmias** as indicated. See Chapters 5 and 43, Bradycardia and Tachycardia, respectively, for specific options.
- **Treat non–life-threatening injuries** as appropriate (ie, control bleeding, splint fractures, etc).
- **Transport to appropriate ED** and ensure patient comfort en route.

Bibliography

Barsan WG and Bain M: Stroke. In Rosen P (ed): Emergency Medicine: Concepts and Clinical Practice, ed 3. Mosby-Year Book, St. Louis, 1992, pp 1825–1839.

Caroline NL: Emergency Care in the Streets, ed 4. Little, Brown & Co, Boston, 1991, pp 559– 580.

Henry GL: Stroke Syndromes and Lateralized Deficits. In Tintinalli JE, Krome LR, and Ruiz E (eds): Emergency Medicine: A Comprehensive Study Guide, ed 3. McGraw-Hill, New York, 1992, pp 793–798.

Notes

CHAPTER 10

Chest Pain

Ritu Sahni, MD

Presentation

The chest pain patient can present in a variety of ways, with a wide range of symptoms—from the healthy 20-year-old patient with a sharp chest pain to the elderly cardiac patient with a crushing chest pain and new-onset congestive heart failure. The diagnosis of acute myocardial infarction (AMI) is easy to make when a patient presents with the classic symptoms: crushing retrosternal chest pain that is unrelieved by nitroglycerin, ECG changes, dyspnea, and diaphoresis along with a known history of heart disease; however, one must not overlook the patient who presents with an atypical story. National statistics show that 5% of all AMIs are actually misdiagnosed and the patient is discharged from the ED. Misdiagnosis of AMI results in the most malpractice dollars spent. Given the difficulty in diagnosing the nonclassical AMI, even with the increased training physicians receive along with the greater resources found in the hospital, it is imperative that all patients with chest pain be evaluated in the ED. At the very least, these patients should receive O_2, ECG monitoring, and have IV access established, even though this may result in some patients receiving treatment who may not require it. It is, however, more prudent to err on the side of treatment rather than to allow the patient with cardiac chest pain to go untreated. The medical control physician can be a valuable consultant for the field EMS provider faced with this diagnostic dilemma.

Immediate Concerns

- **Is the patient hemodynamically stable?** Airway, breathing, and circulation should be assessed in all patients. The airway should be secured and fluid resuscitation initiated if the patient is showing signs of shock.
- **All chest pain is cardiac until proven otherwise.** All

patients with a complaint of chest pain should be monitored, given oxygen therapy, and have an IV started immediately.

Important History

- **What is the character of the pain?** The quality of the patient's pain and what produces it can give you an indication as to the underlying cause. Cardiac pain is often described as a pressure or crushing sensation on the chest. A sharp knifelike pain is more likely to be musculoskeletal or pleuritic, whereas a burning midepigastric pain can indicate gastrointestinal (GI) distress. Pain brought about by exertion is a significant finding. Keep in mind, however, that cardiac pain can, and will, present in any of these fashions.

- **Does the pain radiate and how long has it lasted?** Cardiac pain can radiate into both arms, the neck, jaw, and back. A tearing sensation that is felt into the middle of the back is a hallmark for thoracic aortic dissection. Angina pain generally lasts less than 15 minutes whereas chest pain from MI can last longer than 30 minutes, at rest, without relief. Chest pain lasting for days is generally not cardiac in origin.

- **Is there any accompanying nausea, vomiting, or diaphoresis?** Vagal stimulation caused by an MI can cause emesis and marked diaphoresis.

- **Is the patient short of breath?** Patients with CHF, angina, or MI often have difficulty breathing. Of course, chest pain with a pulmonary etiology can also cause shortness of breath.

- **Is there a history of similar chest pain, heart disease, or other medical problems?** Often, patients with a history of heart disease will know what their cardiac chest pain normally feels like. They will usually be able to indicate any change from previous patterns of pain and other related symptoms. During the history, it is important to find risk factors for heart disease, such as diabetes and hypercholesterolemia. It is also helpful to note that not all patients with AMI exhibit the classic signs and symptoms. People with diabetes, for example, are notorious for presenting with MI in an atypical manner. Elderly patients are less likely to present with chest pain. Other complaints, such as malaise, hypotension, altered mental status, and stroke, become more common indicators of cardiac-related emergencies.

- **Is thrombolytic therapy indicated?** Thrombolytic therapy has been shown to limit infarct size and to reduce both morbidity and mortality. Thrombolytic therapy is indicated in all AMI patients with ST-segment elevations who present within 6 hours of the onset of symptoms, if there are no contraindications. There is some evidence that patients who are up to 24 hours out may also benefit from the use of thrombolytics. Patients with the most to gain have been those with an anterior wall MI, but some positive results have been seen in patients with inferior wall MIs as well. The benefit of thrombolytics decreases with time; therefore, if thrombolytic agents are not available in the prehospital phase, the patient must be promptly transported to the ED.

- **Are thrombolytic agents contraindicated?** The following are absolute contraindications to thrombolytic therapy: GI bleeding, prolonged (greater than 1 minute) or traumatic CPR, recent (less than 2 months) intracranial or intraspinal surgery or trauma, intracranial neoplasm, atrioventricular malformation or aneurysm, history of a previous hemorrhagic CVA, and pregnancy. The relative contraindications are recent (less than 10 days) trauma or surgery, poorly controlled severe hypertension, active peptic ulcer disease, previous CVA, known bleeding disorder, hepatic insufficiency, hemorrhagic retinopathy, and if streptokinase or anisoylated plasminogen streptokinase activator complex (APSAC) is to be used, a prior exposure to streptokinase or APSAC (absolute contraindication if there was a previous allergic reaction).

- **What medications does the patient take?** This can often provide a good clue as to the exact nature of the patient's past history, especially when the patient is a poor historian.

Differential Diagnosis

There are many different organ systems represented in the chest and each one is a possible source of chest discomfort.

CARDIAC DISEASE

- *Angina/Unstable Angina.* Angina is often described as a pressure type of pain that is brought on by exertion and that resolves after 10 to 15 minutes of rest and one or two sublingual nitroglycerin doses. Unstable angina is characterized by a change in the pattern of angina such as an increase in the severity of pain, an increase in the frequency of pain, a change in nitroglycerin requirements, or new-onset angina.

- *Acute Myocardial Infarction.* This most often occurs at rest and the pain usually lasts for longer than 30 minutes. It is most often characterized by a severe, crushing substernal chest pain that is unrelieved by sublingual nitroglycerin. Many times, it is accompanied by severe nausea, vomiting, or diaphoresis. It is important to note that an AMI can have multiple types of presentation and can even be silent.

- *Pericarditis or Pericardial Tamponade.* This pain is usually sharp, retrosternal, and radiating into the jaw. It often has a viral etiology and patients may have a history of recent viral syndrome. Other times there is a pericardial effusion, which is detectable on ultrasound. On cardiac examination, many of these patients will have a pericardial friction rub, narrowing pulse pressure, and jugular venous distention (JVD).

PULMONARY DISEASE

- *Pulmonary Embolus.* This serious life-threatening disease most often manifests as acute shortness of breath with tachycardia. Some patients may also complain of a pleuritic type of chest pain, reproducible with palpation, and increased pain on inspiration. Common symptoms include chest pain in 88% of patients, dyspnea in 84% of patients, and cough in 53% of patients. Common physical findings include tachypnea (respiratory rate greater than 16) in 92% of patients, tachycardia (heart rate greater than 100 bpm) in 44% of patients, and temperature greater than 100°F in 43% of patients. Risk factors of pulmonary embolism include a history of atrial fibrillation, obesity, pregnancy, prolonged immobilization, posttrauma, oral contraceptive use, postsurgery, and cancer.

- *Asthma or Chronic Obstructive Pulmonary Disease.* The shortness of breath experienced by asthmatics is often described as a tightness similar to cardiac chest pain. The history of onset and duration are key points in the history. Generally, if shortness of breath is the initial complaint, a pulmonary etiology is more likely.
- *Spontaneous Pneumothorax.* A sudden onset of chest pain with shortness of breath may also be a spontaneous pneumothorax. These patients are usually tall, thin, relatively healthy men. People with asthma are also at increased risk for pneumothorax.

AORTA

- *Acute Aortic Dissection.* This is often described as a tearing pain that radiates into the back. Most of these patients are hypertensive and can have a marked difference in blood pressure in both arms. This is a surgical emergency.
- *Ruptured Aortic Aneurysm.* The majority of aneurysms are abdominal and produce abdominal or lower back pain. However, there are occasional thoracic aneurysms that may leak. Their presentation is usually similar to that of an aortic dissection. This is also a surgical emergency, and some of these patients may become acutely hypotensive.

GASTROINTESTINAL

- *Gastroesophageal Reflux or Hiatal Hernia.* This pain can closely mimic cardiac chest pain. Often there is a history of the pain occurring for days to months to years. These patients, however, should be treated as cardiac patients until proven otherwise. It is also important to note that patients with cardiac disease have had relief of symptoms after being given a "GI cocktail," a combination of antacid, viscous lidocaine, barbiturate, and antispasmodic agents.
- *Esophageal Spasm.* This is a diagnosis of exclusion that is generally reached after a full workup. This is most often given to relatively young, healthy people with an unexplained source of chest pain. This pain can actually resolve with sublingual nitroglycerin. This diagnosis should never be considered as a working diagnosis in transport, and these patients should be treated like all other patients with chest pain.

CHEST WALL PAIN

- *Trauma.* Rib fractures and bruises secondary to trauma can cause a sharp chest wall pain that is reproducible on palpation. It is also important to consider traumatic visceral injuries, such as pulmonary or cardiac contusion, if the mechanism is suggestive. Also remember that trauma patients can still have AMIs.

Key Physical Examination Findings

- *Initial Assessment.* Assess airway and breathing and look for signs of cardiogenic shock.
- *Vital Signs.* Measure blood pressure in both arms.
- *Neck.* Check for JVD which can be a sign of CHF, pericardial tamponade, or tension pneumothorax.
- *Lungs.* Assess for signs of new-onset CHF (ie, crackles at the bases). Also listen for an absence of breath sounds, indicating pneumothorax.
- *Cardiac Examination.* Listen for a friction rub, indicative of pericarditis, or an S_3 or S_4, another sign of CHF.
- *Abdomen.* Palpate the abdomen for a pulsatile mass, indicative of an abdominal aortic aneurysm.
- *Extremities.* Check for evidence of peripheral edema, a sign of CHF.

Treatment Plan for Patients with Chest Pain Consistent with AMI

- *Patient Assessment.* Reassess patient frequently owing to the potential for a worsening of the hemodynamic status, CHF, or life-threatening arrhythmia. Cardiac monitoring is necessary. Be prepared—a high potential for cardiac arrest exists. Rapid, but safe, transport to the ED is an important component of care, and short scene times are essential if thrombolytic therapy is to be effective.
- Administer O_2, **provide ventilatory support** as needed, and monitor O_2 saturation by pulse oximetry if available.
- **Monitor the ECG** and, if possible, obtain a **12-lead ECG.** Screen for possible use of thrombolytics.
- **Establish IV access** with 0.9% NaCL or lactated Ringer's solution at a KVO rate.

- Consult with medical control physician.
- Give **nitroglycerin, 1/150 grain (0.4 mg) SL** (for systolic BP greater than 90 mm Hg). Dosage may be repeated every 5 minutes.
- If nitroglycerin has been ineffective, give **morphine sulfate 1 to 3 mg IV,** (for systolic BP greater than 90 mm Hg). Dosage may be repeated every 5 minutes as needed.
- If prehospital thrombolytic therapy is available, appropriate, and not contraindicated, use the following agents:
  Streptokinase, 1.5 million units IV over 60 minutes,
  or
  APSAC, 30 units IV over 2 to 5 minutes, or
  rt-PA, 15 mg IV bolus, followed by 0.75 mg/kg up to 50 mg IV infusion over 30 minutes, then 0.5 mg/kg up to 35 mg IV infusion over 60 minutes.
- **Treat symptomatic arrhythmias as indicated.** See Chapters 5 and 43, Bradycardia and Tachycardia, respectively, for specific options.
- **Treat cardiogenic shock** as described in Chapter 38, Shock.
- **If pulmonary edema is present, give furosemide (Lasix), 40 to 80 mg IV** (pediatric dose: 1 to 3 mg/kg IV).

Bibliography

Hafen BQ and Karren KJ: Prehospital Emergency Care, ed 3. Morton Publishing Co, Englewood, CO, 1989, pp 351–362.

Stapczynski JS: Chest Pain. In Tintinalli JE, Krome LR, and Ruiz E (eds): Emergency Medicine: A Comprehensive Study Guide, ed 3. McGraw-Hill, New York, 1992, pp 127–132.

Wayne MA and Carrero R: Chest Pain. In Schwartz GR et al. (eds): Principles and Practices of Emergency Medicine. Lea & Febiger, Philadelphia, 1992, pp 303–317.

Notes

CHAPTER 11

Child Abuse

Rebecca Humes, MD

Presentation

Patterns of child abuse can reflect any form of physical or mental trauma but are usually characterized by unexplained or poorly explained injuries of different ages and delay in seeking medical care.

Immediate Concerns

- **Is there evidence of severe burns, head, or abdominal injury?** Virtually all severe abuse falls into these groups. Consider airway and cervical spine protection if there is a change of mental status present. Abdominal injuries and burns require close monitoring of vital signs and establishment of IV access.

Important History

- **What is the mechanism of injury?** Concerns should be raised by stories that are inconsistent with the injury such as a broken leg caused by falling off a chair. Also consider whether the history matches the age and abilities of the child for example, toddlers cannot get hurt falling off a bicycle they were operating.
- **Is there more than one injury present?** Multiple injuries in different stages of healing are characteristic of child abuse. Often specific lesions (ie, cigarette burns) will also be clustered.
- **What is the home environment like?** As a prehospital EMS provider, your observations of the child's home and any evidence of neglect or abuse may be the only information available to the ED physician, protective services, or the courts. For example, a parent who is more concerned

with why the ambulance was called than the care of the child may be significant.

- **Are there other family members at risk?** Other siblings, the mother or girlfriend, father or boyfriend, and elderly individuals are all potential victims of abuse.

Differential Diagnosis

- ***Bruises.*** Bruises are the most common form of child abuse. These are especially characteristic on the face or genitals. Bruises may have patterns reflecting the item with which the child was struck or may be of different colors or ages.
- ***Burns.*** Only 5% to 10% of burns occur from abuse, but they are nonetheless a serious prognostic sign. In addition to the risks posed by the burn, 40% of children with burns requiring medical care will eventually be killed by their abuser if returned home. Look for locations that would be difficult to accidentally burn (eg, the back of the hand). Be alert for other signs of abuse.
- ***Skeletal Injuries.*** Over 50% of fractures in children under 1 year old are caused by abuse. Rib, skull, and midshaft long bone fractures are virtually always due to abuse. Very few young children are able to generate the force to break large bones unless there is a clear external cause, such as a motor vehicle accident.
- ***Head Trauma.*** This includes blunt trauma and trauma secondary to shaken baby syndrome. Children have very large heads in proportion to their bodies, and shaking may result in whiplash injuries with often fatal subdural hematomas. Seizures are common in these patients and cervical spine injuries may also be present.
- ***Abdominal Injuries.*** These are second only to head trauma in abuse fatalities. There are often no external signs of injury. Look for repeated vomiting, abdominal pain, and distention in a child with other evidence of abuse.

Key Physical Examination Findings

- ***Initial Assessment.*** Look for signs of head injury or shock. Assess the home environment and other potential victims.

- *Skin.* Suspect child abuse when there are burns or bruises of different ages and in unlikely areas for accidental injuries are present.
- *Abdomen.* Look for abdominal tenderness, distention, or hypoactive bowel sounds. External signs of injury are often absent.
- *Orthopedic Examination.* Assess for extremity pain, deformity, or unwillingness to bear weight, as many of these conditions may be evidence of abuse.
- *Neurologic Examination.* Be alrt for seizures, coma, or change in mental status, as many of these conditions are suggestive of head injury in abused children.

Treatment Plan

- **Rapidly evaluate hemodynamic instability and mental status.** Head and abdominal injuries are the major causes of mortality and morbidity among abused children.
- **Assess both patient and home environment. Consider other victims** in the home and evidence suggestive of abuse or neglect.

GENERAL TREATMENT GUIDELINES: HEMODYNAMICALLY STABLE PATIENT

- Administer O_2 and **provide ventilatory support** as needed. Protect cervical spine as indicated.
- **Treat non–life-threatening injuries** as appropriate (ie, control bleeding, splint fractures, etc)
- **Transport to appropriate ED.** Ensure patient comfort en route.

GENERAL TREATMENT GUIDELINES: HEMODYNAMICALLY UNSTABLE PATIENT

- Administer O_2 and **provide ventilatory support** as needed. Protect cervical spine as indicated.
- Place patient in the **shock position** (supine with legs elevated), or use PASG, if indicated. The use of PASG is currently controversial; follow local protocol.
- Establish **large–bore IV access** with 0.9% NaCl or LR; fluid resuscitation at 20 ml/kg

- **Rapid transport to appropriate ED.** Do not needlessly delay patient transport—expedite transport.
- **Treat non–life-threatening injuries** as appropriate (ie, control bleeding, splint fractures, etc)

Supporting Documentation. Clear statements of history, using quotes when possible, and accurate descriptions of injuries in laymen's terms are invaluable in court.

Mandatory Reporting. Depending on state and local laws, medical personnel, including prehospital providers, may be required by law to report any cases of suspected abuse or neglect. Inform both the receiving facility and either the police or state child services agency depending on the local policy in effect. In all states, suspected victims may be held at a medical facility for up to 24 hours without a court order, and medical personnel are immune from any legal action as long as reports are made in good faith.

Bibliography

Berkowitz CD: Child Abuse. In Tintinalli JE, Krome LR, and Ruiz E (eds): Emergency Medicine: A Comprehensive Study Guide, ed 3. McGraw-Hill, New York, 1992, pp 498–501.

Bliss J: Child Abuse. Rourke Corporation, Vero Beach, 1990.

Johnson CF and Showers J: Diagnosis and Management: Physical Abuse of Children. Children's Hospital Child Abuse Program, Columbus, 1985.

Kempe CH and Helfer RE: The Battered Child. University of Chicago Press, Chicago, 1980.

Notes

CHAPTER 12

Cough
Jonathan S. Rubens, MD

Presentation

In disorders of the respiratory tract, cough is often a presenting symptom and may or may not be accompanied by hemoptysis. Cough is a reflex resulting from irritation of the airway and stimulation of the afferent fibers of the cranial nerves IX and X. The purpose of the cough reflex is to keep the respiratory tract clear. Cough can have a psychogenic etiology but most often is the result of stimulation of the airway. Hemoptysis is the ejection of blood from the respiratory tract and lungs. In hemoptysis the blood is bright red, usually unclotted, and often mixed with sputum. Bleeding from other sources, such as the mouth and epistaxis, can masquerade as hemoptysis.

Immediate Concerns

- *Airway.* ABCs are of primary importance as always. Patients with persistent cough may be exhibiting this as a symptom of airway obstruction. In addition, any head and neck bleeding, including hemoptysis, can result in airway compromise. Aggressive airway management in these patients is warranted.

  Remember that an effective cough is the best means of a patient clearing their own airway. This should not be interfered with. If and when the cough becomes ineffective, then aggressive management for airway obstruction or occlusion should be undertaken.

- *Breathing.* In patients with hemoptysis, positioning the patient with the bleeding side down may allow for enhanced airway clearing as well as normal aeration of the unaffected side. Auscultation and percussion may help determine which is which.

Important History

- **Is there a history of fever, immune system compromise, or known infection?** Cough is a common symptom of upper respiratory illnesses and pneumonia. Progression of cough or hemoptysis may herald the worsening of one of these conditions. Patients with immune system compromise (ie, patients with AIDS and those with a history of tumors on chemotherapeutic regimens) are more prone to infectious causes of illness.
- **Is there associated shortness of breath or chest pain?** These symptoms may point to bronchospastic or cardiac causes of the complaint.
- **Is the patient a smoker or does the patient have a history of environmental smoke or fume exposure?** Smoke from any source is a respiratory tract irritant, and therefore may cause cough.
- **Does the patient have any prior lung or heart disease history?** Prior similar episodes or a history of tumors, emphysema, asthma, bronchitis, or cardiac disease are important historical clues to diagnosis and treatment.
- **Has there been any trauma?** Injury to the head, neck, or thorax may produce cough and or hemoptysis.

Differential Diagnosis

The causes of cough and hemoptysis are similar if not identical in many cases. Those conditions also frequently associated with hemoptysis are described in the following text.

UPPER RESPIRATORY TRACT

- **Airway obstruction** is usually manifested by stridor or wheezing in addition to a cough. With upper airway obstruction, stridor is the more common sign. It is a loud, musical sound heard usually only on inspiration. Stridor can be heard to come from the larynx whereas wheezing is usually generated in the chest. The presence of stridor should alert the examiner to a potentially life-threatening cause of the distress, including infections like croup and epiglottitis as well as tumors and inhaled foreign bodies (particularly in children).
- **Asthma** is characterized by reversible airway obstruction

and inflammation and may be a source of cough. Because of the variable degree of ventilation-perfusion changes in each patient with asthma, not all patients will wheeze and, particularly in children, a dry cough may be the only presenting symptom. The patient will usually complain of dyspnea, tightness, or pressure in the chest and show signs of tachypnea. Sputum production is variable and usually greatest as the attack resolves. The findings of a prolonged expiratory phase and wheezes throughout inspiration and expiration help to identify this condition. If severe, the attack can progress to severe respiratory distress, lethargy, hypercarbia with carbon dioxide narcosis, pneumothorax and respiratory failure.

- **Cancer of the larynx** can cause cough and hemoptysis leading to airway compromise. Bleeding from the upper airway is usually from the high-pressure bronchial circulation and may be brisk. Tumors account for approximately 20% of cases of hemoptysis. It is to be strongly suspected in middle-aged to elderly patients with a history of smoking.

- **Infections** such as rhinitis, pharyngitis, and laryngotracheobronchitis cause cough due to direct irritation of the upper airway. History of other upper respiratory symptoms as well as examination of the pharynx may give diagnostic clues to these etiologies.

BRONCHI

- **Bronchitis**, or the inflammation of the tracheobronchial tree, is a common cause of coughing. Acute infectious bronchitis is common in the winter months and can accompany the other signs and symptoms of an acute upper respiratory infection (URI). The cough of bronchitis is initially dry and nonproductive with a sensation of needing to expectorate mucus. Severe coughing can lead to chest pain. Bronchospasm can accompany bronchitis, but otherwise lung findings are usually conspicuously absent in these patients.

- **Bronchiectasis** is an irreversible, chronic focal disease of the bronchial tree often associated with infection. Chronic cough and sputum production are the most common symptoms of this disease. In some patients a recent history of pneumonia with residual cough is obtained. Cough is usually worse in the morning and evening hours with symptom-free time during the day. Hemoptysis can sometimes be the presenting symptom. It can be difficult to diagnose and must be differentiated from cystic fibrosis.

- **Bronchial carcinoma and adenoma** (see cancer of the larynx above).

LUNGS

- *Heart failure.* Pulmonary (low-pressure) venous bleeding may occur in association with pulmonary hypertension and, in particular, when associated with left-sided heart failure. Increased pressures cause congestion and, in some cases leaking, in the pulmonary venous system resulting in cough and hemoptysis (the pink frothy sputum of acute pulmonary edema).

- **Pneumonia** (including tuberculosis and fungal and parasitic infections) can be confined to one area of one lobe of the lung or can involve several segments, lobes, or even both lungs. Pneumonias can be viral or bacterial and the etiologic agents vary greatly with age and other underlying factors, including debility and immune system compromise. Often preceded by an URI, pneumonia can be heralded by a single shaking chill (a common finding in pneumococcal pneumonia—the most prevalent type), high fever, tachycardia, tachypnea, constitutional symptoms, and respiratory distress.

- **Pulmonary hypertension** is caused by reductions in the size of the pulmonary vascular bed due either primarily or secondary to diseases affecting this site. Patients may exhibit the same signs and symptoms seen with left-sided heart failure: cough, dyspnea, wheezing, and hemoptysis. Most of these patients will have some history of exertional dyspnea, chest pain, and frequent syncopal attacks. Most patients will have some knowledge of their diagnosis to help the prehospital care provider; occasionally, they will be seen on initial presentation. Bleeding will be from the low-pressure pulmonary venous system but it can be brisk. Supportive or resuscitative measures may be needed.

- **Pulmonary embolism** (PE) is the sudden lodging of a clot in the pulmonary artery or its branches with obstruction of blood flow to the involved area of lung. Patients with massive PE will usually present in shock or full cardiac arrest and must be differentiated from those with acute myocardial infarction, cardiac tamponade, and other causes of shock. The clinical signs of less severe PE are notoriously vague and nonspecific, so much that this is one of the most frequently missed diagnoses in emergency medicine. Small thromboemboli may be completely asymptomatic. Chest pain, pleuritic pain, low-grade fever, tachycardia, cough, hemoptysis, and a pleural friction rub on auscultation are all potential signs of this condition. It should be suspected in anyone with a sedentary lifestyle; the pregnant patient; and anyone with a hypercoagulable state (ie, cancer, tumors), lower extremity swelling, edema, or recent surgery.

- **Trauma** is the most obvious cause of hemoptysis and the insult is usually readily identified by clinical examination or by history. Remember that cough can be a sign of pneumothorax, pneumomediastinum, or both, and in the trauma patient it must not be overlooked.

Key Physical Examination Findings

- *General Appearance.* Observe the patient for signs of dyspnea at rest. Effort and rate of breathing should be noted. Attempt to define the quality and depth of the cough. Visualize and quantitate any sputum or blood expectorated.
- *Skin.* Is there pallor, flushing, cyanosis, or diaphoresis? The presence of a rash might indicate such causes as an allergic reaction or a specific infectious process.
- *HEENT.* Inspect the nose and mouth for clues to the presence of nasal discharge or bleeding, postnasal drip, and upper airway causes of cough or bleeding.
- *Neck.* Stridor as well as cough may be suggestive of a foreign body or of croup. Note the position of the trachea: is it midline or shifted, suggesting a mass lesion or pneumothorax? Are the neck veins distended, suggesting heart failure? Is the voice hoarse?
- *Chest.* Observe for any evidence of trauma, bruising, or asymmetric movement of the chest wall. Retractions of the sternum and intercostal areas give evidence of the work of breathing. Dullness to percussion or adventitial breath sounds (rales, rhonchi, wheezes, or rubs) may give clues to diagnosis. In addition, asymmetric sounds may point to areas of decreased aeration, which can be due to bleeding.

- ***Cardiac.*** Listen for murmurs and extra heart sounds, often difficult to hear in the field, but that can be evidence of underlying heart disease.

Treatment Plan

- Assess ABCs.
- Administer humidified O_2 and **provide ventilatory support** as needed. Protect cervical spine as indicated. Monitor O_2 saturation with pulse oximetry if available.

  NOTE: Do not interfere with effective coughing.
- Position the patient for ideal air exchange. Patients will breathe more easily when upright with gravity working with the diaphragm. Patients with lobar bleeding will achieve maximal oxygenation with the bleeding side down.
- Inititate **IV fluid resuscitation** with 0.9% NaCl or LR in cases of bleeding or hemorrhage and shock.
- Expedite transport for any patient with a compromised airway or breathing difficulty.

Bibliography

Karasic RB: Cough. In Fleisher and Ludwig et al. (eds): Textbook of Pediatric Emergency Medicine, ed 3. Williams and Wilkins, Baltimore, 1993, pp 140–143.

Mathisen DJ and Head J M: General Thoracic Emergencies. In Wilkins et al. (eds): Emergency Medicine: Scientific Foundations and Current Practice. Williams and Wilkins, Baltimore, 1989, pp 609–630.

Seward C and Mattingly D: Bedside Diagnosis. Churchill Livingstone, London, 1979, pp 166-169 and 223–230.

Notes

CHAPTER 13

Croup and Epiglottitis: Pediatric Laryngeal Edema

Patrick R. Coonan, RN, EdD, CEN, EMT-CC

Presentation

Two common pediatric disorders that present with airway obstruction symptoms are croup and epiglottitis. These disorders are characterized by inspiratory stridor and are often difficult to differentiate in the field.

Croup is caused by a virus and results in edema of the subglottic tissues; it occurs most frequently in the winter months. It rarely progresses to total obstruction and is much more common than epiglottitis. The child usually has a "barking"–like cough, inspiratory stridor, and dyspnea that responds well to humidity and the cool night air.

Epiglottitis must be considered in any child with stridor. It is caused by a life-threatening bacterial infection and occurs more commonly in children 2 to 4 years old, but can occur in younger children and adults. Symptoms develop suddenly, and symptoms of respiratory distress usually last less than 24 hours. High fever is characteristic along with drooling in about 25% to 50% of the patients. Children with epiglottitis are usually quiet and anxious and appear ill. Most prefer to sit up and lean forward with the neck flexed. They rarely have a croupy cough.

Immediate Concerns

- **Assess the degree of airway obstruction and compromise that is present.** If the infant or child is cyanotic and barely breathing, immediate steps to establish an airway are necessary. If there are signs of moderate or severe respiratory distress, oxygen in high flow should be delivered in a way that is nonthreatening or irritating to the child. The patient should be kept as calm as possible.

Important History

- **When was the onset of stridor?** Is there fever present or other associated symptoms, such as poor feeding, drooling, cough, or hoarseness? The presence of underlying medical conditions, use of any medications at home, allergies, and exposure to others with infection is important.

Differential Diagnosis

- **Differentiate between an obstruction due to a foreign body and an obstruction due to laryngeal edema.** This differentiation is important: foreign body obstructions are treated significantly different than are obstructions caused by edema. In general, foreign body obstructions have a more sudden onset, are not associated with fever or infection, and are not accompanied by signs of allergic reaction (see Chapter 33, Obstructed Airway).
- **Determine if the obstruction is partial or complete.** This is another important distinction. Complete obstruction and partial obstruction with poor air exchange must be managed aggressively: perform the obstructive airway techniques as appropriate, ventilate and oxygenate as indicated. Patients with partial obstruction and adquate air exchange should receive supplemental O_2 and observation. If a foreign body is suspected, the patient should be encouraged to cough.
- Determine diagnosis of stridor.
    Infectious conditions: epiglottitis, croup, enlarged tonsils, or abscess
    Noninfectious conditions: foreign body aspiration, spasmodic croup, caustic ingestions, trauma, various congenital disorders

Viral Croup	Epiglottitis
Children less than 2 years of age	Children more than 2 years of age
Common infection	Less common
Viral	Bacterial

Recurrence possible	Recurrence rare
Gradual onset	Rapid onset
Sick, not toxic	Toxic, high fever
Stridor (characteristic)	Stridor (not always)
Barking cough	No or limited cough
Hoarse voice	Muffled voice
Restless	Quiet
Position not important	Patient wants to sit up, lean forward
No drooling	Drooling occasionally

Key Physical Examination Findings

- *Primary Survey.* Look for signs of airway occlusion. Auscultate the chest to hear how well the child is ventilating.
- *Head and Neck.* Do not attempt to examine the oral cavity or to perform painful procedures. These can increase the respiratory distress. If the child has fever, do not attempt to put a tongue blade or other object in the child's mouth, as this has been reported to cause total laryngospasm in some children.

Treatment Plan

This section addresses the therapeutic modalities recommended for the care of patients with croup or epiglottitis. See Chapter 33, Obstructed Airway, for recommendations regarding treatment of foreign body obstruction.

- *Patient Assessment.* Reassess frequently because the potential for acute and rapid airway obstruction exists. The child should be attached to a cardiac monitor and pulse oximeter without irritating the child. Encourage the participation of the family.

ADEQUATE AIR EXCHANGE

- Let the child assume the most comfortable position.
- Transport expeditiously to the ED. Do not use supine position during transport.
- Do not examine the throat; complete obstruction may occur.

- Administer **humidified O₂** immediately.
- Setup, nebulize, and prepare to deliver **racemic epineph-rine** (Vaponefrin) into a face mask. Dosage 0.25 to 0.50 ml in 2.5 ml 0.9% NaCL. May be repeated in 20 to 30 minutes.
- Be prepared to ventilate the patient should complete obstruction occur.

INADEQUATE OR NO AIR EXCHANGE

- **Do not try to intubate a child with epiglottitis in the field** unless you are unable to ventilate the patient. It is extremely difficult and dangerous. Direct visualization is needed. Transport expeditiously to ED.
- Ventilate the patient with high flow O₂ and a BVM. Forceful ventilation with high pressures will be necessary because of the swollen epiglottis. Consider endotracheal intubation.
- If unable to intubate, the child's only hope is an immediate needle crycothyroidotomy.

Bibliography

Caroline NL: Emergency Care in the Streets, ed 4. Little, Brown and Company, Boston, 1991, pp 689–690.

Epiglottitis and Croup. In Nichols D, et al. (eds): Golden Hour: The Handbook of Pediatric Life Support. Mosby–Year Book, St. Louis, 1991, pp 47–63.

Selbst NE and Steve M: Stridor. In Pediatric Emergency Medicine for the House Officer. William and Wilkins, Baltimore, 1988, pp 181–189.

Notes

CHAPTER 14

Diabetic Ketoacidosis and Hyperglycemia

Douglas Barnaby, EMT-P
Thomas J. Rahilly, MS, EMT-CC

Presentation

A true medical emergency, diabetic ketoacidosis (DKA) is most commonly seen in patients with diagnosed insulin-dependent diabetes mellitus between the ages of birth and 19 years. Because the onset of ketoacidosis is relatively slow (12 to 24 hours), the patient may exhibit a variety of symptoms from general malaise to coma. The patient's skin will usually be warm and dry. Because these patients are likely to be suffering from dehydration, they may have flushed skin color, tachycardia, and hypotension. The breath often has a fruity or acetone odor. Deep respirations (Kussmaul's), whether rapid or not, suggest an attempt by the respiratory system to restore normal pH balance through CO_2 elimination. Although not diabetic in nature, alcohol abuse may be the cause of the patient's condition and should not be overlooked. A person with hyperglycemia may report with nonspecific complaints such as concentrated urine, constant thirst, and "sticky" or "heavy" urine. These patients may have a history of diabetes. The only complaint may be tiredness or lack of energy.

Immediate Concerns

- **What is the patient's hemodynamic status?** Dehydration resulting from the production of large amounts of urine and frequent episodes of vomiting must be treated immediately. If the patient is hemodynamically unstable, begin resuscitation efforts at once with oxygen and normal saline via large-bore IV.

- **Are there tall sharply peaked T waves on the patient's ECG?** Metabolic acidosis may lead to high serum potassium (hyperkalemia) requiring treatment with sodium bicarbonate.
- **Does the patient have an altered mental status?** The patient's mental status provides a good index of severity and plays an important role in determining advanced life support field treatment. The alert patient with normal vital signs who provides a coherent history of frequent urination and increased thirst will clearly be treated differently than the patient who is disoriented and hypotensive.

Important History

- **Does the patient have a history of diabetes mellitus?** Ask the patient if he or she is taking insulin. If so, has the medication been taken as prescribed? Has the patient eaten more or less than usual? Many cases of DKA occur from noncompliance with the prescribed insulin regimen or taking the wrong dosage. Failure to follow dietary guidelines may also bring about a ketoacidotic episode. Do not forget to check for medical alert identification devices and insulin kits.
- **When did the patient last eat?** When did the patient take insulin? A patient with diabetes who has eaten, but has not taken insulin, is at risk for hyperglycemia. Conversely, a patient with diabetes who has not eaten, yet has taken insulin, is at risk for hypoglycemia.
- **How long has the patient been like this?** Hyperglycemia and DKA have a slow onset (12 to 24 hours), whereas the onset of hypoglycemia can occur within minutes.
- **Has the patient experienced recent increased urination or thirst?** High glucose levels lead to increased urination. Increased urination leads to dehydration, which in turn results in thirst and hypotension.
- **Has the patient been treated recently for an infection?** An infection may precipitate hyperglycemia. A fever may indicate sepsis and offer an explanation for hyperglycemia when other findings are normal. In addition, an acute inflammation of the pancreas or chronic pancreatitis may be responsible for ketoacidosis.
- **Has the patient experienced a recent emotional upset?**

Stress hormones secreted during a period of heightened emotional distress have anti-insulin effects and may cause ketoacidosis.

- **Is the patient taking any medication?** Concurrent use of medications such as phenytoin, steroids, and phenobarbital may lead a patient to develop ketoacidosis. Bring all medications to the ED.

- **Is there a history of alcohol abuse?** Once thought to be a condition predominantly affecting middle-aged women, alcoholic ketoacidosis is now seen in younger individuals who drink excessively while eating minimal amounts of food. Even first-time drinkers may experience this illness.

- **Are there bystanders present who may have information relative to the patient's condition?** Family members, friends, or coworkers may have pertinent information related to the patient.

- **Is the patient pregnant?** Diabetes can be induced by pregnancy.

Differential Diagnosis

DIABETES MELLITUS

- *Insulin Dependent.* DKA exists when the blood sugar level is greater than 300 mg/dl, high levels of urine ketones are present, and the patient's pH is 7.3 or less. Many prehospital EMS systems are beginning to make use of field blood glucose analysis techniques to determine whether or not the patient is hyperglycemic.

- *Non–Insulin Dependent.* This form of diabetes often occurs in older patients who are obese. These patients are usually hyperosmolar and hyperglycemic with no acidosis and ketone production. These patients have many of the same signs as DKA but will not present with a fruity breath odor. The hyperosmolar nonketotic hyperglycemic patient will be more dehydrated than the patient with DKA.

- *Gestational Diabetes.* Pregnancy may be accompanied by glucose intolerance.

ACUTE STRESS

Patients suffering from stressful events such as sepsis, trauma, or surgery will usually self-correct after the event is over. AMIs can also lead to ketoacidosis, and this condition should be considered in an unconscious patient with signs of hyperglycemia and a history of AMI.

SPURIOUS (FALSE) HYPERGLYCEMIA

If the blood sugar level indicates hyperglycemia and the patient has no signs or symptoms of the illness, repeat the test.

OTHER SOURCES

Exogenous glucose load, pancreatic disease, and Cushing's syndrome are other less frequent causes of DKA.

Key Physical Examination Findings

- *Initial Assessment.* Look for signs of shock, hypovolemia, and altered mental status
- *Vital Signs.* Check for Kussmaul's respirations.
- *HEENT.* Note any fruity, sweet, or acetonelike odor to the breath, which indicates ketoacidosis. Excessive thirst may indicate dehydration.
- *Abdomen.* Evaluate nausea, vomiting, and abdominal pain, which may disguise ketoacidosis as acute abdomen.
- *Skin.* Assess skin temperature and appearence. In ketoacidosis, skin is usually warm and dry.
- *Other.* Note any unusual changes in urine frequency and volume. Excessive urination results in dehydration and hypovolemia. Check for hyperglycemia by using a reagent strip or the patient's portable glucometer.

Treatment Plan

HEMODYNAMICALLY STABLE PATIENT

- Maintain airway, **administer O$_2$,** and **provide ventilatory support** as necessary.
- Monitor patients vital signs and ECG.
- **Draw blood** (red-top tube) and determine blood glucose level. Establish **large-bore IV** with **0.9% NaCl or lactated Ringer's solution** at a KVO rate.
- Transport to appropriate ED.
  NOTE: Field blood glucose testing is controversial; follow local protocol.

HEMODYNAMICALLY UNSTABLE PATIENT

- Administer O_2 and provide **ventilatory support** as necessary and monitor O_2 saturation with pulse oximetry if available.
- Place the patient in the **shock position**.
- **Monitor ECG**. Hyperkalemia may lead physician to order sodium bicarbonate.
- **Draw blood** (red-top tube), determine blood glucose level and establish large-bore IV access and begin fluid resuscitation with 0.9% NaCl (1 liter per hour).
- If unable to determine blood glucose level and patient has altered mental status, administer 50 ml 50% dextrose IV.
- **Administer 1 to 2 mg naloxone hydrochloride** (Narcan) **IV**.
- **Transport expeditiously to ED. DKA is a TRUE EMERGENCY.** Do not needlessly delay transport—expedite transport. When possible, treat patient en route.

Bibliography

Anderson DL: Diabetic Ketoacidosis (Hyperglycemia). In Cosgriff JH Jr: The Practice of Emergency Care, ed 2. JB Lippincott, Philadelphia, 1984, 293–296.

Bledsoe B, Porter R, and Shade B (eds): Paramedic Emergency Care, ed 2. Brady, Englewood Cliffs, NJ, 1991, pp 710–715.

Haist SA, Robbins JB, and Gomella LG (eds): Internal Medicine on Call. Appleton & Lange, Norwalk, CT, 1991, pp 136–142.

Ragland G: Diabetic Ketoacidosis. In Tintinalli JE, Krome LR, and Ruiz E (eds): Emergency Medicine: A Comprehensive Study Guide, ed 3. McGraw-Hill, New York, 1992, pp 615–623.

Ragland G: Alcoholic Ketoacidosis. In Tintinalli JE, Krome LR, and Ruiz E (eds): Emergency Medicine: A Comprehensive Study Guide, ed 3. McGraw-Hill, New York, 1992, pp 624–627.

Stine R and Marcus M (eds): A Practical Approach to Emergency Medicine. Little, Brown and Co, Boston, 1987, pp 147–150.

Notes

CHAPTER 15

Domestic Violence
Deborah Barclay, EMT-P

Presentation

Domestic violence is defined as physical, emotional, or sexual abuse by a partner involved in an intimate relationship. Although most research has focused on women who have been abused by men, the term domestic violence has been chosen to reflect the awareness that any person, man or woman, may be abused by their partner. It is not currently known how well the research on women abused by men may be applied to the abuse that may occur in gay or lesbian relationships, or even when men are abused by women. The EMS provider must be aware of the potential for violence under these circumstances as well.

Just how bad is the problem of domestic violence? It is hard to know the exact magnitude of the problem because many incidents go unreported. However, studies indicate that as many as 2 million women in the United States each year are abused—actual incidents may be twice as high. Approximately 25% of U.S. women will be abused at least once in their lifetime. Almost half of the husbands who beat their wives will do so three or more times per year. It is estimated that more than half of murdered women were killed by present or former partners. Currently we do not know the extent of the problem in gay and lesbian relationships. Regardless, domestic violence is clearly of epidemic proportion.

The patient who is a victim of domestic violence may present to the paramedic with any type of injury. The paramedic may or may not be initially aware that domestic violence is the cause of the injury.

Immediate Concerns

- **Is the scene safe?** Domestic disputes are potentially dangerous situations for prehospital care providers. Aggressive

93

individuals in the domestic dispute are often jealous and overly possessive of the battered partner and will not allow the patient to be separated from them. If the aggressive person is still at the scene, wait for law enforcement assistance.

- **Does the patient have any serious injuries?** Serious injuries should be treated immediately. Minor injuries should be treated in the safety of the ambulance. Try to separate the patient from the aggressor, prior to the treatment.
- **Are there other potential victims in the house?** An abusive partner may experience rage or helplessness and turn on another weaker victim. If the patient is being transported to the hospital, all potential victims of violence, such as children, should be transported as well.

Important History

- **How was this injury obtained?** Abuse victims will often take responsibility for their injury to protect the abuser. Suspect abuse when:
  - The injury is not consistent with the patient's account of how the injury was obtained.
  - The patient has injuries in various stages of healing.
  - The partner is overly concerned, will not be separated from the patient, and answers questions directed toward the patient.
  - The patient has injuries to the head, face, back, chest or breasts, or buttocks.
- **Is there a psychological profile of the battered women that may be used to help identify victims of abuse?** Unfortunately, none currently exists, however, there do appear to be groups of women at increased risk of abuse.
  - Single, separated, or divorced (or planning a separation or divorce) women
  - Women who are 17 to 28 years old
  - Pregnant women
  - Women who abuse alcohol or drugs
  - Partners of substance abusers
  - Women whose partners are excessively jealous or possessive

- **How should the victim of suspected domestic violence be interviewed?** Be sure to maintain a nonjudgmental and supportive attitude. In addition, the patient should be interviewed apart from their partner. Your interview goal is not only to discover the presence of domestic violence, but also to assess the safety of the patient. The following questions should be asked in the EMS provider's own words.
  - Are you in a relationship in which you have been physically hurt or threatened by your partner?
  - Are you in a relationship in which you have been treated badly? In what way?
  - Has your partner ever forced you to have sex when you did not want to?
  - Has your partner ever threatened or abused your children?
  - Do you ever feel afraid of your partner?
  - You have mentioned that your partner uses drugs or alcohol. How do they act when they are drinking or using drugs? Are they ever verbally or physically abusive?
  - Do you have guns in the home? Has your partner ever threatened to use them when angry?

Differential Diagnosis

Remember, the victim of domestic violence is likely to present with a wide variety of injuries. They may conceal that they are a victim. Have a high index of suspicion when the reported mechanism of injury does not seem believable, when there has been a delay in seeking care, when there are multiple injuries in various stages of healing, and when there are repeated or chronic injuries.

Key Physical Examination Findings

Assess as any trauma patient. Remember, the patient may downplay the extent or severity of injury to protect the partner, so a thorough assessment is vital.
- *Initial Assessment.* Look for signs of head injury or shock. Assess the home environment and look for other potential victims.
- *HEENT.* Look for contusions, abrasions, and minor lacerations.

- *Neck.* Look for contusions and other soft tissue injury.
- *Chest.* Suspect abuse when injury to the chest, and particularly to the breasts, is present.
- *Skin.* Suspect abuse when burns or bruises of different ages and in unlikely areas for accidental injuries are present.
- *Abdomen.* Look for abdominal tenderness, distension, or hypoactive bowel sounds. External signs of injury are often absent. Be suspicious of injuries to a pregnant woman.
- *Orthopedic Examination.* Assess for extremity pain, deformity fractures and strains.
- *Neurologic Examination.* Be alert for seizures, coma, or change in mental status as any of these conditions is suggestive of head injury.

Treatment Plan

- Rapidly **evaluate hemodynamic instability and mental status**.
- **Assess both patient and home environment. Consider other victims** in the home and evidence suggestive of abuse or neglect.
- **Even if the patient's injuries do not require transport, consider transport to remove the patient from the violent situation and to present counseling and shelter options.**
- Separate patient from partner when possible to allow the patient to speak freely.
- Provide information for shelters in your area or the telephone number for **National Domestic Violence Hotline—(800) 333-SAFE.**
- Always report your suspicions to the medical control physician or the staff at the receiving ED.

GENERAL TREATMENT GUIDELINES FOR HEMODYNAMICALLY STABLE PATIENT

- **Administer O_2 and provide ventilatory support** as needed. Protect cervical spine as indicated.
- **Treat non–life-threatening injuries** as appropriate (ie, control bleeding, splint fractures, etc).
- **Transport to appropriate ED.** Ensure patient comfort en route.

GENERAL TREATMENT GUIDELINES FOR
HEMODYNAMICALLY UNSTABLE PATIENT

- **Administer O$_2$ and provide ventilatory support** as needed. Protect cervical spine as indicated.
- Place patient in the **shock position** (supine with legs elevated) or use **PASG, if indicated.** The use of PASG is currently controversial; follow local protocol.
- Establish **large–bore IV access** and begin **fluid resuscitation with 0.9% NaCl or lactated Ringer's solution.**
- **Rapid transport to appropriate ED.** Do not needlessly delay patient transport—expedite transport.
- **Treat non–life-threatening injuries** as appropriate (ie, control bleeding, splint fractures, etc).
- **Transport to appropriate ED.** Ensure patient comfort en route.

Supporting Documentation. Clear statements of history, using quotes when possible, and accurate descriptions of injuries in laymen's terms are invaluable in court.

Bibliography

American Medical Association Diagnostic and Treatment Guidelines on Domestic Violence. Arch Fam Med, 39–47, September 1992.

Haven BQ and Karen KJ. Prehospital Emergency Care & Crisis Intervention, ed 4. Prentice Hall, Englewood Cliffs, NJ, 1992.

Notes

CHAPTER 16

Drug Withdrawal Syndrome

Elizabeth Cohn, RN, EMT-CC
Lorraine Hartnet, MD, FACEP

Presentation

Patients experiencing drug withdrawal may range from alert, oriented, and able to exhibit symptoms of an altered mental status or seizures (usually violent). The overall condition and assessment of vital signs will dictate the prehospital treatment of the patient.

Physical findings usually include hypertension, tachycardia, tachypnea, diaphoresis, dilated pupils, agitation, disorientation, and seizures.

Immediate Concerns

- *ABCs.* Airway, breathing, and circulation must take priority over all other treatment.
- *Altered Mental Status.* Drug withdrawal patients with an altered mental status may be difficult to manage medically and physically. They may become violent and exceptionally uncooperative. Extra personnel may be needed to help control the patient and to assist with establishing IV access and administering oxygen and medication.
- *Seizures.* If the patient begins to seize, maintain the airway, administer high-concentration oxygen, and transport. If IV access can be established, do so, but not at the cost of delaying transport.
- *Arrhythmias.* Although seen more commonly in drug overdose patients, cardiac monitoring of the symptomatic patient is warranted.

Important History

Any history obtained from a drug-dependent person should be carefully questioned, and confirmed when possible. Use available family, friends, or bystanders to obtain as much detailed information as possible.

The history should include:

- What drugs are taken on a regular basis?
- How much of the drug was or usually is taken?
- In what form or dose?
- How often is the drug ingested/injected?
- When was the last dose taken?
- How long has the patient been like this?
- Are there any underlying medical problems such as liver disease, bleeding disorders, human immunodefiency virus (HIV) status, or malignancies?

Differential Diagnosis

Drug withdrawal is not usually life-threatening, but many of the differential diagnoses are and, therefore, must be ruled out. Drug withdrawal is a diagnosis of exclusion.

The differential diagnoses include:

- *Hypoxia.* Hypoxia must be ruled out by examination and history.
- *Metabolic Conditions.* Hypoglycemia should be ruled out by history and use of a blood glucose test.
- *Traumatic Injury.* Subdural, epidural, or intracerebral bleeds are commonly seen in drug abusing patients secondary to trauma. Never assume an alcoholic or substance abuse patient is agitated solely due to the abuse of the substance.
- *Toxic Overdose.* Drug overdose can occur with cocaine, amphetamines, hallucinogens, anticholinergics (tricyclic antidepressants), opiates, benzodiazepines, sedative hypnotics, barbiturates, or alcohol. (Delirium tremens [DTs] is a serious and life-threatening form of alcohol withdrawal.)
- *Infection.* Serious infections, such as encephalitis or meningitis, may manifest with symptoms similar to those of drug withdrawal.
- *Seizure Disorder.* Patients with a history of a seizure disorder may present with seizures unrelated to drug withdrawal.
- *Psychiatric Disorders.* Psychiatric patients can experience a wide range of psychiatric conditions that manifest symptoms similar to those of drug withdrawal.

Key Physical Examination Findings

Generally mild signs and symptoms occur early and become

more serious if left untreated. Early diagnosis and treatment is essential.
- *Vital Signs.* Assess for hypertension (may have hypotension or orthostatic hypotension if volume depleted), tachycardia, tachypnea, low-grade temperature, dilated pupils and tearing, yawning, and runny nose.
- *Skin.* Inspect for diaphoresis and piloerection (goose flesh).
- *Abdomen.* Note increased bowel sounds, nausea, vomiting, and diarrhea.
- *Neurologic Examination.* Agitation, confusion, restlessness, insomnia, depression, tremors, muscle fasciculation, disorientation, hallucinations, and seizures.

Treatment Plan

Determine whether the patient is hemodynamically stable or unstable. The patient with stable vital signs may become hypotensive or start seizing suddenly. Continuous reassessment is essential.

STABLE PATIENTS

Stable patients with normal vital signs who are alert, oriented, and are not experiencing seizures:
- Monitor the patient's condition and transport to ED

UNSTABLE PATIENTS

Unstable patients with abnormal vital signs, altered mental status, or seizures:
- **Administer O$_2$ and provide ventilatory support**. Monitor O$_2$ saturation with pulse oximetry if available.
- **Monitor ABCs**.
- **Establish IV access** with 0.9% NaCl or LR
- Consider the administration of the following agents:
  - 25 g D$_{50}$ IV
  - Thiamine 100 mg IM/IV
  - Narcan 0.4 to 2.0 mg IV. Note Narcan administration may precipitate opium withdrawal
- **Transport to appropriate ED**. Ensure patient comfort en route.

Bibliography

Goldfrank L , et al.: Goldfrank's Toxicological Emergencies. Appleton and Lange, Norwalk, CT, 1990, pp 535–546.

Notes

CHAPTER 17

Dyspnea

Walt Stoy, PhD, NREMT-P
Thomas J. Rahilly, MS, EMT-CC

Presentation

Dyspnea is one of the most common medical complaints witnessed in the prehospital arena. Most patients describe it as a sensation of shortness of breath or a feeling of "air hunger" accompanied by labored breathing. Dyspnea may be caused by pulmonary or cardiac disease or by any mechanism that causes hypoxia. Dyspnea may be mild, manifesting as dyspnea on exertion, or severe dyspnea occurring even at rest. This chapter focuses on dyspnea caused by mechanisms other than foreign body obstruction (see Chapter 33) or croup and epiglottitis (see Chapter 13).

Immediate Concerns

- **Is the patient's airway patent and stable?** Look and listen for indicators of airway obstruction. Check for equal bilateral chest movement and cyanosis in the patient's nail beds and mucous membranes. A patient experiencing difficulty breathing may show signs of labored respirations, such as the use of accessory muscles, tracheal tugging, or nasal flaring. Auscultation of the chest should always follow a visual inspection of the neck and chest.
- **What is the rate and depth of the respirations?** Most adults breathe at a resting rate of about 16 breaths per minute. Patients in respiratory distress usually have a rapid (greater than 25 breaths per minute) and deep pattern of breathing. The respiratory rate (RR) may be slow (less than nine breaths) and shallow if the respiratory drive has been depressed. Be alert for respiratory breathing patterns that may indicate central nervous system (CNS) impairment (Cheyne-Stokes respirations) and medical emergencies (Kussmaul's respirations).

- **Is the patient hypoxic?** It is usually not possible to obtain an arterial blood gas in the field; however, pulse oximetry is becoming more available to paramedics. In the absence of pulse oximetry, clinical assessment must be used. The presence of either tachypnea or bradypnea, tachycardia, or cyanosis may suggest hypoxia. Restlessness, agitation, confusion, and occasionally combative behavior may also indicate hypoxia. The absence of cyanosis is not a reliable indicator of adequate oxygenation. Cyanosis occurs when 5 gm% of hemoglobin is unsaturated with oxygen. The normal adult has approximately 12 to 15 gm% of hemoglobin. A severely anemic patient may have significantly less hemoglobin. A patient with 6 gm% of hemoglobin, for example, will not be cyanotic if more than 1 gm% are oxygenated. This patient has a dramatically reduced oxygen-carrying capacity, approximately 40% to 50% of normal and yet will not become cyanotic until they are carrying less than 9% of the oxygen of a normal healthy patient. Do not withhold oxygen from the hypoxic patient.
- **Does the patient produce abnormal breath sounds?** The breathing process is normally quiet. Listen to the chest for abnormal sounds that may indicate the nature of the problem. Absent breath sounds may indicate a pneumothorax or tension pneumothorax. If a tension pneumothorax is present, immediate needle decompression of the chest is indicated. Open pneumothoraces should be sealed immediately (on three sides) with an air occlusive dressing.
- **In what position was the patient found?** Frequently, the patient experiencing dyspnea will be in a sitting or semisitting position. These patients do not tolerate lying flat and should be transported in a position that permits maximal comfort for the patient.

Important History

- **Does the patient have a history of respiratory disease?** Because many of the respiratory diseases are chronic in nature, there may be a history of the current problem. Persons who smoke tobacco products are especially prone to diseases of the respiratory system.
- **Was the onset sudden or gradual?** Cases of dyspnea that have a sudden onset are usually more acute. Pulmonary embolism (PE), pneumothorax, bronchospasm, and acute pulmonary edema have a rapid onset.

- **What brought on this period of dyspnea?** Was it the result of exertion or stress or did the condition develop spontaneously?
- **Does the patient have any history of other medical problems?** Because dyspnea is only a symptom of a particular disease, it is important to determine the underlying problem, so that it may be treated. Respiratory and cardiovascular diseases are the most common causes of dyspnea but other disease processes such as diabetes and AIDS can result in breathing difficulty.
- **Is there chest pain associated with the dyspnea?** Cardiovascular problems will often cause the patient to experience difficulty breathing. Although, not all chest pain is indicative of a cardiovascular event, it is a significant finding and may be the initial complaint.
- **Does the patient have evidence of infection?** Cough (especially a productive cough), fever, and chills may indicate an infectious etiology, such as pneumonia.
- **What medications is the patient currently taking?** Knowing whether the patient takes medication and, if so, the type may help to identify the current cause of the dyspnea. Bronchodilator inhalers indicate an obstructive disease, such as chronic obstructive pulmonary disease (COPD) or asthma.

Differential Diagnosis

NOTE: Upper airway obstruction is covered in Chapter 33 and croup and epiglottitis in Chapter 13.

PULMONARY ETIOLOGIES

- *Acute Asthma.* Acute asthma is a reversible, episodic disease where there is an obstruction from one or more of the three "Ss": spasm, swelling, and secretions. Wheezes, most commonly heard during expiration, may also be heard on inspiration; however, if severe bronchospasm is present, there may be no wheezing. Status asthmaticus is a prolonged and life-threatening form of asthma that cannot be broken with epinephrine.
- *Anaphylaxis.* Wheezing may be a manifestation of anaphylaxis, as histamine release and inflammation lead to narrowing of the airways. Usually, however, other clues are present to indicate an anaphylactic reaction, such as rash, edema, hypotension, and so forth.

- *Aspiration.* Persistent localized wheezing can suggest the diagnosis of foreign body aspiration, especially in individuals who may not protect their airways well. Foreign body aspiration, however, usually produces an obstruction of the upper airway and therefore is more likely to produce stridor (a continuous sound more prominent during inspiration than expiration) than frank wheezing. Aspiration is more likely to occur in young children and older debilitated patients who cannot protect their airway.
- *Chronic Obstructive Pulmonary Disease.* This disorder is characterized by diffuse obstruction to airflow. The most common types are:
  - **Emphysema**, which is best described as distention beyond the bronchioles with destruction of alveolar septa. Patients with emphysema are usually thin due to weight loss and provide a history of dyspnea on exertion. Exhalation is prolonged and difficult, with the lungs still expanded after exhalation, resulting in a barrel-shaped appearance to the chest. Respirations are rapid and breath sounds are distant and difficult to hear. Patient may appear short of breath and purse their lips during exhalation.
  - **Chronic bronchitis**, which is characterized by inflammation, edema, and excessive mucous production in the bronchial tree. Patients with this condition use their neck and chest muscles to assist with their breathing. They usually have a productive cough and a history of repetitive respiratory infections. On examination, they often cough and rhonchi and wheezing can be heard on both inspiration and exhalation. They will appear to be struggling to get air into their lungs.
  - **Pleurisy.** An inflammation of the lining of the chest cavity, pleurisy is often a complication of tuberculosis, pneumonia, trauma, or tumors and can lead to a pleural effusion. The patient with pleurisy will present with sharp chest pain that increases on inspiration and causes them to take short, quick breaths.
- *Pleural Effusions.* Collections of fluid, blood (hemothorax), or pus in the pleural space may cause dyspnea by compressing the lungs. There are many etiologies, including congestive heart failure (CHF), pneumonia, cancer, tuberculosis, and cirrhosis.
- *Pneumonia.* This illness causes lung inflammation and fluid- or pus-filled alveoli, leading to inadequate oxygen-

ation of the blood. Pneumonia is most frequently caused by a bacterial or viral infection, although it may occur after aspiration of fluids, such as vomit, or inhalation of irritants, such as chemicals or smoke.

- *Pulmonary Embolism.* This condition most often involves acute shortness of breath with tachycardia. Some patients may also complain of a pleuritic type of chest pain that may be increased on inspiration. Common symptoms include chest pain in 88% of patients, dyspnea in 84% of patients, and cough in 53% of patients. Common physical findings include tachypnea (RR greater than 16) in 92% of patients, tachycardia (heart rate greater than 100 bpm) in 44% of patients, and temperature greater than 100.04°F in 43% of patients. Risk factors of pulmonary embolism include a history of atrial fibrillation, obesity, pregnancy, prolonged immobilization, post-trauma, oral contraceptive use, postsurgery, and cancer.
- *Pneumothorax.* This condition occurs when air enters the pleural sac surrounding the lungs. The pneumothorax can be caused by trauma or may occur spontaneously. Tension pneumothorax usually results from trauma. It may, however, result from a spontaneous pneumothorax. Physical examination findings may include absent or diminished breath sounds, tracheal deviation away from the tension pneumothorax, and jugular venous distention (JVD).

CARDIAC ETIOLOGIES

- *Acute Myocardial Infarction.* Some patients experiencing an acute myocardial infarction (AMI) may have a primary symptom of dyspnea and, after questioning, may also admit to chest pain.
- *Acute Pulmonary Edema.* Normally associated with CHF, it occurs when an excess of fluid builds up in the extravascular space in the lungs. Pulmonary edema usually results from a fluid overload in the pulmonary circulation due to an AMI-damaged left ventricle. Inadequate cardiac output may cause dyspnea in patients with symptomatic tachycardias or bradycardias. It can also be caused by drowning, aspiration pneumonia, and smoke or toxin inhalation.
- *Pericardial Tamponade.* Persons suffering from this problem often complain of difficulty breathing. It may result from penetrating or blunt trauma to the chest. It may de-

velop over a time period from minutes to approximately 1 week. Muffled heart tones, together with JVD and narrowed pulse pressure, known as Beck's triad, may be found in pericardial tamponade. There are also several atraumatic etiologies, for example, secondary to pericardial effusions resulting from renal disease, acute leukemias, lymphomas, breast cancer, lung cancer, and ovarian cancer.

NONCARDIAC AND NONPULMONARY ETIOLOGIES

- *Hyperventilation.* Usually brought on by psychological stress, this syndrome typically occurs in young, anxious patients but may also be brought on by an overdose of aspirin or the need to compensate for metabolic acidosis. Hyperventilation is characterized by rapid, deep, or abnormal breathing. Although less common, organic causes of hyperventilation should not be excluded from the diagnosis.
- *Anemia.* Anemia, or decreased red blood cell mass, results in a decreased oxygen-carrying capacity. Anemia may result from inadequate red blood cell production, blood loss, or premature destruction of red blood cells. The anemia may be chronic or acute, as in the case of hemorrhage.
- *Carbon Monoxide Poisoning.* This condition may cause hypoxia and therefore dyspnea. Carbon monoxide has an affinity for hemoglobin 210 times greater than oxygen. Its half-life at room air is 4 to 6 hours. If 100% oxygen is given, the half-life is reduced to 60 to 90 minutes. The use of hyperbaric oxygen may decrease its half-life to 15 to 30 minutes.

Key Physical Examination Findings

- *Initial Assessment.* Look for signs of shock.
- *Vital Signs.* Assess for tachycardia and tachypnea, which usually accompany dyspnea. Hypotension may be present in the trauma, anaphylactic, or AMI patient. Fever may be present with pulmonary causes as well as with AMI.
- *Skin.* Look for peripheral cyanosis, patients experiencing dyspnea may be hypoxic.
- *Neck.* Assess the jugular veins for distention, indicating decompensated heart failure or pericardial tamponade.
- *Accessory Muscles.* Observe the patient for use of the neck and chest wall muscles to assist with breathing, a sign that

the work of breathing is too great for the diaphragm alone. Abdominal breathing is an even later sign which indicates that the patient is beginning to tire. The energy required to breathe in this manner is great, and once fatigue sets in, the patient will no longer be able to compensate for the extra airway resistance.

- *Lungs.* Assess for evidence of abnormal breath sounds. Listen to the nature and character of the breath sounds. Beware, however, of being fooled into a sense of security by a previously noisy chest that has become quiet. Often this change is a sign of impending doom because, as the patient tires, the patient cannot generate enough airflow to create wheezes. Usually at this stage, the patient is rapidly deteriorating and steps should be taken immediately to prevent loss of the airway. Evidence of blunt trauma or penetrating trauma should raise suspicion of intrathoracic injury, including pericardial tamponade, tension pneumothorax, and hemothorax.
- *Heart.* Assess for muffled heart tones indicative of pericardial tamponade.
- *Abdomen.* Assess for evidence of diaphragmatic breathing that could indicate a problem with the CNS.
- *Extremities.* Check for peripheral pulses. They may be absent as perfusion decreases which could indicate trauma as a cause of the dyspnea. Assess the fingers for "clubbing" and nailbeds for cyanosis.
- *Mental Status.* Look for signs of altered mental status, which is a sensitive indicator of inadequate cerebral perfusion and hypoxia.
- *Neurologic Examination.* Evaluate for signs of head or spinal injury, which is quite common in the trauma victim.

ECG

All patients with difficulty breathing should receive cardiac monitoring.

Treatment Plan

The goal of the treatment plan is to relieve hypoxia and improve the oxygenation of the patient. Frequent reassessment of the dyspneic patient is necessary owing to the potential for worsening of the respiratory status. Be prepared—potential for respiratory arrest exists.

GENERAL TREATMENT GUIDELINES

- **Administer O_2 and provide ventilatory support** as needed. Monitor O_2 saturation with pulse oximetry if available. This includes relieving upper airway obstructions, suctioning, performing needle-chest decompression of the tension pneumothorax and sealing an open pneumothorax with an air occlusive dressing or endotracheal intubation.
- Place patient in a comfortable position usually the **sitting or semisitting position**.
- Establish an **IV at a KVO rate** with 0.9% NaCl or LR; if the patient is dehydrated run at a faster rate.
- Provide the specific treatment as indicated below for COPD, asthma, or CHF.
- **Transport to appropriate ED**. Ensure patient comfort en route.

SPECIFIC TREATMENT GUIDELINES

Cardiac (Chapter 10, Chest Pain; Chapter 43, Tachycardia; Chapter 5, Bradycardia), croup and epiglottitis (Chapter 13), and traumatic (Multitrauma, Chapter 28) causes of dyspnea should be treated according to the recommendations established for these purposes.

PULMONARY ETIOLOGIES: COPD, ASTHMA, STATUS ASTHMATICUS

- **Measure peak expiratory flow rate (PEFR)**. The PEFR provides the only objective measurement of the degree of airway obstruction and can be used to follow the patient's progress. PEFR depends on the patient's technique and efforts; therefore, the patient must be coached in its use and encouraged to give their best effort.
- **Provide aerosolized albuterol, 2.5 mg in 3 ml 0.9% NaCl via nebulizer** (pediatric dose: younger than 12 years, one half of the adult dose [1.25 mg], older than 12 years, use full adult dose). Dose may be repeated every 6 hours; however, in cases of severe bronchospasm, it may be given as frequently as back to back. More frequent dosing may result in greater incidence of side effects.

  NOTE: You may also consider metaproterenol (Alupent), isoproterenol, Bronkosol or
- **Administer epinephrine 0.3 to 0.5 mg of a 1:1000 solution SC** (pediatric dose: 0.01 mg/kg SC, not to exceed 0.5 mg) if the patient is hemodynamically stable, or

- **Administer loading dose of aminophylline: 5 to 6 mg/ kg IV infusion over 20 to 30 minutes** (pediatric dose: 6 mg/kg IV infusion over 20 to 30 minutes). Dose may be used in patients who are not currently using aminophylline or theophylline. For patients using a theophylline or aminophylline agent, this loading dose should be reduced by one half (2.5 to 3.0 mg/kg).

CARDIAC ETIOLOGIES—CHF

- **Administer nitroglycerin, 1/150 grain (0.4mg) SL** (for systolic BP greater than 90 mm Hg). Dose may be repeated every 5 minutes as needed.
- **Administer morphine sulfate, 1 to 3 mg IV** (for systolic blood pressure greater than 90 mm Hg). May be repeated every 5 minutes as necessary.
- **Administer lasix (furosemide) 40 mg to 80 mg IV** (pediatric dose: 1.0 to 3.0 mg/kg IV). Higher doses may be necessary if the patient is on chronic diuretic therapy at home.

HYPERVENTILATION

Treatment is aimed at restoring the patient's PCO_2 to a normal state. This may be accomplished by either calming the patient or having him rebreathe his own carbon dioxide. Use caution with the rebreathing method, as there is no exact way of monitoring the carbon dioxide and oxygen mixture.

Bibliography

Caroline NL: Emergency Care in the Streets, ed 4. Little, Brown and Co, Boston, 1991, pp 413–446.

Haist SA, Robbins JB, and Gomella LG (eds): Anaphylactic Reaction. In Internal Medicine on Call. Appleton & Lange, Norwalk, CT. 1991, pp 91–94.

Sheehy SB: Pulmonary Emergencies. In Emergency Nursing: Principles and Practices, ed 4. Mosby-Year Book, St. Louis, MO, 1992, pp 501–515.

Notes

CHAPTER 18

Fever

Patrick R. Coonan, RN, EdD, CEN, EMT-CC

Presentation

Patients with fever present in many different ways, depending on the age of the patient, the rate of rise of the temperature, the magnitude of the fever, the etiology of the fever, and the underlying health of the patient. Presentations are quite patient-specific. The patient's skin will be warm to the touch and may be flushed on observation. The patient may also complain of being warm and perspiring. In addition, there may be symptoms of various other problems, depending on the cause of the fever. Flulike symptoms may accompany fevers, but it should not be assumed that fevers with these symptoms are minor, as there may be a serious underlying medical condition.

Immediate Concerns

- **ABCs.** Depending on the source of the fever, the patient may experience respiratory or hemodynamic compromise.
- **How long has the patient been febrile and how high is the temperature?** It is important to know if an elevation in temperature signals the abrupt onset of fever or represents the gradual worsening of a long-term fever. In children, the time and the rate of rise in temperature is significant, as it can signal whether the child may be prone to seizures. In some cases, a rapid rise in temperature is more significant than the fever itself, as a rapid rate of rise is the trigger mechanism for febrile seizures. Any temperature above 104°F requires immediate action to reduce the patient's core temperature. A common error in the treatment of fever is to wrap the patient in multiple layers of clothes or blankets. This only contributes to the rise in temperature.

Important History

- **Does the patient have any other pertinent medical problems or illnesses?** Patients with chronic health problems may tolerate the stress of infection less. Patients who are immunocompromised (ie, transplant patients, diabetic patients, and AIDS patients) are at increased risk of serious infections. Hyperthyroidism and cancer may also cause fevers.
- **Is the patient taking any medications?** Some fevers occur as a reaction to medications.
- **Is this fever related to an environmental exposure?**
- **Are there any associated symptoms?** During the subjective interview, be alert for symptoms such as chills, rigors, rash, myalgias, cough, chest pain, headache, painful urination, abdominal pain, night sweats, and alterations in mental status. This information will be helpful in localizing the source of infection.

Differential Diagnosis

This list is extremely long and will probably not help the advanced emergency medical technicians in their diagnosis, but the major categories are listed for your information.

Infections of all types

Neoplasms, tumors, lymphomas, and other cancers

Connective tissue disease, arthritis, vasculitis, and so forth.

Thermoregulatory disorders, heatstroke, and thyroid problems

Drug fever—some drugs can cause fevers by themselves

Miscellaneous disorders—pulmonary embolus, myocardial infarction, and others

Fever of unknown origin—no definite etiology

Key Physical Examination Findings

- *Vital Signs.* Take the patient's temperature if the equipment is available. Measure pulse rate and blood pressure to assure hemodynamic stability.
- *Skin.* Check for any indwelling catheters. Look for a rash; if one is present, do not touch it without gloved hands.

Make a note of the rash on the patient care report and provide the best description of its appearance.

- *Neck.* Check for neck stiffness. Ask the patient to touch the chin to the chest. If they cannot, it may indicate the patient has meningitis.
- *Lungs.* Listen for rales or signs of consolidation, indicating possible pneumonia.
- *Abdomen.* Palpate and percuss for signs of tenderness and note occurrences.
- *Extremities.* Check for indwelling catheters, joint effusions, or tenderness. Many patients are now on home infusion therapies that, when improperly maintained, can cause fever.

Treatment Plan

- Treat any hemodynamic instability.
- Carefully list all patient medications.
- **Reduce the patient's temperature.** Patients lose heat through four methods:
  1. Radiation (60%): heat loss from the body into the air
  2. Evaporation (25%): heat loss through the evaporation of perspiration, water, or any liquid applied to the body surface
  3. Convection (10%): Heat loss when air currents blow over the skin
  4. Conduction (5%): heat loss through contact with a solid surface

Prehospital EMS providers can facilitate heat loss in a patient using any combination of these methods:

- Unwrapping a bundled child increases heat loss through radiation.
- Rehydrating a dehydrated patient increases heat loss through evaporation.
- Wet sponges or towels also increase heat loss. Only tepid water should be used, however, as alcohol, cold water, or ice cause additional problems.
- Antipyretics, such as Tylenol or aspirin, may be given if allowed by protocol.
- If fever is present with hypotension, it may indicate the patient is in septic shock. Fluid resuscitation should begin immediately with large-bore IV. Place the patient in the

shock position If the patient fails to respond to fluids, dopamine may be considered at 2 to 5 g/kg per minute, or by medical direction or protocol.

Bibliography

Berkowitz C. Fever. In Tintinalli JE (ed): Emergency Medicine: A Comprehensive Study Guide, ed 3. McGraw-Hill, New York, 1991, pp 159–161.

Haist SA et al.: Fever. In Internal Medicine on Call. Appleton and Lange, Norwalk, CT, 1991, pp 98–103.

Notes

CHAPTER 19

Gastrointestinal Bleeding
Owen T. Traynor, MD

Presentation

The patient with gastrointestinal (GI) bleeding may present in several different ways: with shock, syncope, hematemesis, either bright red blood or coffee ground emesis, melena (the passage of black, tarry stool indicating blood in the GI tract), or hematochezia (bright red blood per rectum).

Immediate Concerns

- **What is the patient's hemodynamic status?** If the patient is hemodynamically unstable, immediate resuscitation is warranted, including oxygen administration, establishment of large-bore IV access, IV fluid administration, and possibly military antishock trousers (MAST).

Important History

- **Has there been hematemesis, melena, or hematochezia?** Hematemesis or coffee ground emesis suggests upper GI bleeding. Melena suggests acute upper GI tract blood loss, whereas hematochezia is likely to indicate bleeding in the distal colon or rectum. However, there are exceptions to the these guidelines; massive upper GI bleeding may involve hematochezia. Vomiting and retching before vomiting bright red blood may indicate a Mallory-Weiss tear of the esophagus.
- **Is there a history of GI bleeding?** If the history is positive, determine the nature of previous bleeding. Although bleeding may recur from the same location, it is not uncommon for bleeding to occur from another site. Be sure to ask about a history of diseases associated with GI bleed-

ing, such as peptic ulcer disease, esophageal varices, diverticular disease, colon cancer, polyps, inflammatory bowel disease, hemorrhoids, or other anal disease.

- **Is the patient taking any medication?** Anticoagulants, steroids, and nonsteroidal anti-inflammatory agents, including aspirin, are associated with GI bleeding.
- **Is there a history of alcohol abuse?** Alcohol abuse can cause gastritis and esophageal varices. Patients with cirrhosis have an increased incidence of duodenal ulcers.

Differential Diagnosis

UPPER GI BLEEDING

- *Peptic Ulcer Disease.* The most common cause of upper GI bleeding is peptic ulcer, accounting for up to 50% of all cases.
- *Gastritis and Esophagitis.* These conditions account for up to 20% of upper GI bleeds. Alcohol use, aspirin use, and hiatal hernia are predisposing factors.
- *Mallory-Weiss Syndrome.* This syndrome is characterized by upper GI bleeding due to a longitudinal tear in the mucosal lining of the esophagus. The classic presentation is one of repeated retching followed by bright red hematemesis. It is associated with recent alcohol intake. It causes up to 15% of upper GI bleeds.
- *Esophageal Varices.* Varices result from portal hypertension, in the United States it is most commonly caused by alcoholic liver disease. They account for up to 10% to 15% of all upper GI bleeds. They are prone to rebleed and carry the highest mortality of upper GI bleeds. Many patients with esophageal varices will never bleed. However, patients with documented varices and GI bleeding may bleed from a site other than the varices.
- *Other Sources.* Cancer causes approximately 1% to 2% of upper GI bleeding—look for a history of weight loss. Sources of bleeding from the ears, nose, and throat (ENT) should be investigated, for they can masquerade as GI bleeding.

LOWER GI BLEEDING

- *Upper GI Bleeding.* The most common cause of apparent lower GI bleeding is actually upper GI bleeding.

- *Diverticular Disease.* The most common cause of massive lower GI bleeding is diverticular disease. Diverticulosis is the presence of small outpouchings in the wall of the colon. These may become infected and erode into blood vessels in the wall of the colon, causing painless bleeding (the typical patient is over 50 years of age).
- *Hemorrhoids.* This condition causes most lower GI bleeding; however, it does not usually cause life-threatening hemorrhage.
- *Other Sources.* Vascular malformations of the colon may cause bleeding in the elderly. Cancer and polyps usually do not cause significant bleeding in the lower GI tract. Patients with cancer often present with weight loss, change in bowel habits, or both. Inflammatory bowel diseases, such as ulcerative colitis and Crohn's disease, are an infrequent cause of significant bleeding.

Key Physical Examination Findings

- *Initial Assessment.* Look for signs of shock.
- *Vital Signs.* Include orthostatic vital signs.
- *HEENT.* Look for ENT source of bleeding.
- *Abdomen.* Hyperactive bowel sounds may indicate blood in the upper GI tract. Check for masses, tenderness, and ascites.

Treatment Plan

- *Patient Assessment.* Frequent reassessment is necessary due to the potential for massive hemorrhage and shock. Cardiac monitoring is necessary in patients with blood loss with documented heart disease or risk of heart disease. Potential for vomiting; therefore, be prepared to protect airway.

HEMODYNAMICALLY UNSTABLE PATIENT

- **Administer O_2 and provide ventilatory support** as needed.
- **Treat for shock** (see Chapter 38, Shock).
- **Establish large-bore IV access** and begin fluid resuscitation with 0.9% NaCl or LR.
- **Transport expeditiously to appropriate ED.** Do not need-

lessly delay patient transport—expedite transport.

HEMODYNAMICALLY STABLE PATIENT

• **Transport to appropriate ED.** Ensure patient comfort en route.

Bibliography

Hematemesis, melena. In Haist SA, Robbins JB, and Gomella LG (eds): Internal Medicine on Call. Appleton and Lange, Norwalk, CT, 1991, pp 117–121.

Hematochezia. In Haist SA, Robbins JB, and Gomella LG (eds): Internal Medicine on Call. Appleton and Lange, Norwalk, CT, 1991, pp 121–124.

Overton DT: Gastrointestinal Bleeding. In Tintinalli JE, Krome LR, and Ruiz E (eds): Emergency Medicine: A Comprehensive Study Guide, ed 3. McGraw-Hill, New York, 1992, pp 147–149.

Notes

CHAPTER 20

Headache

Jonathan S. Rubens, MD, FACEP

Presentation

Headache is a common entity, known to most adult patients at some time in their lives. Consequently, the patient presenting to a paramedic with a chief complaint of headache should immediately send a signal that in the patient's perception, at least, this headache is somehow different and or more severe than other headaches experienced before. Associated symptoms of visual, motor, or sensory disturbances; nausea and vomiting; or fever are often a part of the patient's complaint.

Immediate Concerns

- ABCs
- Circulatory status and vital signs
- Disability
- Mental status (alert, response to verbal or painful stimuli, or unresponsiveness)

Important History

- **Time of onset?** This is one of the most important parameters to establish. A severe headache of acute onset with associated symptoms suggests a serious illness, such as hemorrhage. Preceding events can be helpful (ie, trauma, exercise, or exertion). A headache that recurs, has a prodrome, is associated with foods or menstruation, or occurs at the same time of day generally has a less urgent etiology.
- **Location and quality of the pain?** A throbbing, pulsatile headache is usually of vascular etiology and is generally due to vasodilation, hypertension, or fever. The shocklike, transient pain in the distribution of the fifth cranial nerve (the face) is characteristic of trigeminal neuralgia, whereas

the deep, boring, intense, unilateral pain of cluster headaches helps to differentiate them.

- **Are there associated symptoms?** Nausea and vomiting frequently accompany the pain of migraine headache, but they also accompany many lesions, which result in increased intracranial pressure. In cluster headache, unilateral flushing of the forehead, conjunctival erythema, lacrimation, and nasal congestion are diagnostic. Acute onset of severe headache associated with neck stiffness, numbness or progressive alteration of mental status, and sensitivity to light is suggestive of subarachnoid hemorrhage.

Differential Diagnosis

ORGANIC DISEASE

- *Intracranial.* Tumors, abscesses, subdural, and epidural hematomas
- *Meningeal Irritation.* Meningitis, subarachnoid hemorrhage
- *Cranial.* Cranial bone metastases, Paget's disease
- *Scalp.* Herpes zoster, muscle tension
- *Vascular.* Migraine, hypertension, cluster, toxic
- *Extracranial.* Glaucoma, iritis, otitis media, sinusitis, oral lesions

POSTTRAUMATIC

Usually localized to the site of injury, history of trauma, and normal examination.

Key Physical Examination Findings

- *Initial Assessment.* Monitor ABCs.
- *Vital Signs.* Monitor blood pressure and respiratory pattern and rate. Diastolic blood pressure elevations greater than 130 mm Hg associated with mental status changes or other focal neurologic findings is a true neurologic emergency. In cases of cerebral edema and increased intracranial pressure, Cushing's reflex, increased blood pressure associated with a decrease in pulse rate may be found. Changes in respiratory pattern or rate may give evidence of a toxic etiology of the headache.

- *Inspection and Palpation.* Assess pupillary reaction and extraocular movements. Look for redness of the eye or corneal changes to signal an ophthalmologic cause of the pain.
- *Neck.* Assess for nuchal rigidity, which may be found in cases of meningeal irritation.
- *Neurologic Examination.* Include the mental status examination.

Treatment Plan

- *Patient Assessment.* Perform continued evaluation of vital signs and mental status. Changes in any of these parameters may require immediate intervention during transport.
- **Treat shock** (see Chapter 38, Shock) or hemodynamic instability
- **Transport to the appropriate ED.** Ensure patient comfort, offer reassurance.

Bibliography

Henry G: Headache. In Rosen P, et al. (eds): Emergency Medicine: Concepts and Clinical Practice, ed 2. CV Mosby, St. Louis, 1988, pp 279–291.
Tintinalli JE, Krome, LR, and Ruiz E (eds): Emergency Medicine: A Comprehensive Study Guide, ed 3. McGraw Hill, New York, 1992, pp 789–792.

Notes

CHAPTER 21

Human Immunodeficiency Virus Infections

Andrew W. Stern, MPA, MA(PS), NREMT-P

Presentation

A patient infected with human immunodeficiency virus (HIV) or having acquired immunodeficiency syndrome (AIDS) may present in a healthy manner, denying any complicating diseases or infection, or with extensive medical problems. Some of these medical problems may include pneumonia, tuberculosis (TB), wasting, visible sores, and numerous other complications resulting from a variety of opportunistic infections.

Immediate Concerns

- **What is the patient's ABC status?** Evaluate the status of the ABCs. If indicated, clear the airway, assist breathing, and handle hemodynamic instability. Any patient exhibiting poor perfusion should be administered oxygen, have a large-bore IV established, IV fluids given, and temperature monitored.

  NOTE: HIV infection results from a person becoming infected with the virus that causes AIDS. When a person who has HIV infection becomes ill from a specific group of diseases or opportunistic infections, this is referred to as AIDS. An HIV-infected person's immune system does not respond well when it becomes suppressed. The course of the disease process can be quite long. Many of the infections that affect AIDS patients can be controlled or cured. Even though the progression of HIV infection to AIDS can take more than 10 years, in the end stages of most cases the infected person becomes debilitated. Eventually, the majority of these patients die from one of a number of opportunistic infections or related disease processes that are common in AIDS patients.

Important History

- **Signs and symptoms the patient may manifest.** Patients with HIV infection or AIDS manifest a variety of signs and symptoms. These may be attributable to either the HIV infection itself or one of the secondary diseases that complicate HIV illness. In the prehospital care setting, the treatment objective is to provide supportive care. The following is a list of common patient presentations for HIV and AIDS:

    Dyspnea
    Nausea
    Vomiting
    Diarrhea
    Difficult or painful swallowing (dysphagia or
      odynophagia)
    Poor appetite
    Female patients may manifest gynecologic problems,
      such as pelvic inflammatory disease (PID)
    Diminished mental status
    Lassitude and fatigue

- **Opportunistic infections the patient may manifest.** The patient with HIV or AIDS may provide a past medical history that includes a number of opportunistic infections some of which they may currently have. The following is a list of some of the most common infections.

    Tuberculosis (including multidrug-resistant TB)
    Pneumocystis carinii pneumonia (PCP)
    Esophageal candidiasis
    Lymphoma
    Kaposi's sarcoma
    Toxoplasmosis
    Retinitis
    Herpes
    Cytomegalovirus (CMV)
    Mycobacterium avium complex (MAC)

- **Is the patient taking any medications?** Antiretroviral drugs, PCP prophylaxis and treatment, antiviral drugs, antibacterial drugs, antifungal agents, toxoplasmosis therapies, steroids, analgesics, and other medications to deal with the disease process are all readily prescribed.
- **Is there a history of other pre-existing medical condi-**

tions? Patients who become infected with HIV from high-risk behaviors may also have a history of other pre-existing medical problems that are sometimes associated with these same behaviors. For example, a patient with a history of intravenous drug use may report having had hepatitis. As HIV can be sexually transmitted, patients may have a history of sexually transmitted diseases, such as syphilis, gonorrhea, and chlamydia.

NOTE: An HIV-infected patient or a patient with AIDS may not know they are infected. If they know, the patient may not be willing to inform the prehospital care provider of the diagnosis.

Differential Diagnosis

AIDS manifests many different clinical presentations. As a result of the weakened immune system, any body system, has the potential of becoming affected.

- *Flulike Symptoms.* Early stages of HIV disease may include swollen lymph nodes, sore throat, low-grade fever, and other flulike symptoms.
- *Respiratory Distress.* Pneumonia and TB are highly prevalent among patients with AIDS. Approximately 50% of patients with AIDS die from respiratory complications.
- *Hypovolemia.* Dehydration due to vomiting, diarrhea, and profuse diaphoresis. In addition, cases of internal bleeding from various sites that have resulted in significant blood loss.
- *Skin Problems.* Skin problems include skin rashes, fungal infections, large blotches from Kaposi's sarcoma (male patients usually), and weeping sores.
- *Gynecologic Disease.* Women with AIDS may present with a variety of gynecologic disorders, including PID and vaginal bleeding.
- *Psychologic Disorders.* In the later stages of this disease, patients may be demented and their ability to mentate, greatly diminished. The patient may manifest bizarre and difficult-to-understand behavior.
- *Other Disorders.* Patients with HIV or AIDS, particularly in the final stages of the disease process, will present like patients in many other terminal diseases, and they will be weak, with wasting and significant pain.

Key Physical Examination Findings

- *Initial Assessment.* Look for respiratory distress and signs of shock.
- *Vital Signs.* Attempt orthostatic vital signs if patient can tolerate, and check capillary refill.
- *Secondary Survey.* Examine skin and evaluate temperature.
- *Mental Status.* Determine if oriented to date, time, and place.

Treatment Plan

Supportive therapy is the main objective.
- Administer O_2 and **provide ventilatory support** as needed.
- **Treat for shock.** Establish **large-bore IV with 0.9% NaCl or LR.**
- **Treat for chilling or fever** as indicated.
- Provide psychological support.
- **Transport to appropriate ED.** Ensure patient comfort en route.

   NOTE: Patients with AIDS in the end stages of the disease may have a do not resuscitate (DNR) order. If this is the case, observe local and state laws and follow appropriate protocols.

Bibliography

AIDS Institute, New York State Department of Health: Protocols for the Medical Care of HIV Infection, ed 2 rev. December 1992.
Stine GJ: Acquired Immune Deficiency Syndrome (Biological, Medical, Social, and Legal Issues). Prentice Hall, Englewood Cliffs, NJ, 1993.

Notes

CHAPTER 22

Hypertensive Emergencies
Roy E. Cox, Jr, BS, EMT-P

Presentation

Hypertension is a common medical problem. Generally, the patient with hypertension will not require treatment for hypertension in the prehospital phase. However, there are certain hypertensive emergencies that must be treated promptly. A hypertensive emergency exists when there is hypertension and evidence of end-organ injury. The organs most at risk of injury are the brain, the heart, and the kidneys. There is no agreed on minimum BP that will result in injury; therefore, the paramedic must look for evidence that there is end-organ dysfunction associated with high BP. The EMS provider, in most cases, will not be able to determine whether renal dysfunction is present. It may be discovered by careful evaluation, though, that there is injury to the brain or heart.

Immediate Concerns

- **Is there evidence of a cerebral injury?** Patients with a cerebral hypertensive emergency, or hypertensive encephalopathy, may manifest severe headache, nausea, vomiting, neurologic deficits, seizures, or alterations in their mental status. These signs and symptoms may progress rapidly to coma and death. The goal of therapy is to safely reduce the mean arterial pressure (the diastolic BP plus one third of the pulse pressure) in a controlled fashion over 30 to 60 minutes. It may be difficult to determine whether a CNS event, such as an intracerebral hemorrhage, occurred first, causing an elevated intracranial pressure and hypertension, or whether the hypertension has caused the CNS event.

- **Is there evidence of cardiovascular injury?** The patient with a cardiovascular hypertensive emergency may present with chest pain, myocardial ischemia, or pulmonary edema. Hypertension is also the most common cause of a thoracic aortic dissection (aneurysm). Patients with this condition may manifest back or chest pain.
- **Is the patient pregnant?** Pre-eclampsia occurs when the patient is hypertensive, pregnant and has confusion, hyperreflexia, headache, or epigastric pain. Eclampsia occurs when the pre-eclamptic patient has a seizure. The uterine blood flow is markedly decreased in the eclamptic patient, placing the fetus at risk. Definitive treatment requires delivery of the fetus; however, the goals of acute management are to reduce the BP and to prevent seizures.

Important History

- **Does the patient have a history of hypertension?** One out of every four people in the United States has high BP. More than half of those have excessively high pressure, and some of them are unaware of this silent killer that has no clear early signs or warning symptoms.
- **Does the patient have a history of any end-organ injury?** A history of renal disease, cardiac disease, or cerebrovascular accidents suggests a long history of poorly controlled hypertension.
- **Is the patient taking any medications?** The patient with hypertension may be taking diuretics, calcium channel blockers, angiotensin converting enzyme (ACE) inhibitors, vasodilators, or beta blockers. Rapid withdrawal from sympathetic agents may result in a rebound hypertension, precipitating end-organ injury. Monoamine oxidase inhibitors (MAOI), such as phenelzine (Nardil), tranylcypromine (Parnate), and isocarboxazid (Marplan), used for psychiatric illnesses, may cause hypertension if the patient uses any other agent, including cocaine or amphetamines, or eats foods such as aged cheeses or wine, containing the amino acid tyramine.

Differential Diagnosis

- *Hypertensive Encephalopathy.* A life-threatening alteration of the CNS function with high blood pressure. The patient exhibits headache, visual changes, altered mental status, or neurologic deficits. These complaints usually develop gradually over 12 to 72 hours. When the mean arterial pressure is high, the brain loses its ability to keep the blood flow in the brain constant. When the pressure is high, the cerebral blood flow may become dangerously high, resulting in damage to the blood-brain barrier. This allows fluid to infiltrate into the brain, eventually leading to a decrease in blood flow into the brain. There is danger in reducing the longstanding hypertensive patient's BP to "normal." Over time, they have adapted to require higher than normal mean arterial pressure to achieve normal cerebral blood flow. Dropping their mean arterial pressure below 120 mm Hg may cause inadequate cerebral perfusion. Thus a controlled reduction in BP is key to successfully treating these patients.

• **Primary CNS Injury.** Any CNS injury that raises intracranial pressure may cause herniation and injury to the brainstem, resulting in a Cushing response—hypertension and bradycardia. The high BP may be necessary to perfuse the brain in the face of high intracranial pressure. Less aggressive reduction in BP is, therefore, undertaken for fear of extending the injury or stroke by decreasing the perfusion to the brain. Be alert for the possibility of a subarachnoid hemorrhage in patients who describe "the worst headache" of their life. This is a neurologic emergency requiring oxygen, analgesia, reduction of intracranial pressure, and possibly neurosurgic intervention. It is often difficult to differentiate primary CNS injuries, such as CVAs and intracranial hemorrhages, from hypertensive encephalopathies.

• **Myocardial Ischemia.** The etiology of the cardiovascular emergency is related to the excessive afterload the heart must pump against. This causes increased myocardial oxygen requirements and may reduce coronary artery blood flow. These patients may present with the signs and symptoms of ischemic chest pain, ECG changes, and pulmonary edema. Treatment involves the use of oxygen, nitroglycerin, and possibly morphine and diuretics.

• **Aortic Dissection (Aneurysm).** Longstanding hypertension may damage the endothelium of the aorta, with subsequent creation of false channels in the media of the vessel.

The high pressure may cause these false channels to dissect the thoracic aorta. If the dissection extends proximally toward the arch of the aorta, the arch vessels, including the carotid arteries, may become occluded. These patients may have neurologic deficits similar to a CVA, as well as back or chest pain. You should suspect a thoracic dissection in all CVA patients who present with chest or back pain. The dissection may extend even more proximally to cause pericardial tamponade. When the dissection extends distally, there will be different blood flow in the vessels of the arms and legs. The forcefulness of the pulses will be different. A difference in BP of greater than 10 mm Hg in each arm is concerning. The patient with a thoracic aortic dissection is initially hypertensive, but may become hypotensive as the dissection begins to leak. The goal of therapy is prompt recognition and, if the patient is hypertensive, reduction of the blood pressure and force of the pulse wave using nitroprusside and beta blockers. If the patient is hypotensive, fluid resuscitation should be begun immediately.

• *Pre-Eclampsia and Eclampsia.* Also known as the toxemia of pregnancy, this condition may present with a spectrum of findings including hypertension (greater than 140/90 mmHg), peripheral edema, proteinuria, renal failure, seizures, hyperreflexia, and an altered mental status. Until a seizure occurs, the diagnosis is considered pre-eclampsia. The edema and renal failure result from intense vasospasm. Immediate therapy involves reduction of the hypertension and prevention of seizures. Diuretics may be harmful in these patients because, although they have peripheral edema, they are actually intravascularly hypovolemic secondary to the vasoconstriction. Hydralazine is the vasodilator of choice. Fluid resuscitation should be initiated as well. Magnesium sulphate is used to prevent the seizures of eclampsia.

NOTE: Nitroprusside is specifically contraindicated in the gravid patient.

Key Physical Examination Findings

• *Initial Assessment.* Look for signs of altered mental status, respiratory compromise, and hemodynamic instability.
• *Vital Signs.* Be sure that you are using the appropriate size BP cuff—a cuff that is too small will give a falsely high reading, while a cuff that is too large will give a falsely low

reading. Be sure to compare BPs in both arms in the patient who complains of chest or back pain.
- *Lungs.* Assess for evidence of pulmonary edema.
- *Heart.* Assess for muffled heart tones.
- *Abdomen.* Be sure to check gently for the pulsatile abdominal mass found in patients with an abdominal aortic aneurysm.
  NOTE: Do not palpate further if a pulsatile mass is discovered.
- *Peripheral Pulses.* Check evenness of peripheral pulses. Unequal pulses may be found in the patient with a dissecting aortic aneurysm.
- *Mental Status.* Assess for signs of an altered mental status, which is a senitive indicator of inadequate cerebral perfusion.
- *Neurologic Examination.* Assess for facial asymmetry, motor deficits, sensory impairment, pupillary responses, and altered mental status.

ECG

May reveal evidence of myocardial ischemia.

Treatment Plan

- *Patient Assessment.* Perform a rapid and systematic initial assessment and institute treatment as life-threatening problems are discovered. Prompt transport to the appropriate ED is a key intervention. Frequent reassessment of the patient with a hypertensive emergency is necessary owing to the potential for worsening of their cardiovascular and neurologic status. Be prepared—potential for cardiac arrest exists.

HYPERTENSIVE ENCEPHALOPATHY

- **Administer O$_2$ and provide ventilatory support** as needed.
- Place patient in a **head elevated position**, unless spinal immobilization is indicated.
- Monitor the ECG and O$_2$ saturation if pulse oximetry is available.

- **Establish large-bore IV access** with 0.9% NaCl or RL.
- Consider the following interventions:
  Nifedipine, 10 mg po or sl. Onset of action within 10 minutes, with peak effect in 30 to 60 minutes.
  Nitroprusside infusion (50 mg/500 mL 5% dextrose in water) starting at 0.5 µg/kg per minute and titrating to a systolic BP decrease of 30 to 40 mm Hg and a diastolic decrease of 10 to 20 mm Hg. Nitroprusside is the drug of choice for hypertensive encephalopathy because of its short duration of action and the fine control of BP reduction that this IV infusion affords. The patient's blood pressure must be monitored continuously. If the patient's BP falls precipitously, discontinue the infusion and consider a 200 mL fluid bolus.

  NOTE: If the patient has a history of coronary artery disease or is demonstrating evidence of myocardial ischemia, consider pretreatment with nitroglycerin (as noted below) before starting nitroprusside.

- **Nitroglycerin 0.4 mg sl** every 3 to 5 minutes, or
- **Nitroglycerin infusion** (25 mg/250 mL 5% dextrose in water) starting at 10 µg per minute (6 gtts per minute), and titrating by 5 µg per minute (3 gtts per minute) every 5 to 20 minutes until chest pain is relieved, systolic BP is less than 100 mm Hg, or patient shows signs of inadequate perfusion.
- Frequently reassess the patient's hemodynamic and neurologic status.
- Transport to appropriate ED. Ensure patient comfort en route.

THORACIC AORTIC DISSECTION

- **Administer O$_2$ and provide ventilatory support** as needed.
- Place patient in a position of comfort.
- **Monitor ECG and O$_2$ saturation** (if pulse oximetry is available).
- **Establish large-bore IV access** with 0.9% NaCl or RL.
- Consider the following interventions:
  Propranolol, 1.0 mg IV. Repeat 1.0 mg dose as needed to a maximum total dose of 0.1 mg/kg. Stop the administration when the heart rate becomes less than 60 mm Hg.

> **Nitroprusside infusion** (50 mg/500 mL 5% dextrose in water) starting at 0.5 μg/kg per minute and titrating to a systolic BP between 90 and 120 mm Hg.
> **Nitroglycerin, 0.4 mg sL** every 3 to 5 minutes, or Nitroglycerin infusion (25 mg/250 ml 5% dextrose in water) starting at 10 μg per minute (6 gtts per minute), and titrating by 5 μg per minute (3 gtts per minute) every 5 to 20 minutes until chest pain is relieved, systolic BP less than 100, or patient shows signs of inadequate perfusion.

- **Transport to appropriate ED**. Ensure patient comfort en route.

CHEST PAIN, CARDIAC ISCHEMIA, AND PULMONARY EDEMA

- **Administer O_2 and provide ventilatory support** as needed. Monitor O_2 saturation by pulse oximetry if available.
- **Monitor ECG** and, if possible, obtain a 12-lead ECG. Screen for possible use of thrombolytics if permitted by local protocol.
- **Establish large-bore IV access** with 0.9% NaCL or LR at a KVO rate.
- Consult with medical control physician.
- Consider the following interventions:
  > **Nitroglycerin, 1/150 grain (0.4 mg) sL** (for systolic BP greater than 90 mm Hg). Dose may be repeated every 5 minutes. If ineffective,
  > **Morphine sulfate, 1 to 3 mg IV** (for systolic BP greater than 90 mm Hg). Dose may be repeated every 5 minutes as needed.
- **Treat symptomatic arrhythmias per AHA ACLS guidelines**. See Chapter 5, Bradycardia and Chapter 43, Tachycardia.
- **Treat cardiogenic shock** as described in Chapter 38, Shock.
- **If pulmonary edema is present, give furosemide (Lasix), 40 to 80 mg IV** (pediatric dose: 1 to 3 mg/kg IV).

PRE-ECLAMPSIA AND ECLAMPSIA

- **Administer O_2 and provide ventilatory support** as needed. This includes endotracheal intubation, if indicated.

- Place patient in a **left lateral recumbent position**.
- Monitor ECG and O_2 saturation (if pulse oximetry is available), vital signs, and fetal heart rate, if possible.
- **Establish large-bore IV access with 0.9% NaCl or RL at 60 mL per minute.**
- Consider the following interventions:

  Hydralazine, 5 mg IV over 3 minutes. Repeat 5 mg dose as needed every 5 minutes (maximum total dose of 20 mg) until diastolic pressure is between 90 and 100 mm Hg.

  Magnesium sulfate, 4 to 6 gm IV over 5 to 10 minutes if a seizure occurs. After the loading dose, start an IV infusion at 2 gm per hour (40 mg/1000 mL lactated Ringer's solution). Magnesium may decrease both respiratory rate and deep tendon reflexes. If either side effect occurs, or if there are additional seizures or a change or absence in fetal heart tones, the magnesium dose must be reduced or discontinued. Seek medical control guidance.

- Transport to appropriate ED. Ensure patient comfort en route.

Bibliography

Jackson R: Hypertensive Emergencies. In Tintinalli JE, Krome LR, and Ruiz E (eds): Emergency Medicine: A Comprehensive Study Guide, ed 3. McGraw-Hill, New York, 1992, pp 237–246.

Matthews J: Hypertension. In Schwartz GR, et al.(eds): Principles and Practices of Emergency Medicine, ed 3. Lea and Febiger, Philadelphia, 1992, pp 1253–1260.

Notes

CHAPTER 23

Hyperthermia
Mark Scheatzle, MD

Presentation

Hyperthermia, or heat illness, occurs commonly during the hot and humid season. Patients with heat exhaustion will be hemodynamically stable with a normal mental status. Typically, they are nauseated and fatigued with a temperature of 102°F or less. Unlike the heat exhaustion patient, the patient with heatstroke typically presents with hemodynamic instability with an abnormal mental status (ie, bizarre behavior, seizure, coma, confusion).

Immediate Concerns

- **What is the patient's temperature?** The patient with heatstroke will have a temperature above 104°F. This is a medical emergency that necessitates immediate cooling and transport to the nearest appropriate ED. The patient may also be hemodynamically unstable, requiring airway control, oxygen, large-bore IV access, and IV fluids.

Important History

- **What are the circumstances of the event?** Pertinent information includes duration of onset, age, and general health of the patient; and degree of activity at onset. This information will help determine the treatment in the emergency department as well as the prognosis. Heatstroke is commonly separated into classic heatstroke and exertional heatstroke. Classic heatstroke occurs in infants, the elderly, and the chronically ill, who are prone to become severely dehydrated over several days. Their skin will be hot and dry on presentation. Exertional heatstroke occurs in

133

the young, unacclimatized athlete, who is not dehydrated. They will thus be sweating profusely.

- **Is the patient taking any medications?** Medications, both over the counter and prescription, can have a profound impact on a patient's ability to tolerate heat. For example, drugs with anticholinergic properties, tricyclic antidepressants, and cold medications decrease the body's ability to dissipate heat through sweating. Cocaine, amphetamines, and salicylate intoxication increase the body's heat production, as do overdoses of synthetic thyroid hormone. In addition, patients recently begun on neuroleptics, most commonly haloperidol (Haldol), are susceptible to neuroleptic malignant syndrome (NMS). NMS causes the basal metabolic rate to greatly increase, leading to severe hyperthermia.

Differential Diagnosis

- *Fever.* This is an entity separate from hyperthermia with a different pathophysiology and treatment. Fever is best discriminated from hyperthermia by history; however, the distinction is not always clear. Look for evidence of infection: respiratory symptoms, such as cough and runny nose; abdominal complaints, such as diarrhea and pain; urinary tract symptoms, such as burning on urination, foul-smelling urine, increased urinary frequency and hesitancy; and evidence of meningitis, such as stiff neck, photophobia, and an altered mental status.
- *Severe Dehydration.* This is a common cause of hyperthermia. Total body volume depletion leads to vasoconstriction, causing a decrease in the body's ability to dissipate heat through sweating.
- *Medications.* Hyperthermia may occur secondarily to medication use (discussed previously).
- *Hyperthyroidism or Thyroid Storm.* Thyroid storm most commonly occurs in patients with nondiagnosed or undertreated hyperthyroidism. However, it may occur with overdose of exogenous thyroid hormone. Symptoms are identical to the patient with hyperthermia. Physical findings may be subtle and include the presence of a goiter (thyroid nodule in the neck) or exopthalmus (prominent, bulging eyes).
- *Neuroleptic Malignant Syndrome.* This syndrome is a rare

complication of neuroleptic medications. It can occur during early therapy or years later. It is characterized by fever, an altered mental status, and muscular rigidity. Patients are often profoundly diaphoretic. Medicines associated with NMS include phenothiazines (Thorazine, Prolixin, Trilafon, Compazine, Mellaril), butyrophenones (droperidol, haloperidol), and thiothixene.

- *Delirium Tremens.* Delirium tremens (DTs) typically occur 3 to 4 days after cessation of excessive alcohol intake. Symptoms can be identical to heatstroke with a prominence of tremor or seizure activity. History and a careful physical examination provide the best clues in diagnosing DTs.

- *Heat Cramps.* This is a relatively benign condition characterized by painful muscle cramps, usually in the acclimatized patient working in a hot, humid environment. The cramps may begin during or after several hours of exertion. It is caused by inadequate fluid or electrolyte replacement.

- *Heat Exhaustion.* This usually occurs in an unacclimatized person who has worked under hot, humid conditions. There are two varieties of heat exhaustion, water depletion–type and salt depletion–type. The water depletion–type is characterized by thirst, dizziness, fever, confusion, and poor motor coordination. The salt depletion–type is characterized by weakness, headache, muscle cramps, nausea, and vomiting. Patients are usually without thirst or fever. Both varieties of heat exhaustion present with diaphoretic skin, tachycardia, and possibly hypotension. Although there are two varieties of heat exhaustion, most patients present with a combination of the two. Heat exhaustion may progress to heatstroke if untreated.

- *Heatstroke.* The typical heatstroke patient is either very young or elderly. Heatstroke usually has a gradual onset over several days, although it may occur acutely. When the onset is gradual, the patient may be markedly dehydrated. When heatstroke develops acutely, it is usually in the younger unacclimatized patient working under significant heat stress for several hours. Heatstroke patients are tachycardic, tachypneic, hypotensive, febrile (temperature above 104°F) and with an altered mental status. They are usually still able to sweat. All organ systems are damaged by the elevated temperature, with the damage related to both the magnitude of the fever and to the duration of the fever. If the temperature is not rapidly reduced, death may occur. The cause of death is usually caused by disseminated intravascular coagulation (severe clotting abnormality characterized by the widespread formation of microthrombi and by difficult-to-control bleeding), acute renal failure, acute liver failure, or acute respiratory distress syndrome.

- *Central Nervous System Lesions.* Cerebrovascular accidents (CVAs) or tumors, which damage the hypothalamic thermoregulatory center, can cause marked temperature elevations. There will be accompanying neurologic deficits.

Key Physical Examination Findings

- *Initial Assessment.* Look for signs of shock.
- *Vital Signs.* Monitor vital signs, particularly temperature, as they will indicate severity of the disease.
- *Skin.* Inspect for redness and flushing or profuse sweating.
- *HEENT.* Note whether pupils are reactive or fixed and dilated.
- *Neurologic Examination.* Assess for neurologic deficit or decrease in mental status. Hyperthermia with these features indicates heatstroke.

Treatment Plan

- Patient Assessment. Frequent reassessment is necessary as the patient's temperature may continue to increase despite cooling efforts. The patient's mental status may deteriorate, requiring aggressive airway management. In addition, these patients are prone to vomit, seize, or develop hypotension.

GENERAL TREATMENT GUIDELINES

- Remove patient from the heat stress and place in a cool environment.
- **Administer O_2 and provide ventilatory support** as needed

SPECIFIC TREATMENT GUIDELINES

Heatstroke

- Follow general guidelines.
- Continuously monitor the patient's temperature.
- **Institute rapid cooling.** The patient must be placed in a cool environment with removal of clothes. There are several effective methods for decreasing temperature. The most effective is spraying the patient with a mist of room temperature water while constantly fanning. Sponging the patient with water while fanning is also effective. Do not sponge the patient with alcohol. Placing ice packs in the patients groin, axial, and neck may be used; however, this is not as effective as the previous methods.
- **Establish large-bore IV** and begin fluid resuscitation with 0.9% NaCL or lactated Ringer's solution if the patient is hypotensive.
- **If patient is seizing give diazepam (Valium), 5 to 10 mg IV bolus**. Dose may be repeated every 10 to 15 minutes (pediatric dose: 0.2 to 0.5 mg/kg by slow IV bolus, maximum dose: age younger than 5 years, 5 mg; age older than 5 years 10 mg).
- **Transport expeditiously to appropriate ED.** Do not needlessly delay transport—expedite transport. Continue cooling efforts en route.

Heat Exhaustion

- **Establish large-bore IV** and begin fluid resuscitation with 0.9% NaCL or lactated Ringer's solution if the patient is hypotensive.
- Transport expeditiously to appropriate ED as progression to heatstroke can occur.

Bibliography

Schmidt EW and Nichols CG: Heat Illness. In Harwood-Nuss A, et al. (eds): The Clinical Practice of Emergency Medicine. JB Lippincott, Philadelphia, 1991, pp 626–629.

Simon HB. Hyperthermia. In Desforges JF (ed): N Engl J Med 329: 1993.

Yarbrough B: Heat Illness. In Rosen P and Barkin RM (eds): Emergency Medicine: Concepts and Clinical Practice. ed 3. Mosby-Year Book, St. Louis, 1992, pp 944–963.

Notes

CHAPTER 24

Hypoglycemia
Thomas Pangburn, MD

Presentation

The many signs and symptoms that characterize hypoglycemia may be divided into the two broad categories: adrenergic and neurologic symptoms. Adrenergic stimulation, or symptoms related to increased epinephrine levels, include the following:

- Anxiety
- Diaphoresis
- Hunger
- Hypertension
- Pallor
- Palpitations
- Tachycardia

Neurologic symptoms, which result in central nervous system dysfunction from low glucose levels, include the following:

- Blindness
- Coma
- Confusion
- Decreased visual acuity
- Headache
- Seizures
- Visual hallucinations
- Weakness

Immediate Concerns

- **What is the patient's mental status?** If the patient is unconscious, then the routine airway, breathing, and circulation protocol should be followed. During their careers, all prehospital EMS providers will be confronted with an abundance of calls concerning patients with a decreased mental status. A history from a family member or friend can easily help to identify hypoglycemia as a possible diagnosis for the decreased mental status patient. If a clear history cannot be obtained, however, the standard protocol for initial management of decreased mental status should be instituted with a focus on obtaining venous access for administration of glucose, thiamine, and naloxone (Narcan). A blood glucose sample should also be obtained to measure the glucose level.

Important History

- **Is the patient diabetic?** A large number of all hypoglycemic episodes requiring skilled medical treatment occur in people with diabetes that have taken an excessive amount of insulin to meet their required needs. This situation is particularly prevalent during the summer in younger patients, who require less insulin as a result of increased physical activity.
- **Is the patient an alcoholic or has the patient recently consumed alcohol?** Alcoholics frequently present with hypoglycemia as a result of chronic liver damage or starvation. Also, people with diabetes frequently become hypoglycemic when consuming alcohol, because liver production of glucose between meals is inhibited.
- **When was the last meal?** This question can help distinguish certain etiologies of hypoglycemia because many patients who have had gastric surgery become hypoglycemic even after recently eating a meal. The question is more obvious in diabetic and alcoholic patients in whom the lack of a recent meal is the cause for most hypoglycemia.
- **Does the patient have a fever or recent infection?** Sepsis, along with diabetes and alcohol, accounted for 90% of the hypoglycemic cases at Harlem Hospital in New York. Hypoglycemia from sepsis is especially prevalent in the infant and elderly population.
- **Is the patient taking any medications?** Insulin and oral hypoglycemic medications are the most common cause. However, aspirin, Tylenol, beta blockers, antipsychotic drugs and antibiotics such as sulfa-based, tetracycline, and amoxicillin (Augmentin) have been implicated.

Differential Diagnosis

- *Postprandial Hypoglycemia* (after a meal). This form of hypoglycemia occurs in prediabetic patients (patients that someday will require insulin therapy), gastric surgery patients, or patients with enzymatic deficiencies that affect glucose metabolism.

- *Fasting States.* The typical patient who has fasting hypoglycemia is a patient with diabetes on insulin or oral hypoglycemics, but suicide and homicide attempts using insulin or oral hypoglycemic agents have been reported.
- *Organ Failure.* Liver disease, the most common etiology, can be caused by hepatitis, cirrhosis, and passive congestion from heart failure. Renal failure, adrenal failure, and hypothyroidism also cause hypoglycemia.
- *Insulin-Secreting Tumors.* These tumors usually are of pancreatic origin.
- *Pediatric Causes.* Hypoglycemia is especially common in neonates because they have relatively small glucose stores, and require frequent feedings. Also inborn enzyme defects of glucose metabolism may manifest as hypoglycemia.

Key Physical Examination Findings

- *Initial Assessment.* Look for compromised airway, ineffective breathing, and signs of shock.
- *Vital Signs.* Assess for tachycardia, fever, or hypotension.
- *Skin.* Inspect for diaphoresis.
- *Neurologic Examination.* Assess for decreased level of consciousness that may be secondary to hypoglycemia or a postictal state (after a generalized seizure). Note seizure activity, decreased visual acuity, motor weakness, and tremors.

Treatment Plan

- *Patient Assessment.* Perform a rapid and systematic primary survey and institute treatment as life-threatening problems are discovered. Frequent reassessment of the patient with an altered mental status is necessary owing to the potential for worsening of the neurologic status and airway compromise.
- **Administer O$_2$ and provide ventilatory support** as needed.
- Monitor the patients ECG and O$_2$ saturation by pulse oximetry if available.

- Place patient in the **semi-Fowler or Fowler position**. The coma position is also useful to reduce the aspiration risk in patients with a compromised gag reflex or depressed consciousness.
- If hypoglycemia is suspected, or if the patient has an altered mental status of unknown etiology, obtain a blood sample (red-top tube) and test it using an approved method. If the glucose level is low (less than 70 mg/dL), give dextrose.
- **In a conscious hypoglycemic patient with an intact gag reflex, give an oral glucose solution**. If the patient is not able to safely manage an oral solution, then perform the following procedures:
- **Establish large-bore IV access** with 0.9% NaCl or lactated Ringer's solution.
- If the patient has an altered mental status consider the administration of the following agents:

  Dextrose (50%) 25 g IV (pediatric dosage: dilute 1:1 with sterile water or 0.9% NaCl, and give 0.5 to 1.0 g/kg IV). May be repeated, if there is insufficient improvement.

  Naloxone, (Narcan) 0.4 to 2.0 mg IV bolus (pediatric dose: 0.01 mg/kg IV bolus, if insufficient response, increase dose to 0.1 mg/kg). Dose may be repeated in 2 to 3 minutes.

  Thiamine, 50-mg slow IV bolus and 50 mg IM (100 mg IM if no IV available (not recommended for prehospital pediatric use). Thiamine should be administered before 50% dextrose in patients suspected of having a thiamine deficiency—alcoholics and anyone with poor nutrition—in order to prevent precipitating Wernicke's encephalopathy.

- **If immediate IV access is not possible, give glucagon 1.0 mg IM** (pediatric dose: 0.1 mg/kg IM, up to a maximum of 1.0 mg IM per dose). Dose may be repeated in 10 to 30 minutes. Further attempts to establish an IV are advised while awaiting a response from Glucagon. As mental status improves, an oral glucose preparation can be given.
- Evaluate patients who do not respond to the above therapeutic modalities. Evaluate for other causes of altered men-

tal status, including toxic ingestions or cerebrovascular accidents.
• Transport to the appropriate ED.

Bibliography

Clemens RC: Hypoglycemia. In Schwartz GR, et al. (eds): Principles and Practice of Emergency Medicine, ed 3. Lea and Febiger, Philadelphia, 1992, pp 2087–2095.
Finegold DN: Hypoglycemia. Top Emerg Medicine 5:57–63, 1984.
Yealy DM and Wolfson AB: Hypoglycemia. Emerg Med Clin North Am 7:837–848, 1989.

Notes

CHAPTER 25

Hypotension
Myles Greenberg, MD

Presentation

The patient with a low blood pressure may present anywhere along the clinical spectrum from completely asymptomatic to exhibiting profound shock. Most often, you will discover hypotension during your evaluation of the patient.

Immediate Concerns

- **Is the patient hemodynamically stable?** Stability is defined by both symptoms and signs. The primary sign of hemodynamic instability is poor mentation (ie, confusion, agitation or decreased level of consciousness). Signs include cyanosis, poor capillary refill, systolic BP less than 90 mm Hg in both arms, new dysrhythmias, urine output less than 0.5 ml/kg per hour, and tachycardia without another explanation. Any patient who is unstable warrants immediate resuscitation. The type of resuscitation depends on the etiology of the hypotension. All patients, however, should receive oxygen administration, ventilatory assistance if necessary, large-bore IV access, and possibly PASG.

- **Is there any immediately obvious source of the patient's low blood pressure?** Respiratory arrest or hypoventilation should be treated with all necessary measures, including endotracheal intubation if indicated. External hemorrhage should be controlled, including the use of PASG for lower extremity open fractures. Obvious evidence of a hypovolemic cause for hypotension such as gastronintestinal (GI) bleeding or trauma, is justification for immediate, large-volume fluid resuscitation. An unstable cardiac rhythm should prompt the initiation of ACLS protocols.

Important History

- **Does the patient have a history of blood loss or dehydration?** Hypovolemic hypotension is best treated promptly with fluid resuscitation. Search for hypovolemia by asking about a history of recent trauma or bleeding; recent GI bleeding, hematemesis, melena, or hematochezia; previous history of GI bleeding; history of a bleeding disorder; recent history of poor oral intake; a recent history of severe diarrhea or vomiting.
- **Are there any symptoms of cardiac ischemia?** Coronary disease is the primary killer in the United States. Hypotension may occur as a result of ineffective cardiac performance due to pump failure or dysrhythmias.
- **Has the patient been febrile or had other symptoms of an infectious process?** Is the patient immunocompromised or elderly? Hypotension may be the presenting sign of sepsis in certain populations. The elderly, nursing home residents, and HIV positive patients are particularly susceptible to fulminant infections.
- **Is the patient taking any medications that may predispose the patient to hypotension or bleeding?** A large variety of medications, particularly antihypertensives, can cause hypotension. Look for any new medications or recently increased doses. A patient on anticoagulant therapy may be bleeding. Poorly controlled diabetics on insulin may present with hypotension.
- **Is there evidence of allergic reaction?** A patient in anaphylactic shock needs prompt attention to the ABCs as well as specific therapy with epinephrine, antihistamines, IV fluids, and possibly steroids.

Differential Diagnosis

SHOCK

For more detailed information on shock, refer to Chapter 38, Shock.

- *Hypovolemic Shock.* Hypovolemic shock is caused by loss of blood volume secondary to bleeding or dehydration. The most common causes are trauma, GI bleeding, intractable vomiting or diarrhea, and diabetic ketoacidosis. This is by far the most common cause of shock in young patients.

- *Cardiogenic Shock.* Cardiogenic shock is caused by loss of myocardial pumping ability. Myocardial ischemia or infarction causes this loss of pumping action directly or indirectly through the inducement of non–life-sustaining dysrhythmias. This form of shock occurs in older patients, particularly those who have a history of previous cardiac disease or a history of diabetes, hypertension, smoking, hypercholesterolemia, or obesity. Other common causes of pump failure include cardiomyopathies, valvular disease, and prosthetic valve dysfunction.

- *Septic Shock.* Septic shock is caused by loss of vascular integrity and subsequent loss of intravascular volume due to bacterial toxins. This only occurs in the setting of acute infection and is much more common in elderly, debilitated, or immunocompromised individuals.

- *Neurogenic Shock.* Neurogenic shock is caused by loss of vascular tone due to the loss of sympathetic nervous tone. This can occur after high spinal (cervical) trauma. This is a fairly uncommon cause of shock.

- *Anaphylactic Shock.* Anaphylactic shock is caused by systemic release of potent vasoactive substances, particularly histamine, resulting in airway compromise, vascular collapse, and extensive skin reactions. This response can be caused by any substance to which the patient has developed an allergy; often foods and bee stings are the culprits. Patients can also develop allergic reactions that cause hypotension but do not result in shock.

OTHER CAUSES OF HYPOTENSION

All of the processes listed previously under shock can occur in less severe form, causing hypotension without the shock syndrome. Other causes of low blood pressure include:

- *Dysrhythmias.* Bradycardias or tachycardias often cause low blood pressure without progressing to frank shock. Common etiologies are second and third degree heart block, sinus bradycardia, pacemaker failures, sinus tachycardia, atrial fibrillation or flutter, paroxysmal supraventricular (PSVTs), and ventricular tachycardia.

- *Hypovolemia Without Shock.* A multitude of conditions

can cause hypovolemia with hypotension. Bleeding, GI losses (vomiting or diarrhea), renal losses, infection (insensible losses), and adrenal insufficiency are examples.

- *Pulmonary Embolism.* This condition should be suspected in any patient who is tachycardic and tachypneic and has any predisposing factors, such as inactivity, recent surgery, malignancy, and old age.
- *Tension Pneumothorax.* This condition should be considered in the trauma patient and patients with advanced COPD or asthma.
- *Medications.* As mentioned previously, many medications can be the cause of a lower-than-normal BP. Antihypertensives that have recently been started or increased in dosage can cause either orthostatic hypotension or resting hypotension.
- *Vasovagal Response.* Commonly known as fainting, the vasovagal response is caused by stressful situations. The vasovagal response consists of bradycardia and hypotension that often result in syncope. The episode usually resolves quickly after the patient is placed in the supine position.
- *Physiologic Mechanisms.* Some patients, particularly young women and pregnant women, may normally have a low blood pressure. If the patient is asymptomatic and nonorthostatic, a low pressure may be normal.

Key Physical Examination Findings

- *Initial Assessment.* Monitor ABCs. If the patient has ventilatory or circulatory compromise, this must be addressed first.
- *Vital Signs.* Monitor heart rate and rhythm, BP in both arms, temperature, and respiratory effort. All essential to diagnosing the etiology of the patient's low BP.
- *Secondary Survey.* Look for evidence of bleeding or trauma.
- *Neck.* Examine for cervical fractures, which can cause neurogenic shock.
- *Abdomen.* Look for peritoneal signs (ie, extreme tenderness, guarding, rebound) as a source of bleeding or infection.
- *Extremities.* Assess for long bone fractures, which may be a cause of hypovolemia.

- *Neurologic Examinations.* Assess for depressed level of consciousness, which may indicate shock.
- *Skin.* Inspect for hives, pallor, cool temperature, and delayed capillary refill—an indication of allergic reaction.

Treatment Plan

- *Patient Assessment.* Constantly evaluate any hypotensive patient for deterioration to a shock state. All patients should receive cardiac monitoring and frequent reassessments of mental status, which are the best indicators of adequate perfusion. If a specific etiology of the patient's shock is known, institute specific shock therapy as outlined in Chapter 38, Shock. Following are general guidelines for the care of the nontraumatic hypotensive patient.

HEMODYNAMICALLY UNSTABLE
NONTRAUMATIC PATIENT

- **Administer O_2 and provide ventilatory support** as needed. This includes needle-chest decompression of the tension pneumothorax.
- Place patient in the **shock position** (supine with legs elevated) or use **PASG if indicated**. The use of PASG is currently controversial. The controversy centers on some studies that have demonstrated no clear benefit from PASG use, and that PASG inflation can harm some patients with bleeding above the diaphragm.
- **Establish large-bore IV access** and begin fluid resuscitation with 0.9% NaCl or lactated Ringer's solution. If transportation is delayed, or if there is inadequate response to 2 to 3 liters of crystalloid infusion, consider infusing colloid solutions, such as plasmanate or hespan. If there has been inadequate response to ongoing fluid resuscitation, consider using vasopressors such as dopamine 2 to 20 µg/kg per minute IV infusion (pediatric dosing: start at 1.0 µg/kg per minute), titrated to systolic BP greater than 90 mm Hg. Vasopressors are a temporary last-ditch effort to be used only after fluid resuscitation is inadequate. Remember, the patient is not bleeding dopamine.
- **Expeditiously transport to appropriate ED.** Do not needlessly delay patient transport—expedite transport.

HEMODYNAMICALLY STABLE NONTRAUMATIC PATIENT

- **Establish large-bore IV** access with 0.9% NaCl or lactated Ringer's solution.
- **Transport to appropriate ED.** Ensure patient comfort en route.

PATIENT WITH HYPOTENSION SECONDARY TO DYSRHYTHMIA

- Treat the patient with shock secondary to a tachycardia or a bradycardia according to guidelines in Chapters 5 and 43, on Bradycardia and Tachycardia, respectively.

Bibliography

Guidelines for Cardiopulmonary Resuscitation and Emergency Cardiac Care. JAMA, 268:2171–2302, 1992.

Shock. In Tintinalli JE, Krome LR, and Ruiz E (eds): Emergency Medicine: A Comprehensive Study Guide, ed 3. McGraw-Hill, New York, 1992, pp 132–140.

Notes

CHAPTER 26

Hypothermia
Thomas J. Rahilly, MS, EMT-CC

Presentation

Patients experiencing generalized cooling of the body (hypothermia) mostly present in two specific manners. The first is a situation where a person has suffered from direct exposure to a very cold (less than 30°F) environment. The other is a more common finding: the body has been exposed to a more passive cooling condition, one in which the patient has been subjected to relatively warmer temperatures (30°F to 50°F), but for longer periods of time. The very old or very young are especially at risk in this situation, as their ability to generate and conserve heat is less than adequate for their environment. Substance abusers who use central nervous system depressants are at increased risk of hypothermia because of a decreased ability to respond appropriately to a cold environment.

Immediate Concerns

- **What is the patient's hemodynamic status?** Ordinarily this question is not difficult to answer. In the presence of hypothermia, however, it may be more difficult to assess the status of the patient as the body may have instituted several mechanisms in an attempt to counteract the drop in body temperature. For the hypothermic patient, standard resuscitative measures may be inappropriate and even contraindicated. Your immediate concern should be to stop the cooling process by insulating the body from the cold environment. Warmed, humidified oxygen should be administered by mask or bag-valve-mask at a rate of 5 to 10 breaths per minute. Note: Rough handling of a hypothermic patient may precipitate cardiac arrest. Initial measures should be directed at preventing ventricular fibrillation, as the hypothermic myocardium is extremely susceptible to lethal arrhythmias.

Important History

- **What environment has the patient been subjected to in the past 24 hours?** Hypothermia is most common in the patient who has been exposed to temperatures of 30°F to 50°F for several days in an indoor environment. It is not difficult to recognize "accidental" hypothermia due to exposure to the extreme temperatures of the outdoors. However, the patient who presents with an altered mental status and depressed vital signs may be suffering from hypothermia. It is important to note and record the environmental conditions in which the patient is found.

- **Is there a history of a chronic illness?** Patients suffering from a chronic illness may have lost the ability to respond to extremes in temperature as a result of damage to their thermoregulatory functions. Sepsis has been known to cause a change in the hypothalmic temperature set point, which can bring about hypothermia. Suspect hypothermia in any individual with a chronic disease found in an environment that is below 50°F.

- **Is there evidence of a serious infection?** In one study, 41% of the hypothermic patients admitted to the hospital had a serious infection. Pneumonia and urinary tract infections are major causes of these infections. Be sure to make a thorough examination of the respiratory system. Ask the patient if there is any abnormal urination pattern or pain while urinating.

- **Is the patient taking any medication?** Certain medications, such as barbiturates and phenothiazines, can disrupt the thermoregulation of body temperature. Any substance that depresses the central nervous system can impair the ability of the body to respond to the cold. Insulin, thyroid medication, and steroids can do the same.

- **Is there a history of substance abuse?** Any substance that depresses the central nervous system can impair the ability of the body to respond to the cold. Alcohol is most often associated with hypothermia, as it causes vasodilation in addition to depressing the central nervous system.

Differential Diagnosis

It is often difficult for the paramedic to diagnose hypothermia as the thermometers used in the prehospital environment are not capable of measuring a temperature below 94°F.

- *Sepsis.* Because of the large number of these cases (41%) causing hypothermia, sepsis must be given adequate consideration.
- *Environmental Exposure.* Was the patient found outdoors or in a nonheated or poorly heated building? Remember that alcohol may also be a factor.
- *Hypoglycemia.* Patients suffering from hypothermia may have hypoglycemia as either the cause of the problem or as a result of shivering muscles depleting glycogen stores.
- *CNS Dysfunction.* Hypothermia brought about by insult to the central nervous system may be caused by the ingestion of a depressant, by a CVA, head injury, or damage to the spinal cord. Assessment of the patient's neurologic functions is essential.

Key Physical Examination Findings

- *Initial Assessment.* Monitor ABCs.
- *Vital Signs.* There are two grades of hypothermia: moderate and severe. The preferred method of determining whether the patient is suffering from moderate or severe hypothermia is by obtaining a body core temperature with a rectal thermometer capable of measuring lower-than-normal body temperatures.

MODERATE HYPOTHERMIA (90 TO 95°F)

During this stage, the body attempts to compensate for the loss of heat through physiologic adjustments, such as shivering. The patient is alert and responsive. The heart rate is elevated, and the blood pressure, normal.

SEVERE HYPOTHERMIA (LESS THAN 90°F)

As the body temperature falls below 90°F decreased myocardial and cerebral blood flow cause depressed metabolic function, including oxygen use and CO_2 production. Shivering stops while the heart rate slows and the blood pressure falls. Cardiac dysrhythmias appear as the myocardium becomes extremely irritable. Atrial fibrillation or flutter, atrioventricular block, premature ventricular contractions, and asystole may present at any time. A classic electrocardiographic sign of hypothermia is the Osborne (J) wave, a slow positive deflection at the end of the QRS complex. Ventricular fibrillation may be caused by any actions that stimulate the heart, including rough handling of the patient. The pulmonary function will decline and may progress from an initial tachypnea to a declining respiratory rate and tidal volume. Expect the cough and gag reflex to disappear and aspiration pneumonia to result if the airway is not secured.

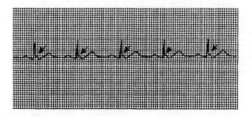

Representation of an ECG strip with a J wave.

- *Inspection and Palpation.* Assess for muscle rigidity and pupillary reaction to light. Muscle rigidity may be present as the core temperature decreases. Pupillary reaction to light stimulus is lost in severe hypothermia
- *Neurologic Examination.* The patient's level of consciousness will gradually decline to a coma state. During this decline, the patient will have difficulty making rational decisions and may actually exhibit behavior that will exacerbate their condition, such as removing clothing.

Treatment Plan

- **Maintain body temperature and prevent further heat loss.** Gently remove any wet clothing and cover the patient with blankets to insulate the patient against heat loss. Avoid measures that will cause rapid rewarming.
- **Secure the airway.** Endotracheal intubation is indicated in the same circumstances as a normothermic patient; how-

ever, it should be performed as gently as possible to avoid causing ventricular fibrillation. **Oxygenate with warm, humidified oxygen** if available.

- **Treat shock or hemodynamic instability**. Because many patients with hypothermia are hypovolemic due to extravascular plasma fluid shifts, a fluid challenge using 0.9% NaCl may improve tissue perfusion.
- **Monitor cardiac electrical activity.** Bradycardia is common. Potentially lethal cardiac dysrhythmias are likely to arise in the patient with hypothermia. Most of these will be self-correcting after rewarming. Dysrhythmias are usually refractory to conventional treatment modalities, such as drug therapy, pacing, and defibrillation. CPR should be performed on patients in cardiac arrest. The medical control physician will determine whether or not aggressive field resuscitation is warranted before rewarming.

NOTE: Hypothermic patients are not dead until they are warm and dead.

- **Transport to appropriate ED.** Field-specific therapy is relatively limited for the patient with hypothermia. Continue to monitor the patient, maintain body warmth, and transport as gently as possible. Passive rewarming may cause "afterdrop," a condition where the body core temperature actually decreases as a result of peripheral vasodilation and subsequent return of cooler blood to the central circulation.

Bibliography

Hypothermia. In Haist SA, Robbins JB, and Gomella LG (eds): Internal Medicine on Call. Appleton and Lange, Norwalk, CT, 1991, pp 180–183

Jones SA, et al. (eds): Advanced Emergency Care for the Paramedic. JB Lippincott, Philadelphia, 1992, pp 623–626.

Tintinalli JE, Krome LR, and Ruiz E (eds): Emergency Medicine: A Comprehensive Study Guide, ed 3. McGraw Hill, New York, 1992, pp 334–338.

Notes

CHAPTER 27

Irregular Heart Beat

Dean Johnson, MD

Presentation

An irregular heartbeat may initially present asymptomatically, as palpitations, as a fluttering, or as a skip in the heartbeat. The patient may seek care for the irregularity or may have another serious illness with the irregular pulse as a sign. The first sign of an irregular heartbeat may be a very rapid heart rate with chest pain, as in the case of atrial fibrillation. It may also be associated with drug reactions, either from an overdose or not taking a medication.

Immediate Concerns

- **Does the patient complain of chest pain?** An irregular pulse may accompany cardiac ischemia—either as a result of the ischemia, or if the heart rate is too rapid or slow, as a cause of the ischemia. Refer to Chapter 10, Chest Pain; Chapter 5, Bradycardia; or Chapter 43, Tachycardia, for more information.
- **Is there evidence of hemodynamic instability?** Hypotension, congestive heart failure, altered mental status, or chest pain indicate that the arrhythmia may need treatment.
- **What is the origin of the arrhythmia?** An irregular pulse can be premature ventricular contractions, runs of ventricular tachycardia, atrial fibrillation, premature atrial or junctional contractions, multifocal atrial tachycardia, sinus arrhythmia, or a transition between rhythms. An ECG tracing may be necessary to identify the treatment modality to be implemented.

Important History

- **Has the patient had recent chest pain, shortness of breath, or heart surgery?** Cardiac ischemia can cause premature ventricular contractions. Shortness of breath can be associated with ischemia or congestive heart failure; either can result in atrial fibrillation with a rapid ventricular response. Multifocal atrial tachycardia is associated with chronic lung disease. Heart surgery can be associated with atrial fibrillation or premature ventricular contractions.

- **What medications is the patient taking?** Medications to look for include antiarrhythmic agents such as digoxin, quinidine, procainamide, and verapamil; diuretics such as lasix, thiazides, and bumetanide (Bumex); as well as coumadin, synthroid, or theophylline.
- **Has the patient had an irregular pulse before?** If so, what was the previous diagnosis? This may be the most useful question during the medical history interview.
- **What medical history does the patient have?** History of atrial fibrillation, valve disease, rheumatic heart disease, thyroid disease, congestive heart failure, chronic obstructive lung disease, medication changes, or being on "blood thinners" suggest the underlying cause of the irregular pulse.

Differential Diagnosis

CARDIOVASCULAR CAUSES

There are many different cardiovascular causes of arrhythmias:
- Atrial fibrillation secondary to ischemia, congestive heart failure, rheumatic heart disease, or valve disease. Atrial fibrillation is commonly idiopathic, particularly in young patients.
- Premature ventricular contractions secondary to myocardial ischemia or digoxin toxicity.
- Second- and third-degree heart blocks secondary to atrioventricular node ischemia and, often, inferior and anterior wall myocardial infarction.
- Sinus arrhythmia in an otherwise healthy young person.
- Premature junctional beats in congestive heart failure, inferior wall myocardial infarctions, and digoxin toxicity.
- Very slow, irregular sinus rates with slow ventricular response can be seen in sick sinus syndrome.
- Irregular rates greater than 200 bpm can be associated with Wolff-Parkinson-White syndrome.

PULMONARY CAUSES

Hypoxia can cause cardiac ischemia and premature ventricular contractions. Chronic obstructive lung disease can be associated with multifocal atrial tachycardia. Pulmonary embolus can cause sudden death from ventricular fibrillation.

ENDOCRINE CAUSES

Thyroid disease can cause atrial fibrillation. Diabetes can be associated with multifocal atrial tachycardia.

METABOLIC CAUSES

Diuretic use can lead to hypokalemia (low serum potassium) and ventricular ectopy. Renal failure may lead to hyperkalemia (high serum potassium), another cause of ventricular ectopy.

DRUG CAUSES

Theophylline, caffeine, cocaine, and sympathomimetics can be associated with premature atrial contractions. Thyroid replacement can be associated with atrial fibrillation. Recent excessive alcohol consumption is associated with the "holiday heart" syndrome of atrial fibrillation.

ECG

Therapeutic interventions often are based upon an analysis of the rhythm. Refer to Chapter 5, Bradycardia, or Chapter 43, Tachycardia, for specific therapeutic interventions.

Key Physical Examination Findings

- *Initial Assessment.* Assess for evidence of altered mental status and pattern of irregularity. An altered mental status is a sign of inadequate perfusion. Is the irregular pulse in a pattern (regularly irregular)? Think regular premature ventricular contractions or second-degree heart block. Is the irregular pulse without any seeming pattern (irregularly irregular)? Think atrial fibrillation or multifocal atrial tachycardia. Is the irregularity associated with breathing? This is often a sinus arrhythmia.
- *Vital Signs.* Monitor pulse and respirations. A very slow irregular rate can indicate a need for atropine or external

cardiac pacing. A rapid rate (over 160 or 170 bpm) can lead to circulatory collapse, because the heart does not have sufficient time to fill between beats. Is the blood pressure adequate? If not, treat the rhythm and hypotension at the same time. Tachypnea is a sign of hypoxia and possible pulmonary edema. Slow respirations can be the cause of hypoxia and ventilations will need to be assisted.

- *Neck.* Note jugular venous distention, which can be a sign of congestive heart failure.
- *Lungs.* Assess for signs of new-onset congestive heart failure (ie, crackles at the bases). Remember that wheezes can be heard in congestive heart failure (cardiac asthma) as well as lung disease.
- *Heart.* The presence of a gallop, either an S^3 (rhythm is "Ken-tuc-ky") or S^4 (rhythm is "Ten-nes-see") may indicate congestive heart failure.
- *Extremities.* Check for evidence of peripheral edema. Does the pulse felt at the wrist correspond to the auscultated heart sound? Premature ventricular contractions may not perfuse because the heart may be only partly full of blood during the contraction. Delayed capillary refill can be one of the most sensitive indicators of tissue perfusion, because the body shunts blood away from the extremities when the vital organs are in trouble.

Treatment Plan

GENERAL TREATMENT GUIDELINES

- **Administer O_2 and provide ventilatory support** as needed.
- Monitor ECG.
- **Establish large-bore IV access** with 0.9% NaCL or lactated Ringer's solution.
- **Transport to the appropriate ED.** Consultation with the medical control physician may prove valuable in the management of the patient with rhythm abnormalities.

SPECIFIC TREATMENT GUIDELINES

Hemodynamically unstable patients

- Identify and treat the underlying rhythm by using the appropriate AHA ACLS protocol.

Hemodynamically Stable Patients

- Treat by following the general principles outlined previously.
- In stable patients with bradycardic rates and second- or third-degree blocks, apply external pacemaker pads as a precaution.

Bibliography

Gewitz MH and Vetter VL: Cardiac Emergencies. In Fleisher GR and Ludwig S (eds): Textbook of Pediatric Emergency Medicine, ed 3. Williams and Wilkins, Baltimore, 1993, pp 552–553.

Levitt MA: Palpitations. In Hamilton GC and Sanders AB (eds): Emergency Medicine: An Approach to Clinical Problem Solving. W.B. Saunders, Philadelphia, 1991, pp 196–213.

Stapczynski JS: Disturbances of Cardiac Rhythm and Conduction. In Tintinalli JE, Krome RL, and Ruiz E (eds): Emergency Medicine: A Comprehensive Study Guide, ed 2. McGraw-Hill, New York, 1988, pp 67–92.

Yealy DM: Dysrhythmias. In Rosen P and Barkin RM (eds): Emergency Medicine Concepts and Clinical Practice, ed 3. Mosby-Year Book, St. Louis, 1992, pp 1199–1249.

Notes

CHAPTER 28

Multitrauma
Patrick R. Coonan, RN, EdD, CEN, EMT-CC

Presentation

Each year, one out of every three Americans sustains a traumatic injury. Trauma is a major cause of disability in the United States and accounts for approximately 140,000 deaths annually. Trauma is the leading cause of death in people under the age of 44 years, accounts for half the deaths in children under 4 years, and 80% of deaths in persons aged 15 to 24 years. The trauma patient varies in presentation based on the type and mechanism of injury. Primarily, the prehospital EMS provider is concerned with five areas in the field: securing the scene to protect both rescuers and patients, conducting the primary survey and managing ABC^4 explained in the following section, extricating the victim rapidly while protecting the cervical spine, and immobilizing and transporting the victim to an appropriate facility.

Immediate Concerns

FIRST PRIORITY

The first priority is to detect obvious injuries and instability of the respiratory and cardiovascular systems. The approach to the trauma patient is based on the same primary survey "ABC" approach used on all patients. In addition, the trauma patient requires an ABC^4 approach: Airway, Breathing, C^1 = Circulation, C^2 = Spine, C^3 = Chest, C^4 = Consciousness.

- On arrival of the EMS team, each patient is rapidly assessed for:
  Altered mental status
  Patient airway
  Labored respirations
  Noisy respirations
  Cyanosis
  Tachypnea

Decreased chest wall motion

Decreased chest wall motion
Pale, clammy skin
Peripheral pulses
Significant external bleeding
- Auscultate the chest for breath sounds.
- Administer 100% oxygen.
- Institute tracheal intubation if indicated.
- Determine pulse quality and rate.
- Control external hemorrhage.
- Monitor blood pressure.
- Establish IV access with 0.9% NaCL or lactated Ringer's solution.
- Use PASG if indicated by local protocol.
- Perform a rapid neurologic assessment on extremities and pupils

If the number of patients exceeds the ability of the EMS response team to immediately assess and treat all patients, refer to Chapter 52, The Multiple Casualty Incident.

INITIAL TRAUMA SURVEY

A = Airway
- Airway adjuncts: oropharyngeal airway, nasopharyngeal airway, esophageal gastric tube airway, endotracheal tube, and cricothyroidotomy. Use the specific modality required for the patient based on the assessment. Head and neck alignment is paramount during airway control, as cervical spine injury cannot be ruled out in the field. Suction should be readily available.

B = Breathing
- Provide supplemental 100% oxygen by non-rebreathing bag mask.
- Use mouth-to-mask, bag-valve-mask, demand valve, or ventilators to assist ventilations.
- Use the appropriate modality for the situation at hand. It is always preferable for professional rescuers to use an adjunctive device rather than the mouth-to-mask method. The mouth-to-mouth method should not be used by prehospital EMS providers.

C^1 = Circulation
- Assess by checking for the presence and quality of carotid or femoral pulses or both. Peripheral pulses may be absent

as a result of direct injury or sympathetic nervous system response. This compensatory mechanism causes peripheral vasoconstriction. Radial pulses are usually present when the systolic BP is greater than 80 mm Hg; femoral pulses indicate a systolic BP greater than 60 mm Hg; and carotid pulses indicate a systolic BP greater than 50 mm Hg.

C^2 = Cervical Spine

• Consider cervical spine injuries in all multiple trauma patients until they can be ruled out by the appropriate medical personnel. The cervical spine should be protected by using a stiff cervical collar, rolled blanket, tape, and backboard, or by using other methods acceptable according to local protocol. Be sure to protect the other areas of the spine by immobilizing the patient from the head to the hips.

C^3 = Chest

• Assess for five types of chest injuries because they may require immediate therapeutic intervention in the field, as any of them may be immediately life-threatening:
  1. Tension pneumothorax
     a. *Signs and Symptoms:* cyanosis, distended neck veins, shortness of breath, deviated trachea, cough, tachycardia, decreasing BP
     b. *Intervention:* needle thoracostomy
  2. Flail chest
     a. *Signs and Symptoms:* paradoxical movement of the chest wall, dyspnea, cyanosis, tachycardia
     b. *Intervention:* Endotracheal intubation, if indicated, 100% oxygen under pressure, controlled fluid administration, stabilization of the flail segment
  3. Pericardial tamponade
     a. *Signs and Symptoms:* increased heart rate, Beck's triad (decreased BP, muffled heart sounds, distended neck veins), dyspnea, paradoxical pulse
     b. *Interventions:* 100% oxygen, high Fowler position, IV line
  4. Sucking Chest Wound
     a. *Signs and Symptoms:* sucking sound, dyspnea, decreased breath sounds tachycardia, hypotension, signs of tension pneumothorax
     b. *Interventions:* occlusive dressing taped on three sides, watching closely for signs of tension pneumothorax

(if signs appear, remove occlusive dressing), 100% oxygen
5. Hemothorax
   a. *Signs and Symptoms:* same as for hypovolemic shock
   b. *Interventions:* hypovolemic shock treatment, 100% oxygen, IV lines for large fluid replacement, rapid transport for definitive treatment

$C^4 =$ *Consciousness*

- Assess neurologic status using Glasgow Coma Scale (see Appendix C). It is advisable to also calculate a trauma score based on the method used in your local jurisdiction (see Appendix D).

Important History

- **What is the mechanism of injury?** An assessment of the mechanism of injury will allow you to detect injuries that may be related to it. Injuries such as cardiac tamponade, tension pneumothorax, and pelvic injury may not be readily apparent on examination but may be assumed to be present based solely on the mechanism of injury.
- **Does the patient complain of specific symptoms?** Obtaining a brief medical history is an important part of the secondary survey.
- **Initiate the secondary survey.** After the primary survey, a more thorough secondary survey should be performed. Begin by re-evaluating the patient's airway and rechecking vital signs. Fractures should be splinted. If possible, discreetly undress the patient and check the patient's back. Systematically assess and treat the head and neck for lacerations, fractures, and deformities.

  Perform a rapid systematic evaluation of the following:
  - *Ears, nose, and throat:* recheck airway; check for fractured larynx, CSF leaks, penetrating objects
  - *Neck:* check for wounds, hematomas, neck vein distention, pulses, deformities, pain, penetrating objects, tracheal shift, subcutaneous emphysema
  - *Eyes:* check pupillary response; check for trauma
  - *Chest:* check for wounds, abrasions, deformities, penetrating objects (in addition to those found on primary survey)
  - *Abdomen:* check for rigidity, pain, tenderness, wounds,

abrasions, hematomas, penetrating objects, eviscerations, distention
- *Spine*: check for deformities, pain on palpation, abrasions, bruises
- *Pelvis and hips:* check for fractures, deformities, femoral pulses, abnormal rotation or flexion of legs
- *Extremities:* check for pulses, neurologic status distal to injury, fractures, dislocations, crepitus, movement, skin color and temperature, capillary refill
- *Perineum:* check for bleeding, urine extravasation
- *Buttocks:* check for wounds, abrasions

Key Physical Examination Findings

UNDRESSING THE PATIENT

Key in the of evaluation of the trauma patient is the ability to perform a complete examination. Without exposing the patient, it is impossible to make a systematic assessment of all the patient's injuries. Although undressing the patient may seem rather benign, there are situations that require special attention:

- **Helmets.** A variety of helmet types are available for sports that recommend head protection. Examples are motorcycling, bicycling, football, flying, and auto racing. The removal of these requires a special procedure.
- **Boots.** Heavy boots create a problem if the patient has sustained an unstable injury to the foot or lower extremity. Some simple techniques make the process of removal less painful. Boots are usually very expensive and removal without cutting is generally appreciated. If cutting must be done, cutting and ripping the seam will usually allow the boot to be repaired.
- **Wet Suits.** In most cases these can be rolled and pulled off the patient, being turned inside out in the removal. If this is not an option, cut wet suit along the seams.
- **Removal of Clothing Without Cutting.** Preserve as much clothing as possible. Undress the uninjured extremity first. Consider the chain of evidence if foul play is suspected, as the clothes or contents may be needed for evidence.
- **Initial Assessment.** See previous discussion
- **Vital Signs.** Assess heart rate and rhythm, breathing, BP.

Tachycardia and tachypnea usually precede hypotension. Hypotension is a late sign of shock.

- *Skin.* Inspect skin: usually cool, pale, and moist in the shock patient

- *HEENT.* Assess for the presence of JVD in the shock patient, which may indicate an obstructive shock—consider tension pneumothorax, pericardial tamponade, and massive pulmonary embolism. Also assess for tracheal deviation.

- *Lungs.* Assess for evidence of tension pneumothorax. Evidence of blunt trauma or penetrating trauma should raise suspicion of intrathoracic injury, including pericardial tamponade, tension pneumothorax, and hemothorax.

- *Heart.* Listen for muffled heart tones.

- *Abdomen.* Assess for evidence of penetrating or blunt trauma, which may indicate intra-abdominal injury. In addition, check for the pulsatile abdominal mass found in patients with an abdominal aortic aneurysm.

- *Peripheral Pulses.* Check for peripheral pulses. These may be absent as perfusion decreases. Radial pulses are usually present when the systolic BP is greater than 80 mm Hg; femoral pulses indicate a systolic BP greater than 60 mm Hg; and carotid pulses indicate a systolic BP greater than 50 mm Hg.

- *Mental Status.* An altered mental status is a sensitive indicator of inadequate cerebral perfusion.

- *Neurologic Examination.* Assess using the Glasgow Coma Scale.

ECG

All trauma patients should receive cardiac monitoring to detect electrical abnormalities in the myocardium.

Treatment Plan

- *Patient Assessment.* Perform a rapid and systematic primary survey, as mentioned in the previous section, and institute treatment as life-threatening problems are discovered. Prompt transport to the appropriate trauma center or ED is a key intervention. A secondary survey should be performed once the primary survey and all primary survey interventions have been accomplished. Frequent reassessment of multiple trauma patients is necessary owing to the potential for worsening of their hemodynamic status.

- *Communications.* Consult with a medical control physician for guidance and institution of appropriate orders, as well as notification of the receiving ED. Such consultation may prove invaluable in the care of the trauma patient.

GENERAL TREATMENT GUIDELINES: HEMODYNAMICALLY STABLE PATIENT

- **Administer O$_2$ and provide ventilatory support** as needed.
- Place patient in the **shock position** (supine with legs elevated), protecting the cervical spine as indicated.
- **Establish large-bore IV access** with 0.9% NaCl or lactated Ringer's solution.
- **Treat non–life-threatening injuries** (ie, control bleeding, splint fractures, etc).
- Transport to appropriate ED. Ensure patient comfort en route.

GENERAL TREATMENT GUIDELINES: HEMODYNAMICALLY UNSTABLE PATIENT

- **Administer O$_2$ and provide ventilatory support** as needed. This includes needle-chest decompression of the tension pneumothorax.
- Place patient in the **shock position** (supine with legs elevated) or use **PASG if indicated**. The use of PASG is controversial. The controversy centers on some studies that have demonstrated no clear benefit from PASG use, and that PASG inflation can harm some patients with bleeding above the diaphragm.
- **Establish large-bore IV access and begin fluid resuscitation** with 0.9% NaCl or lactated Ringer's solution. If transportation is delayed, or if there is inadequate response to 2 to 3 liters of crystalloid infusion, consider infusing colloid solutions, such as plasmanate or hespan. If there has been inadequate response to ongoing fluid resuscitation, consider using vasopressors such as dopamine, 2 to 20 µg/kg per minute IV infusion (pediatric dosing: start at 1 µg/kg per minute, titrated to systolic BP greater than 90 mm Hg).

NOTE: Vasopressors are a temporary last-ditch effort to be used only after fluid resuscitation is inadequate. Remember, the patient is not bleeding dopamine.

• **Transport expeditiously to appropriate trauma center or ED.** Do not needlessly delay patient transport–expedite transport.

Bibliography

Committee on Trauma, American College of Surgeons: Advanced Trauma Life Support Student Manual, ed 5. American College of Surgeons, Chicago, IL, 1993.

Dunham C and Cowley RA: Shock Trauma/Critical Care Handbook. Aspen Publishers, Rockville, MD, 1986, pp 3–6.

Sheehy S: Mosby's Manual of Emergency Care, ed 3. St. Louis, CV Mosby, 1990, pp 544–555.

Notes

CHAPTER 29

Musculoskeletal Trauma

Owen T. Traynor, MD

Presentation

Musculoskeletal and soft tissue injuries are generally non–life-threatening; however, they can be associated with other life-threatening injuries. In addition, they can be limb threatening if not properly managed. Their often obvious and dramatic nature may distract you from treating the immediate life-threatening injuries. A stepwise systematic approach to patient assessment will help the you to avoid transporting a well-splinted, but dead, patient. Early proper management of patients with musculoskeletal and soft tissue injuries can significantly reduce morbidity and mortality.

Immediate Concerns

- **Are there any life-threatening injuries present?** A rapid and thorough primary survey should be performed on all patients before treatment of obvious non–life-threatening injuries. Prompt intervention in cases of life-threatening airway, respiratory, and circulatory emergencies should be carried out as the problems are discovered. Patients who have life-threatening injuries should be expeditiously transported to the appropriate ED, with care continued throughout transport. A secondary survey and treatment of the high-priority injuries may be carried out en route to the ED, if time and patient condition permits. Patients who are not immediate transport patients should receive a thorough head-to-toe secondary survey. Their injuries should then be ranked according to priority and treated before transport.

Important History

- **What is the mechanism of injury?** Often the patient's injuries can be predicted based on the mechanism of injury. Essentially, injury results from the absorption of kinetic energy by the patient's body. A knowledge of the kinetics of the injury can help you search for occult injury. For example, a fall on an outstretched hand can result in injury from the fingers up through the shoulder and neck.

- **What is the age of the patient?** Certain injuries are more common in various ages: greenstick fractures are common in pediatric patients, whereas dislocations are rare. Elderly patients have higher incidences of fractures even without "significant" mechanisms of injury.

- **What is the patient's chief complaint?** Under most circumstances, the patient's chief complaint will lead you to the site of the injury. Exceptions to this rule are when the patient has an altered mental status or has anesthesia on board, either alcohol or other substances, and when there are other significant distracting injuries. The pain of a fractured femur is likely to distract the patient from the pain of a fractured metacarpal bone.

- **What is the patient's past medical history?** The patient's medical history may provide important information about the nature of a patient's injury or predisposition to injury. Patients who have osteoporosis (an atrophy or reduction in bone mass), bone cancer or bony metastases, multiple myeloma, or a history of chronic steroid use are at higher risk of fractures. In fact, a fracture, particularly compression fractures of the spine, may occur in the absence of significant trauma.

Differential Diagnosis

In this section, common or significant musculoskeletal injuries of the upper and lower extremities are reviewed. This is not a comprehensive list of all possible injuries.

UPPER EXTREMITY

- *Shoulder.* The wide range of motion afforded by the shoulder predisposes it to instability and injury. Approximately 15% of all athletic injuries seen in the ED involve the shoulder. Shoulder dislocations account for more than half of all dislocations seen in the ED. The nature of the immature skeletal system in pediatric patients reduces the incidence of shoulder dislocations. Their joint capsule and ligaments

are significantly stronger than their growth plates. Therefore, they tend toward fractures of the growth plate rather
than the dislocations or sprains that adult patients develop.

Fractures

- **Clavicular fractures** are the most common fractures of
childhood. There are three characteristic clavicle fractures:
fracture of the middle third, the most common; fracture of
the lateral third; and the fracture of the medial third clavicle,
the least common. Indirect trauma to the lateral shoulder
can result in fracture at the middle third. Direct trauma to
the top of the shoulder can cause fracture of the lateral
third clavicle. The medial third may fracture when there is
direct trauma to the anterior chest. The patient complains
of pain at the fracture site and presents with the injured
extremity held close to the body. Often, the shoulder will
be slumped downward, inward, and forward. Complications include pneumothorax and injury to the subclavian
arteries and veins and the brachial plexus, a group of nerves
that supply the upper extremity.
- **Scapular fractures** are uncommon, found usually in young
men who have had high-speed auto accidents, falls, or
crushing injuries. There are often other significant injuries
present and therefore scapular injuries are often missed.
Patients with scapular fractures present with their arm held
to the body. There is pain associated with any movement
of the shoulder. Complications include hemothorax,
pneumothorax, pulmonary contusion, and injury to the
axillary arteries and veins, and the brachial plexus.
- **Proximal humerus fractures** occur mainly in the elderly
patient with osteoporosis, resulting from a fall on an outstretched hand. The younger patient with this mechanism
of injury is more likely to develop a dislocation. Often there
can be a fracture-dislocation. Proximal humerus fractures
also occur when there is either direct trauma to the lateral
arm or an axial load transmitted through the elbow. Patients present with the arm held close to the body. Complications include axillary artery and brachial plexus injury.

Dislocations

- **Acromioclavicular joint (ACJ) dislocations,** or shoulder
separations, are commonly caused by direct trauma to the

point of the shoulder with the arm adducted. A fall on an outstretched hand may also produce this injury. Patients present with a spectrum of symptoms from mild tenderness with minimal swelling over the joint to severe pain, obvious deformity, holding their injured limb close to the body with the shoulder hanging downward. Common complications are associated fractures of the clavicle or coracoid process.

- **Glenohumeral joint dislocations** are the most common major joint dislocations. More than 95% of all shoulder dislocations are anterior dislocations. Posterior dislocations account for approximately 4% of dislocations, and inferior and superior dislocations are rare. The typical patient with an anterior dislocation is a either a young man between 20 and 30 years of age or an older woman between 60 and 80 years of age. It can result from either direct or indirect trauma. In the older patient it usually follows a fall on an outstretched hand, whereas in the younger patient it results from a combination of abduction, extension, and external rotation occurring during athletic activity. The patient presents with severe pain and the arm slightly abducted and external rotated. The shoulder appears squared off, with a fullness in the anterior aspect. Common complications include injury to the axillary artery and nerve, radial nerve, or brachial plexus.

HUMERUS AND ELBOW

Injuries near the elbow run the risk of significant complications and disability. Injuries to the median nerve, ulnar nerve, radial nerve, and brachial artery may occur.

Fractures

- **Midshaft humerus fractures** usually result from direct trauma to the arm, but may also occur as a result of a fall on an outstretched hand. This fracture is usually obvious owing to swelling and inability of the patient to use the arm. The most common complication is injury to the radial nerve. Vascular injury may also occur.
- **Distal humerus fractures** may be supracondylar, proximal to the epicondyles, or involving the epicondyles. Supracondylar fractures usually result from a fall on an outstretched hand. The typical patient is younger than 20

years old. Their ligamentous structures are stronger than the bone; therefore, a fracture results. The adult patient, whose bones are stronger, suffers a dislocation. The brachial artery and the median, ulnar, and radial nerves are often injured by the distal bone fragment.

- **Elbow fractures** are actually fractures of the bones that make up the elbow joint: fractures of the distal humerus, including condylar fractures and fractures of the articular surfaces; fractures of the radial head; or fractures of the ulna's olecranon process. These injuries can result from direct trauma, a fall on an outstretched hand, or other mechanisms. Neurologic injuries of the radial, median, or ulnar nerves, as well as injury to the brachial artery, may complicate the fracture. In addition, dislocation of the elbow may be found.

Dislocations

- **Elbow dislocation** refers to the dislocation of the ulna on the humerus or the dislocation of the radius on the ulna. There are often associated fractures due to the tremendous force required to dislocate the elbow. The most common type of elbow dislocation is a posterior dislocation resulting from a fall on an outstretched hand in an adult patient. As mentioned previously under distal humerus fractures, pediatric patients will more commonly suffer a fracture due to this mechanism of injury. Patients with a posterior elbow dislocation often present with the elbow flexed and a prominent olecranon. These injuries may relocate on their own. Neurovascular complications may occur.
- **Radial head subluxation,** or "nursemaid's elbow," is a common childhood injury found most often in pediatric patients aged 1 to 3 years old. This commonly results from a longitudinal pull on the forearm while the arm is pronated. This mechanism stretches the annular ligament, allowing the radial head to slip out of position on the humerus. The patient is reluctant to move the arm with the arm found slightly flexed in a pronated position.

FOREARM AND WRIST

Injuries near the wrist run the risk of injuries to the median, ulnar, and radial nerves. There are eight carpal bones that make up the wrist, each of which can be fractured, dislocated, or subluxed. It is often not possible to differentiate between fracture, dislocation, or subluxation without x-rays. However, it is usually possible to determine that an injury has taken place.

Fractures

- **Radius-ulnar fractures** usually result from direct trauma to the forearm but may also occur as a result of a fall on an outstretched hand. These fractures are often displaced because significant force is required to fracture both of these bones. Fractures of either the radius or ulna may occur alone or with dislocations at either the wrist or elbow.
- **Colles fracture,** a fracture of the distal radius with dorsal displacement of the distal radius, is the most common wrist fracture. It occurs most frequently in adults over the age of 50 years due to a fall on an outstretched hand. The patient usually presents with the "silver-fork" deformity and pain.

Dislocations

Dislocations of the wrist, depending on the bones involved, may cause nerve impingement. These injuries may occur as a result of direct or indirect trauma.

HAND

Fractures of the bones in the hand, including fingers, are common. Complications of both fractures and dislocations can be significant because they may result in dysfunction of the hand.

PELVIS, HIP, AND FEMUR

Pelvic fractures comprise less than 5% of all fractures. These fractures and other associated injuries are a frequent cause of death in the trauma patient. The most common etiologies are secondary to motor vehicle accidents (MVAs), or pedestrian accidents, or falls from heights; however, as many as one third result from minor falls in the elderly. Femur fractures also require significant force and may be associated with other injuries.

Fractures

- **Pelvic fractures** may be associated with hypotension owing to the significant force required to fracture the pelvis.

Consideration of the patient's hemodynamic status is important. There are many different classification systems used to describe these types of fractures. It is sufficient for you to know that there can be fractures of the individual pelvic bones, fractures that disrupt the pelvis ring (usually fractured in two places), and fractures of the weight or non–weight-bearing parts of the pelvis. Pelvic fractures may result from either direct or indirect trauma. Complications include intra-abdominal, retroperitoneal, gynecologic, urologic, or neurovascular injuries.

- **Hip fractures** are actually fractures of the proximal femur. They are characterized by shortening and external rotation of the affected limb. Certain types of hip fractures are associated with hip dislocations. Often the patient is elderly, with osteoporotic bones, and the fracture results from a minor fall. The younger patient with a fractured hip has often suffered a high-energy trauma—other associated injuries should be investigated. The femur may show evidence of significant internal hemorrhage. In addition, neurologic injury may occur.
- **Femoral shaft fractures** are painful and present with a shortened limb. Their presence may distract you from finding other significant coexisting injuries. Significant pain relief occurs when traction is applied to the fracture.

Dislocations

- **Hip dislocations** may be anterior, posterior, or central dislocations. Posterior dislocations are, by far, the most common, accounting for as much as 90% of all hip dislocations. In adults with normal hips, significant force is required to dislocate the hip. It most commonly results during an MVA, after the patient's knee strikes the dashboard, transmitting force along the femur to the hip. Hip dislocations occur with considerably less force in patients with prosthetic hips. In children a hip dislocation may occur rather than a fracture of the proximal femur. The patient with a posterior dislocation presents with a shortened, partially flexed, adducted, internally rotated leg. Neurologic injury to the sciatic nerve may occur, resulting in motor and sensory deficits in the lower leg and foot. Anterior dislocations present with abducted and externally rotated legs. Injury to the femoral vessels and nerve may accompany these injuries.

KNEE AND LOWER LEG

Knee injuries have become more prevalent in our sports conscious society. Most common are ligamentous or meniscal injury. The tibia is the most commonly fractured long bone.

Fractures

- **Patellar fractures** result from direct trauma, a fall on a flexed knee, or a forceful contraction of the quadriceps.
- **Tibial plateau fractures** are produced by direct trauma to the femoral knee. Although both medial and lateral plateaus may be fractured simultaneously, the lateral tibial plateau is most commonly fractured. The patient presents with a painful swollen knee and is reluctant to bend it.
- **Tibial shaft fractures** may result from direct trauma, resulting in a fracture of the fibula as well, or from rotational or indirect forces, resulting in an isolated tibial fracture. Complications include infection (these fractures are often open), compartment syndrome (neurovascular injury caused by swelling in the compartments bounded by fascial sheets, which limits expansion of the leg with increasing edema), and injury to the peroneal nerve if the fracture is near the fibular head.
- **Isolated fibular fractures** are uncommon. Patients are often able to bear weight and walk with these isolated fractures.

Dislocations

- **Knee dislocations** are one of the few true orthopedic emergencies. Vascular and neurologic injury often follow. Traumatic dislocation is uncommon; however, the popliteal artery is often injured. The incidence of vascular injury is approximately 40% with half of these patients requiring amputation. Early reduction of the dislocation is important. This injury may reduce spontaneously, but vascular injury may have occurred and therefore these patients should be transported to the ED.
- **Patellar dislocations** commonly result from a twisting injury to the extended knee. The patella is usually dislocated laterally.

Tendon, Ligament, and Meniscal Injuries

- **Tears of the patellar or quadriceps tendon** may occur during strenuous contraction of the quadriceps. The injury results in the inability to actively extend the knee.
- **Injuries of the collateral and cruciate ligaments** are not uncommon. The majority of these injuries are related to athletic activity. The medial collateral ligament is the most frequently injured ligament. This injury is caused by a force to the lateral aspect of the slightly flexed and internally rotated knee. The lateral collateral ligament is less frequently injured because it is often protected from a medial force by the opposite leg. The anterior cruciate ligament (ACL) may be injured from a sudden deceleration, flexion, and rotation. Injury to the posterior cruciate ligament is rare, because the ligament is stronger than the ACL and the collateral ligaments. It may tear when the knee hits the dashboard in a high-speed MVA. Cruciate injuries are often associated with an audible "pop," buckling of the knee, swelling, and pain.
- **Meniscal tears** are difficult to diagnose, but are associated with a twisting motion in the flexed knee. Pain is worst on weight bearing. The patient may report that the knee is locking up after the initial trauma.

ANKLE AND FOOT

The ankle and foot bear the entire weight of the patient and are subject to significant stress. Injury results in temporary loss of function.

Fractures

- **Ankle fractures, or malleoli fractures,** often result from a rotational force applied to the joint while the foot is fixed in place. The most common malleolus fractured is the lateral malleolus. Significant ligamentous injury may accompany ankle fractures, leaving the joint unstable. Neurovascular compromise should be evaluated.
- **Foot fractures** commonly result from falls and MVAs. The talus bone, responsible for support of the body and distribution of body weight, is rarely fractured. However, it has a limited blood supply and may suffer avascular necrosis if fractured or dislocated. The patient will present with pain,

swelling, and deformity of the ankle. Calcaneal fractures manifest swelling and pain over both the medial and lateral aspects of the bone. A bruise may be present on the sole of the foot. Because this injury follows a fall, one must search for associated axial load injuries—fractures of the lower extremities, hip, and back.

Dislocations

- **Ankle dislocations** are found, most often, in combination with ankle fractures. The most common dislocation is a posterior dislocation of the talus. Ankle dislocations have significant potential for vascular compromise. If not promptly relocated, avascular necrosis of the talus or loss of the foot may occur.

Sprains

- **Ankle sprains** are the most common ankle injury. Sprains of the lateral ligaments occur with the greatest frequency. The mechanism of injury is such that the ankle is internally rotated, inverted, and plantar-flexed. The medial ligaments may be sprained when the foot is everted, dorsiflexed, and externally rotated. The patient presents with pain, possibly ecchymosis, and swelling.

Key Physical Examination Findings

- *Initial Assessment.* Evaluate and treat life-threatening injuries as they are discovered.
- *Vital Signs.* Evaluate for hemodynamic instability.
- *Secondary Survey.* Perform a thorough and systematic examination once life-threatening injuries have been treated. Do not be distracted by obvious musculoskeletal injuries.
- *Lungs.* Assess for evidence of tension pneumothorax. Evidence of blunt trauma or penetrating trauma to the shoulder, clavicle, or scapula should raise suspicion of intrathoracic injury including pericardial tamponade, tension pneumothorax, and hemothorax.
- *Abdomen.* Assess for evidence of penetrating and direct or indirect blunt trauma, which may indicate intra-abdominal injury.

- *Pelvis and Hip.* Assess for deformity, ecchymosis, tenderness, crepitus, loss of range of motion and soft tissue injury.
- *Extremities.* Assess for deformity, ecchymosis, tenderness, crepitus, loss of range of motion, length discrepancies, and soft tissue injury. Be sure to evaluate distal neurovascular status—check distal pulses, capillary refill, and sensory and motor status.

Treatment Plan

- *Patient Assessment.* Perform rapid and systematic primary survey and institute treatment as life-threatening problems are discovered. Prompt transport to the ED is a key intervention. A secondary survey should be performed once the primary survey and all primary survey interventions have been accomplished. Frequent reassessment of the patient with a significant mechanism of injury is necessary, owing to the potential for worsening of the hemodynamic status. It is often difficult for the EMS provider to differentiate between a fracture and a dislocation. Fortunately, the principles of management of these injuries are identical.

GENERAL TREATMENT GUIDELINES: HEMODYNAMICALLY STABLE PATIENT

- **Administer O$_2$ and provide ventilatory support**.
- Management principles for treatment of suspected closed fractures and dislocations:
  - Treat all life-threatening injuries.
  - Ensure that the patient is not a "load and go" patient.
  - Stabilize the injury site to prevent further injury.
  - Evaluate the distal neurovascular status.
  - Controversy exists surrounding whether or not limb alignment should be sought in the field. Some experts maintain that the paramedic should "splint them where they lie," unless there is vascular compromise. In the case of vascular compromise, one attempt at limb alignment or relocation of the dislocation is recommended. Obtaining limb alignment poses the risk of causing additional soft tissue or neurovascular injury. It is often difficult, however, to adequately immobilize an angulated

fracture, thereby risking further injury while transferring the patient from the accident scene to the ED. It is for this reason that some physicians recommend applying in-line traction and obtaining limb alignment.

○ If relocation of a dislocated joint is attempted, consider the use of analgesia before the attempt if the patient is hemodynamically stable and alert.

○ Select the appropriate immobilization device and apply it without causing additional injury.

○ Be sure to immobilize the joint proximal and distal to the injury.

○ Re-evaluate the distal neurovascular status.

• **Management principles for treatment of open fractures.** Treat using the management principles previously recommended for treatment of suspected closed fractures and dislocations, except add the following steps for applying the immobilization device:

○ Irrigate the wound with sterile normal saline.

○ Apply a dry sterile dressing over the wound.

○ Apply a slight compression dressing if the wound is actively bleeding.

○ Reduce swelling by elevating the injury. Apply a cold pack to the injury to decrease pain and swelling.

• **Transport to appropriate ED.** Ensure patient comfort en route.

GENERAL TREATMENT GUIDELINES: HEMODYNAMICALLY UNSTABLE PATIENT

• **Administer O_2 and provide ventilatory support** as needed. This includes needle chest decompression of the tension pneumothorax.

• Place patient in the **shock position** (supine with legs elevated). Use care not to aggravate other injuries, or use PASG if indicated. The use of PASG is currently controversial. The controversy centers on some studies that have demonstrated no clear benefit from PASG use and that PASG inflation can harm some patients with bleeding above the diaphragm.

• **Establish large-bore IV access and begin fluid resuscitation with 0.9% NaCl or lactated Ringer's solution.** If transportation is delayed, or if there is inadequate response to 2 to 3 liters of crystalloid infusion, consider infusing colloid solutions, such as plasmanate or hespan. If there has been inadequate response to ongoing fluid resuscitation, consider using vasopressors such as dopamine, 2 to 20 μg/kg per minute IV infusion (pediatric dosing: start at 1.0 μg/kg per minute), titrated to systolic BP greater than 90 mm Hg.

NOTE: Vasopressors are a temporary last-ditch effort to be used only after fluid resuscitation has failed to restore stable hemodynamics. Remember, the patient is not bleeding dopamine.

- **Rapidly transport to appropriate ED.** Do not needlessly delay patient transport—expedite transport.

Bibliography

Chin HW, Propp DA, and Orban, DJ: Forearm and Wrist. In Rosen P (chief ed): Emergency Medicine: Concepts and Clinical Practice, ed 3. Mosby-Year Book, St. Louis, 1992, pp 588–608.

Cwinn AA: Pelvis and Hip. In Rosen P (chief ed): Emergency Medicine: Concepts and Clinical Practice, ed 3. Mosby-Year Book, St. Louis, 1992, pp 658–683.

Daya M: Shoulder. In Rosen P (chief ed): Emergency Medicine: Concepts and Clinical Practice, ed 3. Mosby-Year Book, St. Louis, 1992, pp 626–657.

Dronen SC and Birrer P: Shock. In Tintinalli JE, Krome LR, and Ruiz E (eds): Emergency Medicine: A Comprehensive Study Guide, ed 3. McGraw-Hill, New York, 1992, pp 132–140.

Gruber JE: Proximal Femur and Femoral Shaft. In Rosen P (chief ed): Emergency Medicine: Concepts and Clinical Practice, ed 3. Mosby-Year Book, St. Louis, 1992, pp 684–707.

Lammers LR and Freemyer BC: Hand. In Rosen P (chief ed): Emergency Medicine: Concepts and Clinical Practice, ed 3. Mosby-Year Book, St. Louis, 1992, pp 544–587.

Magnusson AR: Humerus and Elbow. In Rosen P (chief ed): Emergency Medicine: Concepts and Clinical Practice, ed. 3. Mosby-Year Book, St. Louis, 1992, pp 609–625.

Mayeda DV: Ankle and Foot. In Rosen P (chief ed): Emergency Medicine: Concepts and Clinical Practice, ed 3. Mosby-Year Book, St. Louis, 1992, pp 745–777.

Mayeda DV: Knee and Lower Leg. In Rosen P (chief ed): Emergency Medicine: Concepts and Clinical Practice, ed 3. Mosby-Year Book, St. Louis, 1992, pp 708–744.

Waeckerle JF: Foot Injuries. In Tintinalli JE, Krome LR, and Ruiz E (eds): Emergency Medicine: A Comprehensive Study Guide, ed 3. McGraw-Hill, New York, 1992, pp 1012–1014.

Waeckerle JF: Knee Injuries. In Tintinalli JE, Krome LR, and Ruiz E (eds): Emergency Medicine: A Comprehensive Study Guide, ed 3. McGraw-Hill, New York, 1992, pp 987–998.

Waeckerle JF and Steele MT: Ankle Injuries. In Tintinalli JE, Krome LR, and Ruiz E (eds): Emergency Medicine: A Comprehensive Study Guide, ed 3. McGraw-Hill, New York, 1992, pp 1007–1011.

Waeckerle JF and Steele MT: Leg Injuries. In Tintinalli JE, Krome LR, and Ruiz E (eds): Emergency Medicine: A Comprehensive Study Guide, ed 3. McGraw-Hill, New York, 1992, pp 1004–1006.

Waeckerle JF and Steele MT: Trauma to the Pelvis, Hips and Femur. In Tintinalli JE, Krome LR, and Ruiz E (eds): Emergency Medicine: A Comprehensive Study Guide, ed 3. McGraw-Hill, New York, 1992, pp 987–998.

Notes

CHAPTER 30

Nausea and Vomiting
Jonathan S. Rubens, MD, FACEP

Presentation

The term *vomiting* is defined as the expulsion of the gastric contents through the mouth. Vomiting is a reflex act initiated in the vomiting center located in the fourth ventricle of the brainstem.

Immediate Concerns

- *ABCs.* Any patient who is vomiting and has an altered mental status may not be able to protect their airway sufficiently and may be at risk for aspiration of vomitus. Airway security, as always, is a priority.
- *Circulation.* Evaluate the patient for signs and symptoms of shock. Severe, prolonged vomiting may cause dehydration. Resuscitative measures should be instituted in these patients.
- *Comfort Measures.* Aside from severe pain and trauma, nausea and vomiting are among the most disconcerting symptoms patients may experience. Comfort measures can go a long way toward easing patients' distress.

Important History

- **What is the duration of vomiting and the amount?** Patients with severe bouts of vomiting may be dehydrated and hypotensive.
- **When and what was the patient's last meal?**
- **What is the age of the patient?** Age is often critical because certain entities more commonly occur in specific age groups.
- **Is there any evidence of obstruction?** Signs and symptoms may include pain, obstipation (unable to pass gas) or

constipation, and abdominal distention in addition to vomiting.

- **Are there any other gastrointestinal (GI) symptoms?**
These may include diarrhea, anorexia, or reflux and indigestion.
- **Are there other systemic symptoms?** Pain, fever, and neurologic symptoms such as headache, stiff neck, blurred or double vision, vertigo, and isolated weakness should be considered. Also, look for any history of urinary symptoms or amenorrhea or missed periods.
- **Is there a prior history of GI disease?** Any prior history of peptic ulcers, prior abdominal surgery, diverticulosis, cirrhosis, and gallbladder disease should be elicited.
- **Is there a history of drug or substance abuse?** Include prescription medications.

Differential Diagnosis

A list of the causes of nausea and vomiting would be exhaustive and useless with this context. Rather, the following major system causes should be considered for each patient:

- *Acute Myocardial Infarction.* Acute myocardial infarction, particularly inferior wall MIs, can present with nausea and vomiting (see Chapter 10, Chest Pain).
- *Pericarditis.* Pericarditis may elicit these symptoms owing to diaphragmatic irritation. Patients may also have chest pain and a pericardial "friction rub" on auscultation.
- *Central Nervous System Disorders.* All of the following can cause nausea and vomiting and are discussed in Chapter 20, Headache: migraine, CVA, tumors, and hypertensive emergencies.
- *Inner Ear Disturbances.* Vertigo and labyrinthine disorders are disturbances of sensorium involving the inner ear and positional senses. These patients will often remain free of nausea and vomiting as long and they remain immobile, but with the onset of "dizziness" or with any motion, they will experience these symptoms. Look for associated hearing loss and headache and focal weakness on examination as clues.
- *Endocrine.* The central nervous system effects of the hormonal changes of early (usually first trimester) pregnancy commonly result in severe morning nausea and vomiting.

- *Diabetes Mellitus.* Diabetes mellitus (DM) and its complications are frequently associated with nausea and vomiting. Elevations of blood glucose, including diabetic ketoacidosis, can result in these symptoms. As well, low blood-glucose levels can cause nausea, diaphoresis, and syncope. Complications of this disease, including esophageal dysfunction, gastroparesis, and postural hypotension, are all known causes of nausea and vomiting in the diabetic patient. A history of DM, polyuria, and polydypsia, weakness and weight loss should be elicited. Likewise, the physical examination may reveal dehydration, the "acetone smell" of the ketotic patient's breath, or an abnormally high blood glucose level.

- *Pediatric Disorders.* Gastroesophageal reflux in infants can sometimes be mistaken for vomiting. This can be differentiated by quantifying how much an infant was fed and how much was vomited. Reflux commonly occurs after each feeding and is sometimes improved with positioning the child more erect after feeding. Similarly, milk or food allergies can cause postprandial vomiting. Again, this is usually associated with feeding and with certain foodstuffs in particular. Feeding history will help differentiate this.

Other less common causes of vomiting in children include: malrotation, infections (ie, meningitis and sepsis), and intussusception (telescoping of the intestine within itself). With intussusception, the child classically has periods of severe distress, with an intermittently tender and crampy abdomen. These episodes can last from several minutes to hours, with intervening periods during which the child appears in no distress at all and looks well. The passage of a "currant-jelly" or clotlike stool can also help in the diagnosis.

- *Eating Disorders.* Anorexia nervosa and bulimia are eating disorders resulting from disordered self-image resulting in fasting (anorexia) or bingeing (bulimia) and self-induced vomiting to avoid weight gain.

- *Psychological Disorders.* Neurosis and irritable bowel syndrome are two psychogenic disorders that result in abnormal stimulation of the autonomic nervous system and can produce nausea and vomiting. Emotional upset, stress, and anxiety are usually precipitating factors.

- *Pneumonia.* Pulmonary patients with pneumonia, due to

irritation of the diaphragm and pleural effusions may complain of nausea and vomiting. Look for a history of respiratory distress, tachypnea, cough with sputum production, and fever as clues. Adventitial sounds (rhonchi, rales, wheezes) may be heard on auscultation of the chest.

- *Drugs.* Many classes of drugs, in particular nonsteroidal anti-inflammatory drugs, erythromycin, aspirin, and codeine, as well as chemotherapeutic agents, can cause nausea and vomiting due to direct irritation of the gastric lining. Likewise, many other substances (including food and bacterial toxins and pesticides) are known to have these effects on the GI system. Searching for a history of ingestion or exposure to these substances is the best way to identify these causes.

All of the following causes of nausea and vomiting are discussed in Chapter 1, Abdominal Pain:

Gastrointestinal gastritis (alcoholic and nonalcoholic), ulcer, appendicitis, obstruction, food poisoning, gastroenteritis

Hepatic and pancreatic hepatitis, cholecystitis, cholelithiasis, pancreatitis, cirrhosis.

Key Physical Examination Findings

- *ABCs.* Monitor vital signs, including temperature, when possible.
- *General Appearance.* Observe the patient for pallor, icterus, and diaphoresis. Patients with central causes of their symptoms and those with appendicitis usually allow very little unnecessary movement, whereas those with kidney stones may elicit signs of restlessness. Does the patient look sick? If the patient is pediatric, are they consolable or irritable? Is there a fever or signs of dehydration?
- *Abdomen.* Are there signs of obstruction, distention, and decreased or high-pitched bowel sounds? Is there costovertebral angle tenderness? Is the abdomen firm or soft?
- *Chest.* Are the breath sounds clear and equal? Is the cardiac rhythm normal?
- *Neurologic Examination.* Are there any signs of neurologic dysfunction or altered mental status?
- *Skin.* Is there a rash?

Treatment Plan

- *Monitor ABCs.* Remember, vomiting with altered mental status may lead to aspiration. An alert patient or secure airway are essential. If signs of dehydration and circulatory compromise are present, or if the history suggests a prolonged illness or associated hemorrhage with vomiting, IV fluid resuscitation should be initiated.
- *Monitor.* Monitor all patients in whom there exists a potential for cardiac disease, either as a cause for their illness or as a coexistent condition.
- *Transport to Emergency Department.* Expedite the transport of critical patients, those with hemorrhage or abnormal vital signs. Ensure patient comfort en route.
- *Adiminister Antiemetics.* These drugs may reasonably be requested by the prehospital care provider, particularly with long transport times and persistently symptomatic patients. Keep in mind that most of these agents will have some effect on the patient's mental status and, for this reason, may be contraindicated until the definitive cause for their symptoms has been determined.

Bibliography

Bledsoe BE: The Acute abdomen. In Bledsoe BE, Porter RS, and Shade BR (eds): Paramedic Emergency Care. Prentice-Hall, Englewood Cliffs, NJ, 1991, pp 745–777.

Henretig FM: Vomiting. In Fleisher and Ludwig (eds): Textbook of Pediatric Emergency Medicine, ed 3. Williams and Wilkins, Baltimore, MD, 1993, pp 506–513.

Seward C and Mattingly D: Bedside Diagnosis. Churchill Livingstone, London, 1979, pp 126–135.

Notes

CHAPTER 31

Near Drowning

Gregg Margolis, MS, NREMT-P

Presentation

Drowning and near drowning can occur in any body of water. Swimming pools are the most common site of drowning. Lakes, ponds, and bathtubs are common sites for aquatic emergencies. When responding to a near-drowning emergency, the prehospital care provider will generally find the patient with one of three presentations: without vital signs, unconscious with vital signs, or conscious. This progression is generally reflective of the degree of hypoxemia secondary to submersion.

Immediate Concerns

- **Is the patient in the water?** If so, an immediate plan for the safe rescue of the patient is the first concern.
- **Is the patient conscious?** If the patient is unconscious, immediate resuscitation and aggressive patient management, including intubation, ventilation, and oxygenation is needed.

Important History

- **Has there been any trauma involved?** If there is any possibility that the patient may have struck his head on the way into the water (on a diving board, etc), on the bottom, or on anything floating in the water, cervical spine precautions must be taken immediately. Any patient found unconscious in the water should be assumed to have a cervical injury until proven otherwise.
- **Is the patient in immediate danger?** Any patient still in the water is in immediate danger. If the patient is submerged, the patient must be recovered immediately. If the patient is found floating on the surface, the patient is in

danger and should only be handled by individuals trained
in water rescue or lifeguarding.
- **Was there a loss of consciousness?** Unconsciousness is
a significant finding in any near-drowning emergency. Some
patients regain consciousness relatively quickly once their
airway is opened and they are ventilated. Obviously, the
prognosis worsens the longer the patient is unconscious.
- **What are the characteristics of the water?** Survival from
submersion incidents is improved in clean, fresh water.
Many patients, especially the young, have survived prolonged submersion in cold water. Resuscitation should be
initiated in any patient who has been rescued within 60
minutes in water with a temperature below 70°F.

Differential Diagnosis

The assessment of the near-drowning patient is usually straight-
forward. Be alert for the following:
- *Traumatic Injuries.* Many drownings occur as divers strike
the bottom of a pool or a diving board. Injuries are much
more common in shallow water. You should assume that
any patient found unconscious in the water has a cervical
spine injury until proven otherwise.
- *Pre-Existing Medical Emergency.* Be aware that there may
be a possibility of a pre-existing medical problem.
- *SCUBA Diving Injury.* Consider the possibility of pulmonary barotrauma, or decompression sickness, or both, in
anyone who has taken a breath of pressurized gas under
water.

Key Physical Examination Findings

- *Mental Status.* Establish baseline level of consciousness
as soon as possible.
- *Airway.* Check for airway obstruction from vomitus and
fluid in the airway.
- *Breathing.* Assess the rate and work of breathing. Be sure
to assess lung sounds.
- *Circulation.* Note any circulatory compromise, which is
generally secondary to a respiratory insult.
- *Trauma.* Observe for signs of head injury, which indicates
the need for cervical spine immobilization.

Treatment Plan

- **Remove the patient from the water.** The first priority in the management of the near-drowning patient is to safely remove the individual from immediate danger. The patient will most often have been rescued by lifeguards, family, or bystanders. If the patient is still in the water, they should be removed as quickly as possible by trained rescuers. Be sure to consider the possibility of cervical spine trauma in any unconscious patient.

- **Secure an airway.** The swallowing of large amounts of water into the stomach makes regurgitation and aspiration a major concern in the management of near-drowning patients. If the patient is not conscious, the protection of the airway by an endotracheal tube is a high priority.

- **Ventilate and oxygenate the patient.** The primary insult in drowning is profound hypoxemia. As a result, hyperoxygenation with 100% oxygen is the main priority of management.

- **Provide cardiovascular support.** If the patient is pulseless, provide immediate cardiopulmonary resuscitation. Remember that the circulatory insult is secondary to hypoxemia. Provide aggressive resuscitation aimed as reversing hypoxia and respiratory acidosis.

- **Prevent heat loss.** Obviously, drowning patients are going to be wet. Water conducts heat from the body many times faster than air. As a result, you must make every attempt to keep the patient normothermic, even in warm environments. Removal of wet clothes and covering the victim with a thermal blanket should suffice in most cases. In cases of hypothermic near drowning, prevent further heat loss but do not spend an inordinate amount of time concerning yourself with rewarming.

- **Establish intravenous access with 5% dextrose in water at a KVO rate.**

- **Bronchodilation.** As a result of the bronchial irritation, many drowning patients suffer from considerable bronchoconstriction. Inhaled β 2 agonists, such as aerosolized albuterol, (0.5 ml in 3 ml saline) are the best short-term therapy for this situation. Remember that these agents can be nebulized directly into an endotracheal tube in the intubated patient.

Bibliography

American Red Cross: Lifeguarding. American National Red Cross, 1990.

Bledsoe BE: Paramedic Emergency Care, ed 2. Prentice-Hall, Englewood Cliffs, NJ, 1993.

Bove AA and Davis JA: Diving Medicine, ed 2. WB Saunders, Philadelphia, 1990.

Environmental Emergencies. Emerg Med Clin North Am, WB Saunders, Philadelphia,

Stewart CE: Environmental Emergencies. Williams & Wilkins, Baltimore, 1990.

Notes

CHAPTER 32

Obstetric Emergencies
Thomas J. Rahilly, MS, EMT-CC

Presentation

The vast majority of human births are not emergencies. In fact, there are probably more births occurring outside of a medical facility, with little or no professional medical assistance, than those that occur in a delivery room. The term emergency childbirth has been used by prehospital EMS systems to describe a labor and delivery attended to by EMTs in the field. Emergency childbirth is more accurately defined as an obstetric emergency with complications that compromise the health of the mother or infant. This chapter focuses on these situations only. It may be worthwhile to review the prehospital care for the mother and infant during a "normal" childbirth, which can be found in all basic EMT textbooks.

Immediate Concerns

- **What is the patient's hemodynamic status?** If the patient is hemodynamically unstable, immediate resuscitation is warranted, including immediate transport, oxygen administration, large-bore IV access, PASG inflation (leg sections only) if indicated, and fluid resuscitation. If the patient is in compensated shock, prompt transport, as well as the these treatments, is necessary. Pregnancy can also cause severe hypertension that is uncontrollable in the field.

The primary efforts of the prehospital EMS provider during an obstetric emergency should be dedicated to supporting the respiratory and cardiovascular functions of the mother. Although the fetus is quite vulnerable during this period, the mother is the life-support system for the fetus and, until the birth occurs, will provide the unborn infant with all of its life-sustaining nutrients, including oxygen. It is, therefore, imperative that all women who may potentially be pregnant receive ventilatory support with supplemental oxygen and careful monitoring of the cardiovascular system, with treatment as necessary.

Important History

Before the 12th week of gestation, the abdomen of the woman will most likely not reveal the signs of pregnancy by either visual examination or palpation. For this reason, all women of childbearing age who present with vaginal bleeding or abdominal or pelvic pain should be presumed to be pregnant until a pregnancy test by the appropriate medical professional positively rules it out.

To determine the type of obstetric problem the women is experiencing, it is essential to conduct a good history. For the woman who has not been diagnosed as being pregnant, the subjective interview may indicate that the she has experienced mistimed, light, or absent menstrual periods; has noticed tenderness of the breasts; is fatigued; and has unexplained nausea or reports more frequent urination. Pelvic or abdominal pain may indicate an ectopic pregnancy, which is a life-threatening emergency that requires prompt action by a surgical team (see Chapter 35, Pelvic Pain).

Women who have experienced pregnancy in the past may relate that they "feel" pregnant. For those who are known to be pregnant, recent changes may include pain or cramping; vaginal discharge; vital signs, including body temperature; or fetal activity. Any changes in the characteristics of the pregnancy will be valuable in diagnosing the woman's condition. Complications during previous pregnancies, such as abortion, pre-eclampsia, or eclampsia, may be useful for determining the current problem.

Differential Diagnosis

- **Is the patient aware that she is pregnant?** Many woman presenting with an acute abdomen are not aware that they may be pregnant. Any woman of childbearing age must be considered pregnant until proven otherwise.
  - *Ectopic Pregnancy.* Ectopic pregnancies are also called "tubal" pregnancies because 95% of all ectopic pregnancies involve one of the fallopian tubes. Known as the

"great imitator," ectopic pregnancy can mimic a ruptured ovarian cyst, acute appendicitis, pelvic inflammatory disease (PID), or complete or incomplete abortion. A ruptured ectopic pregnancy manifests with acute abdominal pain that may radiate to one or both shoulders and signs and symptoms of shock from intraperitoneal bleeding. An unruptured ectopic pregnancy involves little or no pain and no shock. Either case may produce profuse bleeding, spotting, or no vaginal bleeding.

- **Is there any vaginal discharge?** Blood or other fluids discharged vaginally may indicate a serious threat to the fetus as well as the mother. Approximately 4% of all woman have third trimester bleeding. Placentae previa or abruptio placentae is the cause of the bleeding in about one half of these patients. Any vaginal bleeding, especially in the third trimester, should be considered emergent until proven otherwise.
  - *Abortion.* Some vaginal bleeding occurs in approximately 50% of all pregnancies. An abortion may be complete or incomplete, and there may or may not be an expulsion of the products of conception.
- **In which trimester of pregnancy is the woman?** If the patient is known to be pregnant, determine the month of gestation. As the pregnancy progresses, the number of problems and their negative effects on the fetus and mother grow larger.
  - *Placenta Previa.* If the placenta attaches to the lower uterus and fails to "migrate" upward as the fetus grows, it can lead to premature separation. It is clinically distinguished by bright red bleeding with no pain, usually around the 8th month. Bleeding is intermittent at first, progressing to a heavier flow over 1 to 2 weeks. Seen in less than 0.5% of all pregnancies, it is most commonly seen (75%) in other than first pregnancies.
  - *Abruptio Placentae.* The premature separation of the placenta from the uterus, occurring in about 1% of all pregnancies, may cause painful uterine bleeding that is either mild (less than 25% separation accounting for about 90% of the cases) or severe (greater than 50% separation). Bleeding may be evident or occult depending on the position of the fetus' head and type of separation. Severe abruptio placentae results in moderate to

severe pain as well as fetal and maternal (shock syndrome) distress. Mild abruptio placentae may progress into the severe form rapidly.

○ *Pre-Eclampsia and Eclampsia.* Also known as hypertensive disorders of pregnancy, pre-eclampsia and eclampsia occur during the 3rd trimester in 5% to 8% of all pregnancies and carry a 5% mortality. Both conditions can be characterized by hypertension (BP greater than 160/110 mm Hg), poor urinary output (less than 400 ml in 24 hours), headaches, visual disturbances, abdominal pain, massive edema, and cyanosis. Eclampsia occurs when the above conditions combine with seizures or coma.

○ *Postpartum Hemorrhage.* Almost 5% of all woman experience postpartum hemorrhage, with approximately 150 ml of blood loss. The loss of 250 ml of blood after delivery of the fetus, which may be caused by lacerations during delivery or incomplete separation of the placenta, is considered excessive. Bleeding can also be delayed for up to 14 day's postpartum.

• **Has the delivery of the fetus begun?** If the woman has begun to deliver the fetus and there is evidence that this will be an abnormal delivery, a decision must be made to either deliver the infant at the scene (breech only) or transport the woman to the ED.

○ *Breech Presentation.* Buttocks (65%), sitting position (25%), or one or both feet (10%) is the presenting part. This is the only type of abnormal delivery that may be safely accomplished in the prehospital setting with assistance from the EMS provider.

○ *Transverse Presentation.* The fetus lies crosswise in the uterus, and the presenting part is an arm. This type of delivery must take place in the hospital.

○ *Prolapsed Cord.* The umbilical cord presents before delivery of the fetus in 0.5% of all deliveries.

Key Physical Examination Findings

Provide the woman with privacy to the extent possible.
• *Initial Assessment.* Look for signs of shock or hypertension.

- *Vital Signs.* Monitor vital signs, particularly BP and pulse rate. Pregnancy usually results in mild hypotension during the 3rd trimester. A 15-mm increase in the mother's known systolic pressure should be considered suspect. A pregnant woman will have an increased heart rate and may have a resting pulse rate of 100 bpm in her 3rd trimester.
- *Skin.* Inspect for cyanosis, indicating poor perfusion.
- *HEENT.* Observe for the presence of jugular venous distention (JVD) in the pregnant patient, which may indicate that patient is hypertensive.
- *Lungs.* Assess for evidence of pulmonary edema, a sign of pre-eclampsia.
- *Heart.* Listen for muffled heart tones.
- *Abdomen.* Assess for pelvic pain or the pain of labor.
- *Mental Status.* An altered mental status is a sensitive indicator of inadequate cerebral perfusion and fetal perfusion.
- *Neurologic Examination.* Inquire about headaches and cerebral or visual disturbances. The eclamptic woman may have headaches and cerebral or visual disturbances. Also, inquire about any seizure activity.
- *Vaginal Examination.* Examine the vaginal opening for bleeding, presenting parts, or in the case of abortion, fetal tissue.
- *Extremities.* Check the extremities for signs of edema. Although most women (about 75%) experience some edema during pregnancy, excessive or a notable increase in edema may indicate pre-eclampsia.

ECG

Because of the stress associated with obstetric emergencies, the woman should receive cardiac monitoring for electrical abnormalities of the myocardium.

Treatment Plan

Although there will be a great deal of concern for the fetus, it is essential to concentrate on treating the mother for shock.

HYPOTENSIVE PATIENT

- **Treat for shock** (see Chapter 38, Shock), and follow the following guidelines for specific obstetric problems.

- **Monitor the fetal heart rate.** A fetal heart rate of less than 120 bpm indicates fetal distress. Expeditious transport to the ED is indicated with support to the mother.

Hypertensive Patient

- Because the administration of hypertensive medications requires careful titration and monitoring of the patient's blood pressure, treatment is best initiated in the ED.

SPECIFIC OBSTETRIC TREATMENT

Prepartum

- *Ectopic Pregnancy.* Transport expeditiously to ED.
- *Abortion.* Gently remove any protruding tissues. Transport to ED.
- *Third-Trimester Bleeding.* Regardless of the cause, place these patients in the left lateral recumbent position and transport to ED.
- *Eclampsia and Pre-Eclampsia.* Place the patient in a left lateral recumbent position to relieve pressure on the vena cava. Anticipate seizures; medication orders may include diazepam (Valium), 5 to 10 mg slow IV, or magnesium sulfate 10%, 2 to 4 g slow IV. NOTE: This is controversial for seizure prophylaxis.

Active Labor

- *Breech Presentation.* If the delivery of the baby has begun, allow the buttocks and trunk to deliver spontaneously. While supporting the baby's body, lower the body slightly so that the remainder of the delivery is assisted by a majority of the baby's own weight. When the head is almost completely delivered (hairline is visible), gently raise the baby upward, and the head should deliver.

  NOTE: If the head does not deliver within 3 minutes, place a gloved hand in the vaginal opening (palm toward the baby's face), and with your fingers, form a **V** on either side of the baby's nose. Exert gentle pressure against the vaginal wall to provide an oxygen supply.
- *Leg Presentation.* This presentation is not deliverable in the field. Transport rapidly to ED.
- *Transverse (Arm) Presentation.* This presentation is not deliverable in the field. Transport expeditiously to ED.

- **Prolapsed Cord.** This is an absolute emergency. Relieve the pressure of the baby's head from the umbilical cord as you transport the mother and undelivered baby to the ED. Elevate the supine mother's hips to the extent possible. With two fingers of a gloved hand, gently push the baby back up the vagina without pushing the cord with it. Cover the vaginal opening with a sterile drape, maintain gentle upward pressure, and transport.

Postpartum

- **Postpartum Hemorrhage.** Gently massage the uterine fundus and place the baby at the mother's breast to help control postpartum bleeding after delivery. Oxytocin (Pitocin), 10 U (1 ml in 1 liter normal saline), titrated at less than 30 mini drops per minute.

  NOTE: Make certain that all fetuses have been delivered before you even consider oxytocin.

Bibliography

Benson MD: Obstetrical P•E•A•R•L•S. FA Davis, Philadelphia, PA, 1989.

Caroline NL: Emergency Care in the Streets, ed 4. Little, Brown and Company, Boston, MA, 1991.

Hockberger RS: Obstetric Emergencies. In Tintinalli JE, Krome LR, and Ruiz D (eds): Emergency Medicine: A Comprehensive Study Guide, ed 3. McGraw-Hill, New York, 1992, pp 515–524.

Sheehy SD, McCall P, and Varvel: Obstetric and Gynecologic Emergencies. In Sheehy SD (ed): Emergency Nursing: Principles and Practices, ed 3. Mosby–Year Book, St. Louis, MO, 1992.

Notes

CHAPTER 33

Obstructed Airway

Mike Yee, BS, EMT-P

Presentation

Airway obstruction is one of the most readily treatable yet immediately life-threatening emergencies faced by prehospital providers. Patients may present with any degree of obstruction from simple hoarseness cleared with a cough to complete obstruction requiring a surgical airway, such as cricothyrotomy. Significant airway obstruction can occur at any time. Early recognition and treatment is essential to successful outcome. Because of this, it is important to distinguish this problem from more serious conditions that cause sudden respiratory failure, but are treated differently.

Immediate Concerns

- **What is the status of the patient's airway?** The assessment must be more sophisticated than merely noting whether the airway is open, it must consider whether the airway will remain open; and the danger of aspiration. Airways that are endangered must be secured and protected. Positioning of the airway, suctioning, and the use of oropharyngeal or nasopharyngeal airways, as well as endotracheal intubation, should be accomplished early.

- **Is the airway obstructed?** If the patient is not ventilating or cannot be mechanically ventilated then airway obstruction is present. The mechanism causing the obstruction must be promptly discovered. Sudden onset of obstruction is likely to be caused by a foreign body. However, anaphylaxis may occur suddenly as well. A history of fever, chills, or sore throat may point to an infectious etiology; croup and epiglottitis must be considered. The cause is usually readily apparent. If a foreign body obstruction is responsible, the BLS airway obstruction techniques should be employed. If an anatomic obstruction, perhaps caused

199

by angioneurotic edema, infection in the upper airway, or obstruction by a mass or expanding hematoma, is present, the BLS airway obstruction techniques will not be helpful. When it is not possible to know the mechanism of the obstruction, employing the BLS airway obstruction techniques is recommended; foreign body obstruction is more common and is likely to be relieved by these techniques.

- **Is the airway obstruction complete or partial?** Complete obstructions and partial obstructions with poor air exchange are best managed as discussed previously. Partial obstructions with good air exchange are best managed by having the patient continue to cough forcefully and expel the foreign body. Patients with good air exchange need to be monitored; the potential for worsening obstruction is great.

Important History

- **Does the patient have a history that suggests a decreased ability to protect the airway?** Patients who have a depressed mental status are often at increased risk of aspiration. The use of alcohol and other central nervous system depressants also increases the risk of foreign body obstruction.
- **Does the patient have a history of oral or throat cancer?** Airway obstruction may result from a tumor obstructing the airway, bleeding, or swelling.
- **Is there a history of sore throat or fever?** The presence of sore throat should alert you to the possibility of croup or epiglottitis, particularly in children.

Differential Diagnosis

The differential diagnoses presented here are causes of obstruction of the upper airway and therefore do not include lower respiratory causes of respiratory distress, such as pneumothorax, hemothorax, pneumonia, and so forth.

- *Foreign Body Obstruction.* Approximately 3000 deaths occur each year in the United States by choking. Most of these deaths are in children younger than 4 years of age. In adults, the history of a foreign body aspiration is usually readily available from the patient or from bystanders. In children, you should consider the possibility of foreign body aspiration in any patient who presents with ongoing respiratory distress or resolved respiratory distress. The child may have a history of a sudden onset of respiratory distress with choking and cough, by an absence of symptoms and then followed by delayed stridor or wheezing. This cycle occurs when the foreign body is not cleared from the airway but passes distally into the smaller airways. In children, a foreign body may also lodge in the esophagus, causing stridor.

- *Croup.* Croup is usually a relatively benign viral illness occurring in patients 6 months to 3 years of age. The patient usually presents after several days of an upper respiratory infection with a barking cough, stridor, and dyspnea. The patient often improves with humidified or nebulized oxygen. (See Chapter 13, Croup and Epiglottitis: Pediatric Laryngeal Edema.)
- *Epiglottitis.* Epiglottitis, in children, is a life-threatening emergency. The typical patient is between 2 to 7 years of age and presents with several hours of worsening sore throat, a high temperature, drooling, and stridor. The patient is often sitting quietly with the neck slightly extended and chin forward. No attempt should be made to examine the airway: laryngospasm and complete obstruction may occur. Should a complete obstruction occur, the patient with epiglottitis is usually able to be ventilated with a bag-valve-mask device. Epiglottitis may occur in teenagers and adults, with the development of the disease occurring over a period of days. These patients are less likely to develop complete obstruction acutely. (See Chapter 13, Croup and Epiglottitis: Pediatric Laryngeal Edema.)
- *Angioneurotic Edema.* This condition is characterized by a sudden onset of edema due to an allergic reaction in the upper airway, which may involve the uvula, tongue, palate, epiglottis, or larynx. It most commonly occurs in patients who have a history of allergies. It should be treated in a fashion similar to anaphylaxis.
- *Traumatic Obstruction.* This may occur after direct trauma to the neck or throat. A direct injury to the larynx may cause paralysis of the vocal cords, leading to obstruction.
- *Chemical or Thermal Injury.* Chemical or thermal injury to the airway may cause obstruction secondary to the soft tissue injury and swelling.

- *Abscesses.* Abscesses located in the upper airway, such as retropharyngeal and peritonsillar abscesses, may cause obstruction secondary to swelling and mass effect. The history is usually one of prior infection, either upper respiratory infection or tonsillitis, possibly fever, drooling, and trismus (a painful spasm of the muscles of mastication or chewing).
- *Tumors and Cysts.* Tumors and cysts of the upper airway may manifest as airway obstruction. Although these are generally chronic and slow growing, they may manifest as an acute obstruction.

Key Physical Examination Findings

- *Initial Assessment.* Be alert for upper airway compromise; stridor or hoarseness may be present. Respirations may be ineffective. Look for the universal choking sign. Assess the patient's ability to cough or speak.
- **Vital Signs.** Assess for the presence of tachycardia and tachypnea.
- *Skin.* Inspect for generalized erythema (redness), pruritus (itching), urticaria (hives), and angioedema (swelling of the hands, face, neck, and upper airway). Flushing, cyanosis, chills, and diaphoresis may occur.
- *HEENT.* Note the presence of drooling, trismus (inability to open mouth due to spasm), stridor, or angioneurotic edema. Do not attempt to examine the airway of pediatric patients suspected of having epiglottitis.
- *Neck.* Examine the neck for enlarged lymph nodes or masses, or any evidence of trauma.
- *Lungs.* Check breath sounds for signs of broncoconstriction—wheezing and prolonged expiratory phase. A foreign body that has moved into the smaller airways may have localized wheezing rather than the diffuse wheezing found in asthma or anaphylaxis. Look for retractions and use of respiratory accessory muscles.
- *Mental Status.* Impaired mentation, general mental status, or altered consciousness, which may indicate significant respiratory compromise and the need for immediate respiratory support.

Treatment Plan

The goals of the treatment plan are to relieve the obstruction, if possible, and to improve the oxygenation of the patient. Frequent reassessment of the patient with an airway obstruction is necessary owing to the potential for worsening of the respiratory status. Be prepared—potential for respiratory arrest and cardiac arrest exist.

GENERAL TREATMENT GUIDELINES

- **Administer O$_2$ and provide ventilatory support** as needed. This includes relieving upper airway obstructions, suctioning, or endotracheal intubation if indicated. Protect cervical spine as necessary.
- If BLS treatments are not effective, transport expeditiously to the ED.

SPECIFIC TREATMENT GUIDELINES

Foreign Body Obstruction

- Follow AHA guidelines for relieving foreign body obstructions. BLS techniques will likely be effective.
- If BLS techniques are ineffective, perform direct laryngoscopy and, if a foreign body is visualized, use the Magill forceps to remove the object.
- If a foreign body is not visualized or cannot be removed from the airway, attempt endotracheal intubation and ventilation.
- If ventilation is not possible after endotracheal intubation, consider expeditious transport and transtracheal jet insufflation, cricothyrotomy, or advancing the ET tube to push the obstruction into the right mainstem bronchus. Withdraw the tube to a point above the carina, thus allowing both lungs to be ventilated.

Epiglottitis: Pediatric Patients

- **Do not do anything that may precipitate complete obstruction.** Do not examine the airway, do not draw blood. Transport the child in a comfortable position, with the parent present.
- **Provide supplemental O$_2$ and use blowby O$_2$** rather than a mask to provide less noxious stimuli.
- **Transport expeditiously to the appropriate ED.** Do not needlessly delay patient transport. Ensure patient comfort en route.
- **If air exchange is inadequate, ventilate the patient.** Do not attempt endotracheal intubation unless unable to me-

chanically ventilate the patient. A surgical airway may be required if endotracheal intubation is impossible—consider needle cricothyrotomy. (See Chapter 13, Croup and Epiglottitis: Pediatric Laryngeal Edema.)

Epiglottitis: Adult Patients

- **Provide supplemental O$_2$.**
- **Transport expeditiously to the appropriate ED.** Do not needlessly delay patient transport. Ensure patient comfort en route.
- **If air exchange is inadequate, ventilate the patient.** Attempt endotracheal intubation if indicated. A surgical airway may be required if endotracheal intubation is impossible—consider needle cricothyrotomy.

Croup

- Provide supplemental humidified oxygen.
- Transport in a comfortable position.
- If patient is in distress **administer 3 ml of nebulized 0.9% NaCl**—this is often treatment enough and avoids potential for rebound after racemic epinephrine.
- Consider **nebulized racemic epinephrine, 0.25 to 0.5 ml in 2.5 ml of 0.9% NaCl.** Dose may be repeated every 20 to 30 minutes.
- **If air exchange is inadequate, ventilate the patient.** Do not attempt endotracheal intubation unless unable to mechanically ventilate the patient. A surgical airway may be required if endotracheal intubation is impossible—consider needle cricothyrotomy. (See Chapter 13, Croup and Epiglottitis: Pediatric Laryngeal Edema.)

Bibliography

Bledsoe BE, Porter RS, and Shade BR (eds): Paramedic Emergency Care, ed 2. Prentice-Hall, Englewood Cliffs, NJ, 1994, pp 236–233.

Guidelines for Cardiopulmonary Resuscitation and Emergency Cardiac Care. JAMA 268: 2191–2194, 1992.

Marlowe FI: Otolaryngolic Emergencies. In Tintinalli JE, Krome LR, and Ruiz E (eds): Emergency Medicine: A Comprehensive Study Guide, ed 3. McGraw-Hill, New York, 1992, pp 842–845.

Notes

CHAPTER 34

Overdose And Poisoning

Clifton W. Callaway, MD

Presentation

Almost any substance in excess, including medications, can result in poisoning. The appearance of poisoned patients varies depending on the poison, the dose, the route of exposure, and the time of exposure. For example, patients who initially appear normal may rapidly lose consciousness or develop seizures as an ingested substance is absorbed from the gut. Possible manifestation include altered level of consciousness, nausea or vomiting, respiratory depression, or cardiac dysrhythmias. However, many patients are initially asymptomatic.

Immediate Concerns

- **Is the source of the poisoning removed?** Some toxins are absorbed through the skin (insecticides, industrial solvents) or by inhalation (vapors). To stop the poisoning process, remove contaminated clothing and cleanse the skin to prevent further absorption. Decontamination of the stomach after a toxic ingestion is not indicated routinely in the prehospital setting.
- **Is the patient's airway secure?** Decreased level of consciousness increases the patient's risk for aspiration and may be accompanied by respiratory depression. Because the acutely poisoned patient is likely to become worse rather than better, intubation should be considered sooner rather than later.
- **Is the patient hemodynamically stable?** Some poisons produce life-threatening hypotension or hypertension. Supportive therapy with IV fluids or antihypertensive drugs can convert a lethal poisoning into a survivable one.
- **Is the patient at risk for lethal dysrhythmias?** Cardiac dysrhythmias accompany many medication and recre-

ational drug overdoses. Cardiac monitoring is indicated during transport of overdose patients.

Important History

- **What was the poison? What was the dose?** The patient may or may not provide this information. Bring any medications or containers found at the scene to the medical facility. Recreational drug paraphernalia will aid in diagnosis. If pills were taken, attempt to locate any pills or fragments of pills that the patient has spilled or vomited. The emergency department often will subtract the remaining tablets from the total number in the original package in order to estimate the severity of an overdose.
- **How long ago was the exposure?** Depending on the poison, different symptoms can be expected at different times. Furthermore, some oral medications will pass through the stomach more quickly than others. The emergency department will use this information in deciding whether or not to irrigate the stomach.
- **Was the overdose or poisoning accidental?** Assessing the psychological state of the patient may be difficult in the prehospital setting. However, any attempted suicide warrants transport for psychiatric evaluation, even if the patient is medically stable. Local law and custom dictates transport against the patient's wishes. Police involvement is usually required to transport a nonconsenting patient.

Differential Diagnosis

Particular constellations of signs and symptoms characterize overdose or poisoning with different classes of drugs. Depending on the dose and time of poisoning, few or many of the following signs and symptoms may be present.
- *Stimulants.* Tachycardia, hypertension, hyperthermia, agitation, paranoia, dilated pupils, seizures. Stimulants (such as cocaine, amphetamine, diet pills, or caffeine) may be ingested, injected, smoked, or sniffed.
- *Depressants.* Bradycardia, hypotension, hypothermia, respiratory depression, stupor (or alcohol-like intoxication), dilated or pinpoint pupils. Depressants are usually taken as pills (benzodiazepines, barbiturates) or injected (opiates).

- *Anticholinergic and Antidepressant Agents.* Tachycardia, hyperthermia, delirium, dilated pupils, blurred vision, dry mouth, difficulty urinating, flushed skin. Cardiac dysrhythmias are possible. Anticholinergics include antihistamines, antiemetic medicines, neurologic medications, and psychiatric medications.
- *Cardiac Medications.* These can induce hemodynamically stable or unstable cardiac dysrhythmias. Many of these medications also depress the central nervous system.
- *Solvents, Alcohols, and Cleaning Solutions.* Nausea or vomiting, fruity odor on breath, stupor, or unconsciousness. These substances are usually ingested or inhaled.
- *Insecticides.* Bradycardia or tachycardia, increased bronchial secretions, salivation, nausea or vomiting, diarrhea, diaphoresis, pinpoint pupils, tremulousness. Many insecticides are absorbed through the skin or are inhaled.

Key Physical Examination Findings

- *Initial Assessment.* Assess for respiratory depression or apnea and signs of shock.
- *Vital Signs.* Assess for changes in heart rate, respiratory rate, and body temperature, which provide clues to the type and severity of poisoning.
- *Lungs.* Note unusual breath odors (organic poisons). Listen for rales (pulmonary edema).
- *Skin.* Look for rash (red-flushed skin, hives). Look for signs of IV drug abuse.
- *Neurologic Examination.* Note mental status and behavior, pupil size and reactivity, nystagmus, tremor, and seizures.

Treatment Plan

- *Patient Assessment.* Provide continual reassessment because of ongoing toxin absorption and metabolism. Initially stable patients can deteriorate rapidly. Cardiac monitoring is appropriate in patients with decreased level of consciousness or altered vital signs and in all patients with pre-existing heart disease. Patients ingesting any cardiac medications also should be monitored.

UNCONSCIOUS OR DECREASED LEVEL OF CONSCIOUSNESS

- **Administer O$_2$ and provide ventilatory support.** Anticipate vomiting. Intubate for airway protection if positive pressure ventilation is required.
- Establish **IV access.** Check blood glucose level if protocols allow.
- **Administer 50 ml of 50% dextrose IV, thiamine, 100 mg IM/IV, and naloxone (Narcan), 2 mg IV** to reverse hypoglycemia and the effects of narcotic overdose.
- Begin **fluid resuscitation with 0.9% NaCl or lactated Ringer's solution** if patient is hypotensive.
- Consider antihypertensive medication for severe hypertension (esmolol, labetalol, nitroprusside).
- Treat seizures with diazepam (5 mg increments).
- Treat cardiac dysrhythmias per ACLS protocols.
- **Transport expeditiously** to the emergency department; treat en route.
  NOTE: Never give syrup of ipecac to patients with a decreased or changing level of consciousness.

CONSCIOUS AND ALERT

- Establish **IV access.** Check blood glucose level if protocols allow.
- Treat cardiac dysrhythmias per ACLS protocols.
- **Transport expeditiously** to the emergency department; treat en route.

  NOTE: Giving syrup of ipecac to induce vomiting after ingestion of toxic substances is controversial and not generally recommended in the prehospital setting. Vomiting increases risk of aspiration and can delay administration of activated charcoal in the emergency department. For patients with long transport times, phone or radio consultation with the medical control physician or the nearest poison center is appropriate.

Bibliography

Eilers MA and Garrison TE: General Management Principles. In Rosen P and Barkin RM (eds): Emergency Medicine: Concepts and Clinical Practice. Mosby-Year Book, St. Louis, 1992, pp 2470–2503.

Vance MV: General Management of the Poisoned Patient. In Tintinalli JE, Krome LR, and Ruiz E (eds): Emergency Medicine: A Comprehensive Study Guide, ed 3. McGraw-Hill, New York, 1992, pp 545–550.

Notes

CHAPTER 35

Pelvic Pain
Jonathan S. Rubens, MD, FACEP

Presentation

As this book is organized in a fashion that corresponds to calls as they go out to prehospital EMS providers, this chapter may be somewhat of an anomaly. That is to say, it is rare that a call will go out as "pelvic pain." More likely, the patient's complaint will be recorded as abdominal pain, and it is left to the examiner to determine the more specific location of the patient's discomfort. Most of the topics covered in this chapter are also included in Chapter 1, Abdominal Pain. Thus, discussion in this chapter will be limited to those complaints of the female patient specifically relating to the genitourinary and reproductive systems. For conditions of the male patient please refer to Chapter 1.

Immediate Concerns

- *ABCs.* Although difficult to obtain in the field, include fetal heart tones (FHT) if appropriate. Precipitous bleeding from many genitourinary sources may result in circulatory compromise. Abnormal vital signs and signs of shock warrant aggressive immediate resuscitative measures.
- **Is the patient pregnant or is there a possibility of pregnancy?** The causes of pelvic pain differ significantly in the gravid (pregnant) and nongravid patient. Obstetric emergencies can be missed without the benefit of this important information (see Chapter 32, Obstetric Emergencies).

Important History

- **When was the patient's last menstrual period?** In the presence of a history of abnormal, irregular, or late menses, pregnancy should be strongly considered, if not assumed. The precise date of the last menstruation is always helpful in the gravid patient to determine parameters for examination and fetal viability.

- **What is the patient's current or past medical history?** Has the patient had similar symptoms in the past? Is there a history of sexually transmitted disease exposure or treatment? Ovarian cysts? Prior miscarriage?
- **What is the character of the pain?** Its onset? Acute onset of pain is characteristic of ovarian cyst rupture. Patients will often give precise histories of the onset of their symptoms with this condition. In the gravid patient, ruptured ectopic pregnancy and abruptio placentae should be considered with acute onset of pain. Insidious onset or steadily increasing pain may suggest infectious processes or progressive bleeding.
- **Are there other associated symptoms?** Vaginal bleeding, vaginal discharge, fever, hematuria, or abnormal urinary symptoms are just a few symptoms associated with pelvic pain. In the gravid patient, a history of quickening (the sensation of fetal movement) or its absence in relationship to the onset of the pain may be volunteered by many patients. Edema and abdominal pain may indicate preeclampsia.

Differential Diagnosis

The causes of pelvic pain are divided here into two groups: those pertaining to the gravid and the nongravid patient. Note that these are in many cases artificial distinctions, and several of these diagnoses can exist in both types of patients. For a more complete listing of diagnoses refer to Chapter 1, Abdominal Pain.

The Gravid Patient

Abruptio placentae
Ectopic pregnancy
Labor
Preeclampsia or eclampsia
Premature labor
Spontaneous abortion
Threatened abortion
Ureteral calculi
Urinary tract infection

The Non-Gravid Patient
Bladder spasm
Dysmenorrhea
Endometriosis
Genital foreign body
Imperforate hymen or oligomenorrhea (pediatrics)
Neoplasms (uterine and ovarian)
Ovarian cyst and rupture
Pelvic inflammatory disease (PID)
Sexual assault
Trauma
Urinary retention
Urinary tract infection

Key Physical Examination Findings

- **ABCs.** Although difficult in the field, when possible, monitor FHTs as part of any gravid patient's vital signs. Remember that gravid patients have a different physiology and may not exhibit signs of hypovolemia or shock until later in the progression of this disease.
- **General Appearance.** Check the abdomen for signs of the peritoneal irritation. "PID shuffle" or other guarding of movement of the abdomen and its contents, is common with peritoneal irritation.
- **Abdomen.** Inspect for signs of pregnancy. Also look for distention of the abdominal cavity. On palpation, areas or structures of maximal tenderness may be identified. Assess for firmness, guarding, and rebound tenderness suggestive of peritoneal irritation.
- **Genitourinary.** Inspect the perineum of the gravid bleeding patient. Pelvic pain from labor may herald a precipitous delivery, especially in the multiparous patient (more than one delivery). Inspection of the perineum is essential to ruleout impending delivery, crowning, or a prolapsed umbilical cord, and to identify the presenting part if visible. In the case of bleeding, amount and rate may be quantitated by inspection.

Treatment Plan

- **Monitor ABCs.** Although patients with pelvic pain will unlikely have airway or breathing compromise, supplemen-

tal oxygen should be administered to these patients and
may be of particular benefit in the gravid patient.
- **Treat for shock and circulatory compromise** (see Chapter 38, Shock). If the patient is indeed 20 weeks pregnant,
she should be laid on her left side to maximize blood return to the central circulation, which may otherwise be
compromised by the weight of the gravid uterus compressing the inferior vena cava. IV lifelines should be established
for resuscitation from shock and hemorrhage.
- **Transport to the appropriate ED.** Patients should be transported in a comfortable position except the gravid patient
who requires special positioning as noted previously. Expedite transport in any patient with abnormal vital signs,
hemorrhage, or labor. Patients with impending or inevitable delivery may be better treated on the scene and transported after the second stage of labor is complete. **NOTE:**
It is an extremely rare occurrence that patients in active
labor are transferred between institutions.

Bibliography

Stewart C (ed.), Genitourinary Emergencies. Emerg Med Clin North
Am, 6(3). August 1988.
Willson JR, Carrington ER, et al. (eds): Obstetrics and Gynecology,
ed 7. CV Mosby, St. Louis, 1983.

Notes

CHAPTER 36

Rape and Sexual Abuse
Gary T. Ferrucci, EMT-CC

Presentation

The patient who has experienced the trauma of rape or sexual abuse may present in a variety of ways. Physical trauma may be evident along with emotional trauma, which is so prevalent in these situations. In other cases, emotional trauma may be the only presenting problem. Prehospital EMS providers may be thrust into the role of mediator, buffer, or confidant. They may even be subject to violent aggression on the part of the victims or their families.

Immediate Concerns

As always, the safety and well-being of the EMS team should remain paramount. Even though a patient may be visible and in need of immediate care, rescuers must ensure that they do not inadvertently become victims in a hostile or violent situation.

- When dealing with the concerns of the victim, the confidentiality and modesty of the victim should always be considered. The care of the patient always takes precedence and should never be compromised to gather information on possible suspects or perpetrators. The primary investigation of the incident is the responsibility of law enforcement agencies.
- Injuries associated with sexual assault may vary widely. They can be as subtle as slight pain or discomfort or as grossly evident as either debilitating or disfiguring trauma. The victim's injuries may not be obvious or visible on first inspection. Some may deny the injuries and relate untruthful information regarding the occurrence. You must develop and foster rapport with the victim to gain the victim's confidence, so that accurate information can be obtained.

Important History

Unfortunately, rape and sexual abuse are not only confined to the adult population. Rape and sexual abuse can occur in infants, children, adolescents, and the elderly. Rape and sexual abuse are not confined to any one sex or race either. The history offers the best indicator that rape or sexual abuse has occurred. The prehospital provider may be in the best position to observe the patient at the scene of the rape or abuse. A bit of "detective work" on the part of the caregiver may be necessary. The information uncovered from this detective work may be very helpful to those who must investigate any complaint and maybe even more so, in the case of the victim of rape or repeated sexual abuse who is too fearful to report the assaults.

Detectives are trained to be extremely observant. EMS personnel can use their training to identify the abused patient if they take the time to observe all of the elements of a possible rape or sexual abuse case. Take care to record any information about the incident that may assist the victim and law enforcement officials at a later time. Keep in mind that if the incident results in an arrest and subsequent trial, you may be called to provide testimony. Remember, never jump to conclusions, either "pro or con." Be supportive, but remain neutral and concentrate primarily on the physical and emotional care of the patient. Pay particular attention to these five areas:

1. *Recurring Injuries.* "Hospital shopping," that is, patients not wanting to frequent the same hospital or medical facility for fear of detection of possible abuses, usually becomes obvious. An astute emergency medical services staff will recognize this type of activity. Naturally, the fearful victim, be it the parent of an infant, a juvenile, adult, or elderly person who cannot explain the injuries, or if the injuries are not consistent with the scenario as it is reported, should be carefully evaluated. Without being accusatory, follow local protocols and statutes for reporting these incidents. Avoid confrontation with either the patient or bystanders.

2. *Abuses Committed by an "Unknown" Person.* Too often, these situations are ongoing and committed by a family member or someone close to the victim. It goes without saying that neighbors, friends, relatives, immediate family, or even parents can perpetrate rape or

sexual abuses. Therefore, always maintain an open mind. The investigation of any crime is not the responsibility of the EMS system. Assisting the investigators, however, is both a moral requirement and, in many states, a legal one.

3. *Withdrawal or Hostility.* A person who has been subjected to these types of assaults may be hostile to your inquisition. A child may completely regress and may not be able to relate the facts of the incident. Keep in mind that your actions and words play a great part in whether or not you can initiate a dialogue with the patient. Be firm, professional, and caring. Maintain an acute awareness of your attitude and demeanor, as well as that of the entire EMS team. Choosing words or phrases containing innuendoes such as, "Honey," "How did it feel?" "Was this your first time?" can only alienate you from the victim. Again, choosing your words and your actions can work both for and against you. Be sensitive and empathetic when in contact with a victim of any crime.

4. *Confidentiality.* When the victim begins to trust you and the other members of the emergency response team, vast amounts of pertinent information may be thrust forward. Your duty is to listen and reassure the victim and to provide appropriate treatment. These persons may have certain legal rights to privacy during conversations with medical providers. As with any patient contact, never discount "volunteered" information. Often times, the victim in these cases will seek assistance of a professional group or person; you may be that person, so be fair, honest, and concerned. This is considered an "immediate outcry," which is often therapeutic in nature.

5. *Need for Emotional Support.* In the case of a violent confrontation, some victims may seek out a "mentor," someone whom that victim can relate to and will seek refuge. Do not consider the victim's requests to seek an "equal" (ie, equal sex or gender) as an insult to you. What the victim may need most at this point is a "confidant" rather than a medical provider. This is a common occurrence and in some cases can be a great asset to the well-being of the patient. In some documented

cases, this interaction facilitated the apprehension of the perpetrator. This is not a negative reflection on your ability or competency as an EMS provider.

Injuries

Injuries resulting from rape and sexual abuse incidents will vary on a case-by-case basis and may include any of the following:

- *Physical Trauma.* Lacerations, punctures, avulsion, traumatic amputations, and in some isolated cases, human or animal bite injuries may be observed. Each injury should be carefully evaluated and treated. Objects inserted into a body cavity can cause injury and may become foreign bodies in the anatomic structure.
- *Emotional Injuries.* These are usually prevalent in this type of incident. As described previously, they can vary from slight to extreme in nature. Never discount the emotional status of your victim.
- *Respiratory Status.* Your concerns for the patient's respiratory system should never be overlooked. As always, ABCs must be assessed initially and as required thereafter for every patient.

PATIENT–EMS PROVIDER INTERACTION

Your demeanor and attitude will be tested regularly when dealing with victims of rape and sexual abuse. These forms of sexual abuse, which apply to both male and female victim, are among those that you will most frequently encounter:

Rape: unwanted sexual intercourse by another participant.

Sodomy: unwanted, and oftentimes aggressive, deviant sexual activity where the victim is forced to conduct acts of deviant sexual activity or is the recipient of such activity (eg, the forceful insertion of the penis into the mouth of another person).

Sexual abuse: the unwanted feeling, fondling, or probing of the genitalia by a second person.

Sexual abuse, however, is not limited to the genitalia. It can also encompass the other "private parts" of the victim that do not meet the definition of sodomy.

Treatment Plan

Although the patient must be treated for any injury associated with the rape or sexual abuse, care should be taken to preserve any evidence that will be required by law enforcement authorities. Injuries can include rectal bleeding and painful itching, or swollen genitals. Sodomy victims may also have injuries to the mouth and eyes. You must ensure you are properly protected from any sexually transmitted diseases that may be present.

- *Monitor ABCs.* Trauma to the mouth can compromise the airway. Patients in respiratory distress should receive oxygen. The emotional trauma of a sexual assault can result in cardiovascular emergencies.
- *Treat Lacerations.* Apply direct pressure and sterile packing, provide intravenous cannulation, administer oxygen therapy, and transport to the appropriate ED.
- *Treat Avulsions.* As lacerations, skin flaps should not be removed; if intact, apply and secure sterile dressings.
- *Manage Amputations.* Follow local trauma protocol for the amputated part.
- *Treat Puncture Wounds.* Follow same procedure as for the treatment of lacerations. Evaluate the site for impaled objects; secure any objects in place without removing.
- *Provide Emotional Support.* Assist the victim. Be calm; do not accuse or make light of the incident. Continue to monitor and support the patient during transport to the medical facility.
- *Evaluate Fractures at the Injury Site.* Is the fracture consistent with the reported incident? Stabilize and immobilize as necessary.

SPECIAL CONSIDERATIONS

Although your primary function as an EMS provider is the protection of the victim while providing prehospital medical care, the following are a few things to remember:

- In the case of rape, have the victim refrain from showering or washing before the hospital physical examination. This is a natural reaction after a rape and a great deal of sensitivity is required. Valuable medical and forensic information and evidence can be destroyed if the victim is permitted to engage in any personal hygiene activities.

- It is also a good idea that the clothing worn at the time of the incident be retained and transported to the hospital with the victim in a brown paper bag; do not use plastic. This again will provide important information for both institutions.

Criminal Reporting

As for all other incidents, EMS providers will be required to complete pertinent forms and necessary paperwork to document the complaint of a sexual assault. In the case of rape or sexual abuse, the professional healthcare provider may be "duty bound" in some jurisdictions to report the incidence of sexual assault to the authorities. But it is not usually a requirement that the EMS provider do so. Most EMS personnel, however, take the responsibility and initiative to report to local authorities what they believe to be true abuse, either formally or informally. The criminal reporting requirements will vary according to state and local statutes. EMS providers must keep abreast of the laws pertaining to their EMS system.

Bibliography

Angelton SS: Sexual Assault Among Teenagers. Heath and Co, Washington, DC, 1987.

Finkelhor D: Child Sexual Abuse. The Free Press, Division of MacMillan, Detroit, 1984

New York State Penal Law Sections: 130.00; 130.05; 130.16; 130.25–35; 130.38–40; 130.45–70, Looseleaf Law Publications, 1993 Edition, Chapters 1–717 of The Regular Session of The State Assembly.

Notes

CHAPTER 37

Seizure

Micelle Haydel, MD

Presentation

Seizures are a condition in which abnormal electrical discharges of neurons in the brain cause paroxysmal events in the rest of the body. The patient exhibits these paroxysmal events by a disturbance of movement, altered mental status, alteration in sensation, or behavior change. The grand mal (also known as generalized or tonic-clonic) seizure starts with an aura (an altered sensation), which is followed by loss of consciousness and rigid extension of the muscles of the body, apnea, urinary or fecal incontinence, and alternating contraction and relaxation of the extremities. The seizure ends with a period of flaccidity (postictal) in which the patient's level of consciousness slowly improves from unresponsiveness to confusion and, finally, to a cleared sensorium. Complications of seizures include death from anoxia and aspiration, trauma due to loss of consciousness, encephalopathy due to hypoxia, acute renal failure due to muscle breakdown (rhabdomyolysis), and respiratory arrest caused by medications.

Immediate Concerns

- **Does the patient have a patent airway?** Any time there is a decreased level of consciousness, the patient is not able to adequately maintain a patent airway, and a nasopharyngeal airway should be inserted. The patient may not able to clear secretions and should be positioned on the side, with suction equipment easily accessible.
- **Is the patient ventilating adequately?** The period of apnea is usually short and resolves spontaneously; however, supplemental oxygen by non-rebreather mask or bag-valve-mask (BVM) is necessary as ventilations during a seizure are usually ineffective and may result in hypoxia.
- **Does the patient have adequate circulation?** Seizures

can be associated with circulatory collapse and, if the patient is hemodynamically unstable, immediate resuscitation is warranted.

- **Is the patient's safety maintained?** During any phase of seizure activity, the patient is not able to provide for personal safety. Move any potentially hazardous objects away from the patient. Bite blocks may be used to prevent the seizing patient from biting the tongue if the teeth are not yet already clenched.

  NOTE: A bite block should never be forcefully inserted into a seizing patient's mouth.

- **How long has this seizure lasted?** If the patient is still seizing when the EMS providers arrive, it is important to find out how long the seizure has lasted or if this is a second seizure. Status epilepticus must be suspected if the patient has had two or more seizures without regaining consciousness, or if the seizure has lasted for longer than 20 minutes. The patient should be transported as soon as possible, because the longer a seizure lasts, the more refractory it becomes to medical therapies and the risk of complications increases.

Important History

- **Has the patient ever had a seizure before?** Seizures commonly occur in a patient with a known seizure disorder who is not adequately controlled on medications. Patients with a known seizure disorder may have a medical alert tag or bracelet that may help you determine whether this seizure is different from other seizures. If so, the cause may also be different. But remember, medical alert devices are useful but not always definitive.

- **Is the patient taking seizure medications as prescribed?** Commonly, seizures (including status epilepticus) occur in a patient who is noncompliant with medications or needs adjustment of medication dosage or intervals. Common seizure medications include phenytoin (Dilantin), phenobarbital (Luminal), ethosuximide (Zarontin), carbamazepine (Tegretol), valproic acid (Depakene), and clonazepam (Clonopin).

Differential Diagnosis

SEIZURE TYPES

- *Grand Mal.* This seizure (also known as generalized or tonic-clonic), starts with an aura (an altered sensation), followed by loss of consciousness and rigid extension (tonic phase) of the muscles of the body. These signs are followed by apnea, urinary or fecal incontinence, and alternating contraction and relaxation of the extremities (clonic phase). The seizure ends with a postictal phase in which the patient's level of consciousness slowly improves from unresponsiveness to confusion and finally to a cleared sensorium.

- *Petit Mal.* This seizure (also known as absence seizure) is more common in children, manifesting as 10 to 30 seconds of apparent staring, blank expression, or daydreaming. The patient has no loss of consciousness or jerking of the extremities and is often unaware of the seizure.

- *Jacksonian.* This seizure (also known as simple partial seizure) involves no loss of consciousness, but the patient experiences jerking of a distal extremity, which may proceed proximally. The Jacksonian seizure can precede a grand mal seizure.

SEIZURE ETIOLOGIES

- *Hypoxic Seizures.* Seizures can be caused by inadequate airway or ventilation. As in any situation, airway, breathing, and circulation are the priority.

- *Hypoglycemic Seizures.* Seizures can be caused by alterations in electrolytes, such as glucose, sodium, magnesium, and calcium. Low blood glucose levels are treated with 50% dextrose in water. Diabetics may wear a medical alert tag or bracelet. Other electrolyte imbalances cannot be diagnosed and treated in the field.

- *Alcohol or Drug-Induced Seizures.* Seizures are often associated with alcohol and drug intoxication or withdrawal. Pertinent history of alcohol or drug abuse or signs of overdose should be obtained.

- *Intracranial Insults.* Seizures can be due to infections, trauma, strokes, or tumor in the central nervous system. These situations are thought to cause ectopic neuronal firing, which lead to seizure activity.

- *Febrile Seizures of Childhood.* Children who have underlying systemic infections and fevers can have febrile seizures. These are usually self-limiting, but complications can occur and, therefore, should be treated like other seizure disorders.

- *Eclampsia (Toxemia of Pregnancy).* Pre-eclampsia (hypertension after 20 weeks' gestation, edema, and proteinuria) occurs in about 5% of pregnancies and may lead to life-threatening eclampsia, which is a seizure or coma in the pre-eclamptic patient. Seizures during pregnancy are life-threatening to the mother as well as to the baby, and transportation for definitive care should be expedited. Magnesium sulfate is used for treatment or prevention of seizures in the severe pre-eclamptic patient (continuous magnesium sulfate infusions may have been instituted before interhospital transfers). Magnesium overdose causes respiratory depression and cardiac standstill, which are treated with calcium chloride.
- *Unknown Etiology.* Most patients with a seizure disorder will have no known etiology. This diagnosis, however, is one of exclusion.

Key Physical Examination Findings

- *Initial Assessment.* Airway, breathing, and circulation are the priority in all patients, including the actively seizing patient. Life-threatening complications must not be neglected because of the distracting seizure activity.
- *HEENT.* Look for signs of trauma as the patient may have sustained injuries such as tongue or buccal lacerations.
- *Extremities.* Look for traumatic musculoskeletal injuries, which are common due to loss of consciousness. Cervical spine precautions should be taken if injury is suspected. True posterior shoulder separations can occur in this context.
- *Neurologic Examination.* Assess level of consciousness. Serial mental status examinations may be required in postictal patients. Look for any progressive decline in mental status and for any focal weakness.

Treatment Plan

- *Patient Assessment.* Perform a rapid and systematic primary survey and institute treatment as life-threatening problems are discovered. Frequent reassessment of the seizure patient with an altered mental status is necessary owing to the potential for respiratory compromise and worsening of the neurologic status.

- Administer **O₂** and provide **ventilatory support** as needed. This includes insertion of nasopharyngeal airways and endotracheal intubation. Monitor O₂ saturation with pulse oximetry if available.
- Place patient in the **semi-Fowler or Fowler position**. The coma position is also useful to reduce the aspiration risk in patients with a compromised gag reflex or depressed consciousness.
- Establish **IV access** if the patient is still seizing or has an altered mental status.
- If the patient is in status epilepticus consider **diazepam (Valium) 5 to 10 mg IV bolus**. Dose may be repeated every 10 to 15 minutes. (Pediatric dose: 0.2 to 0.5 mg/kg by slow IV bolus. Maximum dose: age younger than 5 years, 5 mg; age older than 5 years, 10 mg.) Lorazepam (Ativan) may also be considered at 0.1 mg/kg slow IV push at a rate not to exceed 2 mg per minute.
- If the patient has an altered mental status consider the administration of the following agents:
    Naloxone (Narcan), **0.4 to 2.0 mg IV bolus**. Dose may be repeated in 2 to 3 minutes.
    Thiamine, 50 mg IV and 50 mg IM. Give 100 mg IM if IV cannot be established.
    50% dextrose, 25 g IV if the patient is hypoglycemic, or if hypoglycemia is suspected in a patient with diabetes.
- Treat symptomatic arrhythmias as indicated. (See Chapter 5, Bradycardia, and Chapter 43, Tachycardia, for specific options)
- If a specific etiology of the seizure is known (eg, hypoglycemia, arrhythmia, hypoxia, fever, etc.) treat the underlying illness as well.
- **Treat non–life-threatening injuries** (ie, control of bleeding and splinting of fractures).
- **Transport to appropriate ED.** Ensure patient comfort en route.

Bibliography

Husk GT: Seizures and Acute Confusion. In Kravis TC and Warner CG (eds): Emergency Medicine: A Comprehensive Review. Aspen Systems, Rockville, MD, 1983, pp 669–675.

Sacks C: Seizures and Status Epilepticus in adults. In Tintinalli JE, Krome LR, and Ruiz E (eds): Emergency Medicine: A Comprehensive Study Guide, ed 2. McGraw-Hill, New York, 1988, pp 563–568.

Notes

CHAPTER 38

Shock

Owen T. Traynor, MD

Presentation

Shock is often defined as a state of inadequate tissue perfusion. This may result in acidosis, derangements of cellular metabolism, potential end-organ damage, and death. Although there are many possible causes of shock, it is helpful to think of the following classes of shock:

- Hypovolemia—caused by hemorrhage, burns, or dehydration.
- Distributive shock—maldistribution of blood, caused by poor vasomotor tone in neurogenic shock, sepsis, anaphylaxis, severe hypoxia, or metabolic shock.
- Pump failure—caused by necrosis of the myocardial tissue, or by arrhythmias.
- Obstructive shock—caused by impairment of cardiac filling, found in pulmonary embolism, tension pneumothorax, or cardiac tamponade.

Early in the shock process, patients are able to compensate for the decreased perfusion by increased stimulation of the sympathetic nervous system, leading to tachycardia and tachypnea. Later, compensatory mechanisms fail, causing a decreased mental status, hypotension, and death. Early cellular injury may be reversible if definitive therapy is delivered promptly. It is not always possible for the advanced EMT to provide this level of care. Therefore, early transportation to the appropriate emergency department is required. Most studies that examine the outcome of patients who experience shock secondary to trauma find that the most significant predictor of outcome is the time spent on the scene. Longer on-scene time is directly related to a higher degree of mortality. Although not always considered to be so, prompt transport is a highly effective treatment modality and should remain a high priority in the patient care plan. The prehospital standard of care for the patient in shock is rapid as-

226

sessment, aggressive treatment of life-threatening injury or illness, and expeditious transport to the appropriate emergency department.

Immediate Concerns

- **What is the patient's hemodynamic status?** If the patient is hemodynamically unstable, immediate resuscitation is warranted, including immediate transport, oxygen administration, establishment of large-bore IV access, PASG inflation if indicated, and fluid resuscitation. If the patient is in compensated shock, prompt transport, as well as the previous treatments, is necessary. Those patients in cardiogenic or arrythmogenic shock require ECG monitoring and may require pharmacologic or electrical therapy.
- **What is the patient's mental status?** Anxiousness, agitation, or confusion may indicate inadequate cerebral perfusion. Continued resuscitation and prompt transport are indicated.
- **Does the patient have a tension pneumothorax?** Immediate needle decompression of the chest is warranted and should result in significant rapid improvement. Continued resuscitation and prompt transport are indicated.

Important History

- **What is the mechanism of injury?** Knowledge of the mechanism of injury will allow you to look for and treat hidden injuries such as spinal injury, cardiac tamponade, tension pneumothorax, fractures, pelvic injury, and intra-abdominal injuries. Be sure to consider the medical causes of shock in patients who do not present with a traumatic mechanism of injury. Examples of these causes are myocardial infarction, arrhythmias, GI bleeding, ruptured or leaking abdominal aortic aneurysm (AAA), ectopic pregnancy in women of child-bearing age, and severe hypoxia.
- **Does the patient complain of any specific symptoms?** Obtaining a medical history is still important. The treatment of the patient whose chest pain is a result of a minor motor vehicle accident may be markedly different than the treatment of the patient whose chest pain is the result of trauma to the chest.

- **Is the patient taking any new medications?** A patient's hypotension may be a result of a new antihypertensive agent.

Differential Diagnosis

HYPOVOLEMIC SHOCK

- *Hemorrhagic Shock.* In the context of severe trauma, acute blood loss is usually obvious; however, patients can lose a great deal of blood into the thoracic, abdominal, and pelvic cavities. A thorough examination of the patient can be a life-saving measure in itself. GI bleeding may be less obvious if it has been gradual ask about melena, hematemesis, and hematochezia. Consider the diagnosis of ectopic pregnancy in all women of child-bearing age if there is a complaint of abdominal or pelvic pain. The burn patient losses massive amounts of fluids and can easily be hypovolemic.
- *Other Fluid Losses.* Severe diarrhea, vomiting, diuresis, or some combination of these features, may lead to dehydration and hypovolemia.

DISTRIBUTIVE SHOCK

Distributive shock may result from poor vascular tone or the maldistribution of blood. Specific examples of this type of shock include sepsis, anaphylaxis, severe acidosis, or CNS injury in the case of spinal shock.

PUMP FAILURE

Pump failure may result from any illness or injury that causes a decrease in the heart's ability to pump, such as heart wall damage from an AMI or arrhythmias. The common pathway is a drop in cardiac output that causes decreased tissue perfusion. If an arrhythmia is the cause, then treatment of the arrhythmia may result in a dramatic improvement in the patient's hemodynamic status. Cardiogenic shock is a clinical syndrome characterized by hypotension and inadequate perfusion in the setting of an injury to the heart; most often, an AMI is the underlying cause. It is generally agreed that when 40% or greater of the left ventricle is infarcted, the heart has difficulty maintaining an adequate cardiac output. This is manifested by hypotension. The patient in cardiogenic shock has a poor prognosis, with mortality greater than 80%. This is due, in part, to the failure of the normal compensatory mechanism, mediated by the sympathetic nervous system, to compensate for poor perfusion (tachycardia and increased peripheral vascular resistance). In addition, an increased work load on the heart and, therefore, an increase in myocardial oxygen demand, exacerbates the shock syndrome. The increase in oxygen demand may potentially increase the infarct size and further decrease myocardial function; thus the poor prognosis.

OBSTRUCTIVE SHOCK

Obstructive shock results from impaired filling of the heart. There are three major causes:

- *Tension Pneumothorax.* This usually results from trauma. It may, however, result from a spontaneous pneumothorax. Physical examination findings may include absent or diminished breath sounds, tracheal deviation away from the tension pneumothorax, and jugular vein distention (JVD).
- *Pericardial Tamponade.* This may result from penetrating or blunt trauma to the chest. It may develop over a time period from minutes to approximately 1 week. Muffled heart tones, together with JVD and narrowed pulse pressure, known as Beck's triad, may be found in pericardial tamponade. There are also several atraumatic causes, for example, secondary to pericardial effusions resulting from renal disease, acute leukemias, lymphomas, breast cancer, lung cancer, and ovarian cancer.
- *Pulmonary Embolism.* This is an important cause of obstructive shock. Risk factors of pulmonary embolism include a history of atrial fibrillation, obesity, pregnancy, prolonged immobilization, posttrauma, oral contraceptive use, postsurgery, and cancer. Common symptoms include chest pain in 88% of patients, dyspnea in 84% of patients, and cough in 53% of patients. Common physical findings include: tachypnea (respiratory rate greater than 16 breaths per minute) in 92% of patients, tachycardia (heart rate greater than 100 bpm) in 44% of patients, and temperature above 100°F in 43% of patients.

Key Physical Examination Findings

- *Initial Assessment.* Look for signs of shock
- *Vital Signs.* Assess for tachycardia and tachypnea, which

usually precede hypotension. Hypotension is a late sign of shock.

- **Skin.** Inspect for temperature, appearence, and signs of moisture or dryness. Skin is usually cool, pale, and moist in the shock patient; however, the skin may be warm and dry in the patient with spinal shock or septic shock.
- **Neck.** Check for the presence of JVD. In the shock patient, this may indicate an obstructive shock—consider tension pneumothorax, pericardial tamponade, and massive pulmonary embolism. Assess for tracheal deviation.
- **Lungs.** Assess for evidence of tension pneumothorax. Evidence of blunt trauma or penetrating trauma should raise suspicion of intrathoracic injury including pericardial tamponade, tension pneumothorax, and hemothorax.
- **Heart.** Assess for muffled heart tones.
- **Abdomen.** Assess for evidence of penetrating or blunt trauma, which may indicate intra-abdominal injury. In addition, check for the pulsatile abdominal mass found in patients with an AAA.
- **Peripheral Pulses.** Check for peripheral pulses. They may be absent as perfusion decreases. Radial pulses are usually present when the systolic BP is greater than 80 mm Hg, femoral pulses indicate a systolic BP greater than 60 mm Hg, and carotid pulses indicate a systolic BP greater than 50 mm Hg. Unequal pulses may be found in the patient with an AAA.
- **Mental Status.** An altered mental status is a sensitive indicator of inadequate cerebral perfusion.
- **Neurologic Examination.** Assess for head or spinal trauma. The trauma victim may also have a head or spinal injury.

ECG

Cardiac monitoring is most helpful when treating shock caused by pump failure; however, all shock patients should be monitored.

Treatment Plan

- **Patient Assessment.** Perform a rapid and systematic initial assessment and institute treatment as life-threatening problems are discovered. Prompt transport to the appropriate ED is a key intervention. A secondary survey should be performed once the primary survey and all primary survey interventions have been accomplished. Frequent reassessment of patients in shock is necessary due to the potential for worsening of their hemodynamic status. Be prepared—potential for cardiac arrest exists.

- **Communications.** Consult with a medical control physician for guidance and institution of appropriate orders, as well as for notification of the receiving ED. Such consultation may prove invaluable in the care of the patient in shock.

GENERAL TREATMENT GUIDELINES: HEMODYNAMICALLY STABLE PATIENT

- Administer O_2 and **provide ventilatory support** as needed. This includes needle-chest decompression of the tension pneumothorax if indicated.
- Place patient in the **shock position** (supine with legs elevated). Protect the cervical spine as indicated.
- **Treat non–life-threatening injuries** (ie, control bleeding, splint fractures, etc).
- Establish **large-bore IV access with 0.9% NaCl or lactated Ringer's solution**.
- **Transport to appropriate ED.** Ensure patient comfort en route.

GENERAL TREATMENT GUIDELINES: HEMODYNAMICALLY UNSTABLE PATIENT

- Administer O_2 and **provide ventilatory support** as needed. This includes needle-chest decompression of the tension pneumothorax.
- Place patient in the **shock position** (supine with legs elevated) or use **PASG, if indicated**. The use of PASG is controversial; follow local protocol.
- Establish **large-bore IV access with 0.9% NaCl or lactated Ringer's solution and begin fluid resuscitation**. If transportation is delayed, or if there is inadequate response to 2 to 3 liters of crystalloid infusion, consider infusing colloid solutions, such as plasmanate or hespan. If there has been inadequate response to ongoing fluid resuscitation, consider using vasopressors such as dopamine 2 to 20 μg/kg per minute IV infusion (pediatric dosing: start at

1 µg/kg per minute), titrated to systolic BP greater than 90 mm Hg. Vasopressors are a temporary "last-ditch" effort to be used only after the patient does not respond to fluid resuscitation.

- **Expeditiously transport to appropriate ED**. Do not needlessly delay patient transport—expedite transport.

SPECIFIC TREATMENT GUIDELINES

Anaphylaxis

The anaphylactic patient should be treated using the guidelines above, with the addition of the following therapeutic modalities:

- **Maintain a patent airway.** A high flow of oxygen via nonrebreathing face mask is indicated. Immediate endotracheal intubation may be required but may be extremely difficult if angioedema or severe laryngospasm is present. Use caution to prevent trauma during the attempted intubation.
- Administer **epinephrine, 0.3 to 0.5 mg of a 1:1000 solution SC** (pediatric dose: 0.01 mg/kg SC, not to exceed 0.5 mg) if the patient is hemodynamically stable, or
- Administer **epinephrine 0.3 to 0.5 mg of 1:10,000 solution IV** (pediatric dose: 0.1 mg/kg IV, not to exceed 0.5 mg) if the patient is hemodynamically unstable. Dose may be repeated every 5 minutes.
- Administer **diphenhydramine (Benadryl), 10 to 50 mg slow IV bolus or deep IM injection** (pediatric dose: 2 to 5 mg/kg IV or deep IM, usual dose is 10–30 mg).
- Administer **hydrocortisone, 100 to 500 mg IV or IM** (pediatric dose: 0.16 to 1.0 mg/kg IV or IM), or
- Administer **methylprednisolone (Solumedrol), 100 to 200 mg IV or IM** (not recommended for prehospital use in pediatric patients).
- Provide **aerosolized albuterol, (0.5 ml in 3 ml saline)** to manage bronchospasm.
- **Transport expeditiously to appropriate ED.** Do not needlessly delay patient transport. Ensure patient comfort en route.

Pericardial Tamponade

- Treat the patient with tamponade using the previous general shock treatment guidelines. A surgical procedure, pericardiocentesis, is necessary to relieve the tamponade. Pericardiocentesis should only be performed by a physician skilled in its use. You should begin fluid resuscitation and transport to the appropriate ED.

Cardiogenic Shock

- The most effective means of managing cardiogenic shock is to prevent it by attempting to limit the infarct size in patients with AMIs. Treat tachycardias, symptomatic bradycardias, and hypertension occurring in the context of an AMI. The administration of O_2, nitrates, analgesia, beta blockers, and aspirin is instrumental. These modalities are covered in Chapter 10, Chest Pain.
- Administer O_2 and **provide ventilatory support** as needed. Endotracheal intubation may be required.
- Establish **IV access**. Although most patients in cardiogenic shock will have pulmonary edema, those who do not may benefit from small 0.9% NaCl fluid boluses.
- If a fluid challenge is not effective or not indicated, vasopressors should be given. Managing the patient's hypotension and hemodynamic status is difficult without the benefit of the Swan-Ganz catheter and arterial lines available in intensive care units. These two modalities are commonly used:

Dobutamine, 2.5 to 10 µg/kg per minute IV infusion (not recommended for prehospital use in pediatrics), titrated to systolic BP greater than 90 mm Hg. If the response is inadequate, add **dopamine, 2 to 20 µg/kg per minute IV infusion** (pediatric dosing: start at 1 µg/kg per minute), titrated to systolic BP greater than 90 mm Hg, or

- **Transport expeditiously to appropriate ED.** Do not needlessly delay patient transport—expedite transport. Ensure patient comfort en route.

Arrhythmogenic Pump Failure

- Treat the patient with shock secondary to a tachycardia or a bradycardia as outlined in the Chapters 5 and 43, Bradycardia and Tachycardia, respectively.

Bibliography

Committee on Trauma, American College of Surgeons: Shock. In Advanced Trauma Life Support Student Manual, ed 5. American College of Surgeons, Chicago, 1993, pp 75–94.

Dronen SC and Birrer P: Shock. In Tintinalli JE, Krome LR, and Ruiz E (eds): Emergency Medicine: A Comprehensive Study Guide, ed 3. McGraw-Hill, New York, 1992, pp 132–140.

Hockberger RS: Pulmonary Embolism. In Tintinalli JE, Krome LR, and Ruiz E (eds): Emergency Medicine: A Comprehensive Study Guide, ed 3. McGraw-Hill, New York, 1992, pp 233–236.

Jorden RC: Cardiogenic Shock. In Harwood-Nuss A, et al. (eds): The Clinical Practice of Emergency Medicine, ed 1. JB Lippincott, Philadelphia, 1991, pp 858–860.

Mattox KL, et al.: Prospective MAST Study in 911 Patients. J Trauma 29:1104–1112, 1989.

McSwain NE: PASG: State of the Art 1988. Ann Emerg Med 17:506–525, 1988.

Notes

CHAPTER 39

Sickle Cell Crisis
Owen T. Traynor, MD

Presentation

Sickle cell disease, a genetic disease that produces abnormal hemoglobin, affects approximately 8% of black persons in the United States. A single amino acid substitution in the hemoglobin molecule accounts for the change in behavior of the molecule, leading to abnormally shaped (sickle-shaped) red blood cells. The sickling occurs under conditions that cause deoxygenation of the hemoglobin. When the red blood cells become sickle-shaped, they can no longer easily pass through capillaries causing the formation of thrombi and subsequent destruction (hemolysis) of the red blood cell. Multiple thrombi and hemolysis lead to ischemia, infarction, and anemia. Because multiple organs are typically involved, the presentation varies from completely asymptomatic to severe pain, dyspnea, blindness, poor healing, infection, and severe anemia.

Immediate Concerns

- **What is the patient's respiratory status?** Multiple thrombi in the pulmonary vasculature can cause a clinical picture consistent with pulmonary embolism. Patients with sickle cell disease also have an impaired immune system that predisposes them to pulmonary infections. Severe anemia may also lead to dyspnea. Pulse oximetry should be employed, as well as the administration of supplemental oxygen. The increase in oxygenation may help the sickled cells return to their normal shape.
- **What is the patient's mental and neurologic status?** Central nervous system manifestations occur primarily as a result of vascular occlusion. Severe anemia, narcotic overdose, or withdrawal also may be responsible for an altered mental state.

Important History

- **Are the patient's current complaints similar to a previous sickle cell crisis?** Different presenting complaints may indicate that something other than a sickle cell crisis may be responsible. Patients with sickle cell disease are at risk for most of the diseases that affect patients without sickle cell disease.
- **Are there any crisis precipitating factors present?** Often, these crises are preceded by infection: pneumonias, urinary tract infections, and pharyngitis. Dehydration, cold exposure, acidosis, and trauma may also predispose toward a crisis.

Differential Diagnosis

This section will focus on sickle cell disease and its manifestations. Remember, however, that patients with sickle cell disease can have myocardial infarctions, appendicitis, strokes, and other serious illnesses. Consult the medical control physician to help differentiate clinical situations.

Sickle cell disease is a genetic disease of hemoglobin. Genes for hemoglobin are contributed by both parents. When both parents contribute the sickle cell gene to their offspring, sickle cell anemia is present. When a person receives only one sickle cell gene, they are said to carry the sickle cell trait. The final class of sickle cell variants are those patients who have one sickle cell gene and one gene for another abnormal hemoglobin.

- *Sickle Cell Anemia.* Patients with sickle cell disease have two genes for sickle cell hemoglobin and therefore have the most severe disease of the sickle cell spectrum. During a severe crisis more than 75% of the hemoglobin may be in the sickle state. This form of sickle cell disease is, in most cases, discovered during childhood (before the age of 15 years).
- *Sickle Cell Trait.* Patients with sickle cell disease have one normal hemoglobin gene and one sickle cell gene, resulting in partial expression of the abnormal gene. Less than 50% of the circulating hemoglobin are abnormal, and therefore the amount of sickling hemoglobin is low. These patients do not have severe crises or anemia.

- **Sickle Cell Trait and Another Abnormal Hemoglobin Trait.**
  Patients with sickle cell trait and another abnormal hemoglobin trait may be without significant crises or may have severe manifestations depending on the type of abnormal hemoglobin present. Diagnosis may be delayed until these patients are in their twenties or thirties.

There are four types of crises that are found in sickle cell disease:

1. Vaso-occlusive crises are caused by the formation of multiple thrombi within capillary beds. This is, by far, the most common type of crisis. Symptoms include constant pain, weakness, and anxiety. The pain commonly occurs in bones, joints, abdomen, back, and chest. The pain may be mild or severe, lasting hours or longer. It may respond to administration of oxygen, IV fluids, and pain medicine. Narcotic analgesia is often required.

2. Hemolytic crises are caused by the premature destruction of red blood cells. Patients in hemolytic crises exhibit symptoms of anemia and jaundice.

3. Aplastic crises are characterized by inadequately low red blood cell and white blood cell counts. This results from bone marrow suppression caused by concurrent infection or folic acid depression.

4. Sequestration crises result from the entrapment of blood cells within the liver and spleen. Patients in sequestration crises exhibit abdominal pain and an enlarged liver or spleen. In addition, their white and red blood cell counts are low. Children in a sequestration crisis may even be in shock.

Complications of sickle cell disease include:

- Increased risk of CVAs
- Pulmonary embolism
- Hepatitis secondary to transfusions
- Hepatic infarction
- Chronic anemia
- Narcotic dependence
- Blindness
- Pulmonary infarcts
- Vascular occlusion
- Hematuria
- Predisposition to infection
- Priapism

- Congestive heart failure
- Pulmonary infections
- Splenic infarction
- Bone infarctions, osteomyelitis (bone infections)
- Seizures
- Mild dehydration secondary to decreased ability to concentrate urine

Key Physical Examination Findings

- *Initial Assessment.* Be alert for respiratory compromise. Look for signs of inadequate perfusion.
- *Vital Signs.* Assess for the presence of tachycardia, tachypnea, fever, and hypotension.
- *Lungs.* Assess breath sounds for pneumonia.
- *Abdomen.* Look for enlarged, tender liver or spleen.
- *Extremities.* Assess for inadequate circulation, swelling or trauma.
- *Mental Status.* Assess for altered mental status and neurologic deficits, which may indicate CNS involvement, severe anemia, narcotic abuse, or withdrawal.

Treatment Plan

- *Patient Assessment.* Perform a rapid and systematic initial assessment and institute treatment as life-threatening problems are discovered. Prompt transport to the appropriate ED is a key intervention. A secondary survey should be performed once all the primary interventions have been accomplished. Be sure to consider alternative diagnoses, such as ischemic heart disease, CVA, and acute abdomen, when appropriate.
- Administer **supplemental O_2** to prevent or reduce additional sickling. Nasal cannula oxygen may be given to all nonhypoxic sickle cell crisis patients. Give high-flow O_2 to hypoxic patients.

  NOTE: Normal pulse oximetry readings may give a false indication of the patient's true O_2 level as the hemoglobin count is abnormally low.
- If the patient is hemodynamically unstable, place in the **shock position** (supine with legs elevated) and use **PASG,**

as indicated. The use of PASG remains controversial; follow local protocol.

- Establish a **large-bore IV with 0.9% NaCl or lactated Ringer's solution**. Fluid resuscitation is a key component of ED treatment, because many of these patients are mildly dehydrated. Fluid resuscitation, however, is often not needed in the prehospital phase.
- Analgesics will likely be used in the ED. Meperidine (Demerol) and morphine are most commonly used. Field use is uncommon, however.
- **Transport to appropriate ED.**

Bibliography

Esposito D: Sickle Cell Anemia. In Tintinalli JE, Krome LR, and Ruiz E (eds): Emergency Medicine: A Comprehensive Study Guide, ed 3. McGraw-Hill, New York, 1992, pp 773–774.

Hamilton GC and Braen GR: Anemia and White Blood Cell Disorders. In Rosen P (ed): Emergency Medicine: Concepts in Clinical Practice, ed 3. Mosby-Year Book, St. Louis, 1992, pp 1865–1867.

Notes

CHAPTER 40

Smoke Inhalation
Bernard Beckerman, MD, FACEP

Presentation

Patients suffering from smoke inhalation may present in many different ways. At one extreme are those found in cardiorespiratory arrest. At the opposite extreme are patients with mild conjunctival and upper airway irritation with no respiratory insufficiency. These latter patients may rapidly become asymptomatic after removal from the source of the smoke.

Immediate Concerns

- **What is the cardiorespiratory status of the patient?** If severe respiratory distress is a presenting symptom, then complete cardiorespiratory collapse may be imminent and immediate resuscitative efforts must be started.
- **What is the mental status of the patient?** A clear mental status in a patient after smoke inhalation gives you the opportunity to carefully plan for their evaluation and treatment. Confusion, combativeness, lethargy, or some combination of those features, are indications that a more severe exposure has occurred, and immediate action is necessary, particularly airway management.

Important History

- **Is the patient's medical history available and is it related to an increased risk of a debilitating outcome?** Patients with underlying cardiac or pulmonary disease are at increased risk from smoke inhalation. Pregnant women and young children also fall within this category of high risk. The following questions, when answered, will give the prehospital and hospital EMS providers valuable information as they develop a treatment plan for the patient.

  ○ How prolonged was the exposure to smoke and/or toxic products of combustion?
  ○ Was the patient hindered in escaping from the scene because of physical or mental handicaps and did these handicaps worsen the clinical picture?
  ○ Is there any indication that the victim is under the influence of alcohol or other drugs (both legal and illicit)?

Differential Diagnosis

Is the patient truly suffering from smoke inhalation or are other entities masquerading as smoke inhalation? These can include the following:

Carbon monoxide poisoning
Inhalation of various toxic substances
Myocardial infarction
Cerebrovascular accident (CVA)
Cyanide poisoning

Key Physical Examination Findings

- Look for signs of carbonaceous (black) sputum in the mouth and nose.
- Look for singed nasal hair, eye lashes, or eyebrows.
- Look for facial or neck burns.
- Check for signs of potential airway burns and pending laryngeal edema and airway compromise.
- *Initial Assessment.* Assess the patient's cardiorespiratory function and search for signs of airway and hemodynamic compromise (shock).
- *Vital Signs.* If the patient appears stable during the initial evaluation, then obtain complete vital signs, and, when possible, orthostatic vital signs. Search out other medical or surgical problems that may contribute or cause the problem (such as the existence of CVA or associated multiple trauma, etc).

Treatment Plan

Repetitive evaluation of the smoke inhalation victim is mandatory because the patient's physical condition may deteriorate rapidly. The longer the transit time to the hospital, the more often re-evaluation should be performed.

HEMODYNAMICALLY UNSTABLE PATIENT

- Administer O_2 and **provide ventilatory support** as needed. Prepare for intubation if tracheal burns or other symptoms of inhalation are present.
- Place patient in **shock position** if shock is apparent. Apply and inflate **PASG** following local protocol for this device.
- Establish **large-bore IV access with 0.9% NaCL or lactated Ringer's solution** and begin immediate fluid resuscitation. Obtain venous blood specimens for laboratory analysis.
- **Transport expeditiously to the appropriate ED.** Burn units and hyperbaric facilities may be considered by medical control physician or be part of standing orders.
- Do not needlessly delay transport—expedite transport. Treat associated injuries en route. Ensure patient comfort en route.

HEMODYNAMICALLY STABLE PATIENT

- Administer O_2 regardless of severity of symptoms (even in patients with COPD).
- Establish **large-bore IV access with 0.9% NaCL or lactated Ringer's solution**. Obtain venous blood specimens for laboratory analysis.
- **Transport expeditiously to the appropriate ED.**
- Do not needlessly delay transport—expedite transport. Treat associated injuries en route. Ensure patient comfort en route.
- Re-evaluate the patient from head to toe on a regular basis, especially when the transit time is prolonged.

Bibliography

Beckerman B and Brody G: Smoke Inhalation. Emerg Med 24:49–56, 1992

Price DP, Silverman H, and Schwartz G: Smoke Inhalation. In Schwartz G et al. (eds): Principles and Practice of Emergency Medicine, ed 3. Lea & Febiger, Philadelphia, 1992, pp 2862–2870.

Respiratory Burns and Smoke Inhalation. In Berman RE, Kliegman RM, et al. (eds): Nelson's Textbook of Pediatrics, ed 14. WB Saunders, Philadelphia, 1992, pp 1088–1089.

Speizer FE: Environmental Lung Disease. In Isselbacher KJ et al. (eds): Harrison's Principles of Internal Medicine, ed 13. McGraw-Hill, New York, 1994, p 1181.

Notes

CHAPTER 41

Sudden Infant Death Syndrome

R. Todd Kiskaddon, MD

Presentation

Sudden Infant Death Syndrome (SIDS) is defined as a previously healthy child who dies unexpectedly during the 1st year of life, and at the time of autopsy, no apparent cause for the death can be found. Current protocols also require a detailed death-scene investigation to rule out environmental causes. SIDS usually occurs during the 1st few months of life. It affects anywhere from 0.9 to 2.0 births per 1000 infants. The child is often discovered in cardiorespiratory arrest by parents after the baby fails to awaken at a regular time.

Immediate Concerns

- **Should cardiopulmonary resuscitation (CPR) be performed?** Although these infants are in cardiopulmonary arrest by definition, infants with a presumptive diagnosis of "crib death" may be apneic, bradycardic, or both. Vigorous resuscitation is indicated in these situations. SIDS is a retrospective diagnosis. As such, all infants should receive standard resuscitation management without regard to this presumptive diagnosis. In some cases, however, infants may meet criteria for pronouncement of death in the field. Because of the often volatile surroundings and the emotional needs of the family, rapid transport with basic life support is often recommended for these patients.
- **What is the emotional state of the family?** SIDS is an unexpected phenomenon. Family response to this shock-filled episode is intense and often unpredictable. Parents may feel anger, panic, denial, or guilt in addition to the

more expected grief and shock. Prehospital personnel should be reassuring and accommodating to the psychological needs of surviving family members. Parents should be encouraged to express their grief and be reassured that this incident was not a result of neglect and that everything possible is being done for their child.

Important History

- **Is there a history of previous apneic events?** The role of previous episodes of respiratory "pauses" has not been clearly established in SIDS cases. A variety of causes including cardiac, primary respiratory, central nervous system, and anatomic airway abnormalities, have been suggested as risk factors. Infants with previous episodes of apnea or "near-SIDS" most probably have definable pathology and are believed to be at greater risk for cardiac arrest.
- **Does the infant have any chronic, congenital, or recent illnesses?** Known previous illness may be the focus of the resuscitative effort (ie, cardiac or respiratory abnormalities primarily). Recent respiratory illness could precipitate significant bronchospasm, hypoxia, pneumonia, and ultimately sepsis. Sepsis in infants can result in severe hypoglycemia and cardiovascular shock.
- **Has there been a recent injury?** The surrounding environment and recent history may suggest the need for trauma management.
- **When was the infant last seen and what was the infant doing?** This may give some indication of the duration of pulselessness and potential success of the resuscitation effort. It should be remembered that presumed "downtime" is not a criterion for failure to initiate CPR. Prearrest activity may give a clue to the cause of cardiac arrest, such as aspiration, fall or trauma, accidental drug overdose or ingestion, or poisoning.
- **Has there been bystander CPR?** Although this is a standard and necessary piece of history, it should be ascertained in a way that does not make parents feel neglectful if CPR was not promptly instituted.

Differential Diagnosis

- *Foreign Body Obstruction or Aspiration.* The presence of vomitus requires aggressive clearing of the airway, suctioning, and ventilatory assistance. Gastroesophageal reflux is not uncommon in the very young.
- *Asphyxiation.* Objects in the crib may present a risk of asphyxiation. Prone sleeping has also been implicated as a major risk factor in SIDS cases, presumably because of the risk of suffocation.
- *Hypothermia.* Inadequate heating or infant covering can result in rapid heat loss in an infant due to the large body surface area-to-mass ratio. It may be difficult to resume a regular cardiac rhythm until adequate rewarming has occurred.
- *Sepsis.* A major cause of cardiac arrest in previously healthy infants is overwhelming sepsis in the presence of an immature immune system. Consider meningitis and pneumonia as primary causes.
- *Toxic Ingestion.* Consider overdoses of medicines or accidental ingestions. Carbon monoxide poisoning is a greater risk during the winter months.
- *Trauma.* Seldom occult in crib deaths, a recent history may reveal an earlier shaking or fall.
- *Abuse.* One study has implied that anywhere from 7% to 19% of infant cardiac arrests may be intentional suffocation or strangulations. The epidemiologic characteristics for these infants tend to be different from those of SIDS babies; therefore, curious behavior, such as inappropriate detachment, should be noted and reported if required by statute.

Key Physical Examination Findings

- *Initial Assessment.* Pay particular attention to possible sources of airway obstruction, as hypoxia is the most common cause of infant cardiac arrest.
- **Assess effectiveness of CPR efforts.**
- *Secondary Survey.* Is there evidence of trauma?
- *Crib Examination.* Look for vomitus, stuffed animals with buttons, balloons, and other objects that could cause foreign body airway obstruction or asphyxia. Include an en-

vironmental assessment (eg, room temperature, electrical hazards, smell of gas, etc).

Treatment Plan

- *Patient Assessment.* Establish apnea, pulselessness, or both. The infant may be cool and cyanotic. In some cases, rigor mortis may be present.
- **Institute Basic Life Support (BLS).** It may be most appropriate to remove the infant from the scene at this point and initiate advanced life support (ALS) in the ambulance or rapidly transport to the ED, while providing BLS en route.
- **Establish an airway,** including suctioning and endotracheal intubation.
- **Establish a route for drug and fluid administration,** either **intravenous or intraosseous**. Drugs may also be given via the endotracheal tube (at different doses and strengths; see Appendix E).
- **Institute ALS** (per American Heart Association guidelines; see Appendix F).
- Give a **fluid bolus of 20 ml/kg of 0.9% NaCL**.
- Administer **50% dextrose, half strength 2 to 4 ml/kg IV**.
- Consider persistent hypoxia and acidosis, tension pneumothorax, or cardiac tamponade.
- **Ensure** that **adequate rewarming** is ongoing.
- Attend to emotional needs of the parents. Assure them that everything possible is being done. Do not be overly optimistic or falsely encouraging. Grief is a normal response. Do not deny the family this emotion. Encourage them to express their feelings and empathize with their suffering. **Direct the family to the hospital chaplain or social worker on arrival at the hospital.**

Bibliography

Guntheroth WG, et al: Sleeping Prone and the Risk of Sudden Infant Death Syndrome. JAMA 267:2359, 1992

Meadow R: Suffocation, Recurrent Apnea and Sudden Infant Death. J Ped 117:351, 1990

Mellins RB and Haddad GG: Sudden Infant Death Syndrome (SIDS). In Behrman RE, Vaughan VC, and Nelson WE (eds): Nelson Textbook of Pediatrics, ed 13. WB Saunders, Philadelphia, 1987, p 1480.

Pediatric Advanced Life Support. JAMA 268:2262, 1992

Notes

CHAPTER 42

Syncope
Carol Johnson, RN, MSN

Presentation

The patient with true syncope presents with a history of a brief, self-limiting episode of unconsciousness. The episode is usually no longer than 15 to 20 seconds. The patient may be nauseated and appear pale and diaphoretic. Bystanders may report that the patient fainted (swooned or fell out). Reports of brief episodes of myoclonic activity or eye rolling are common and are not indicative of a seizure.

Immediate Concerns

- **Is this episode of syncope a symptom of a more serious medical condition?** True syncope is most frequently caused by a change in vasomotor tone, is self-limiting, and requires only supportive care. However, it may be a presenting symptom for a more serious condition that is not immediately obvious. These include, but are not limited to, cardiac arrhythmias, diabetes, neurologic problems, or covert trauma.

Important History

- **Has the patient experienced a strong emotion or witnessed an unpleasant sight?** Syncope is often a physiologic response to a psychological or an environmental cause, such as grief, anger, fear, or sight of blood.
- **What was the length of unconsciousness?** Episodes of unconsciousness in excess of 15 to 20 seconds are indicative of other problems. Even if the patient awakens in this time, other medical problems must be investigated.
- **What was the patient's position before the event?** Prolonged standing in one place may lead to venous pooling

in the lower extremities and a subsequent decrease in cerebral perfusion, leading to syncope. Sudden changes in position (lying or sitting to standing) may have a similar effect.

- **Is the patient taking any medications that may precipitate hypotension?** Medications those prescribed for hypertension, such as beta blockers, calcium channel blockers, vasodilators, and even nitrates, may cause hypotension or postural hypotension.
- **Was there any associated myoclonic activity?** Myoclonic activity of more than a few seconds, evidence of incontinence, or a postictal state would indicate a seizure, not syncope.

Differential Diagnosis

- *Cardiovascular Causes.* Syncope secondary to myocardial infarction, dysrhythmia (Stokes-Adams syndrome), carotid sinus stimulation, postural hypotension, pulmonary embolism, or cardiac arrest.
- *Hemorrhagic Disorders.* Syncope may be the first indication of unrecognized hemorrhage. Consider the potential for GI bleeding, leaking aortic aneurysm, ruptured ectopic pregnancy, ruptured spleen, or other occult trauma.
- *Dehydration.* A history of nausea, vomiting, and or diarrhea may lead to changes in orthostatic vital signs and syncope. Poor oral intake in the elderly or debilitated patients may cause dehydration.
- *Neurologic Disorders.* Syncope is associated with stroke or intracranial bleeding and may be the result of spinal cord injury where there is a loss of peripheral vasomotor tone.
- *Heat Illness.* Dehydration, heat exhaustion, and heat stroke may precipitate syncope.
- *Toxicologic Causes.* Poisonings, drug or alcohol overdose (including hypertensive medications), and carbon monoxide poisoning manifest syncope at advanced stages.
- *Metabolic Disorders.* Hypoglycemia, hyperglycemia, and sepsis may manifest with syncope
- *Iatrogenic Causes* (caused by treatment).

Key Physical Examination Findings

- *Initial Assessment.* The patient is usually lethargic but is now awake and alert after brief, self-limiting unconsciousness.
- *Vital Signs.* Include orthostatic vital signs if practical and possible.
- *History.* Ask about possible psychological causes and the patient's activity before the event. Did any physical or emotional events trigger this response?
- *Physical Examination.* Suspect syncope as a symptom of a more serious medical problem and perform a SAMPLE history and complete secondary survey.

Treatment Plan

- *Patient Assessment.* Assess need for transport. In cases of true syncope the patient may refuse transport. Obtain appropriate signed release form. If syncope is due to an underlying condition, encourage the patient to accept further evaluation in the hospital. Consult medical control physician for guidance and initiation of appropriate orders if the patient's presentation is unclear.

GENERAL TREATMENT GUIDELINES: HEMODYNAMICALLY STABLE PATIENT

- Administer O_2 and **provide ventilatory support** as needed.
- Place patient in the **shock position** (supine with legs elevated), protecting the cervical spine as indicated.
- **Treat non–life-threatening injuries** as appropriate (ie, control bleeding, splint fractures, etc).
- Monitor the patient's condition for changes
- **Transport to appropriate ED.** Ensure patient comfort en route.

GENERAL TREATMENT GUIDELINES: HEMODYNAMICALLY UNSTABLE PATIENT

- Administer O_2 and **provide ventilatory support** as needed.
- Place patient in the **shock position** (supine with legs elevated), or use **PASG, if indicated**. The use of PASG is controversial; follow local protocol.

- Establish **large-bore IV access with 0.9% NaCl or lactated Ringer's solution.**
- **Begin fluid resuscitation.**
- **Treat for shock** (see Chapter 38, Shock).
- **Expeditiously transport to appropriate ED.** Do not needlessly delay patient transport—expedite transport. Ensure patient comfort en route.

Bibliography

Goldman JM: Cardiac Syncope. In Harwood-Nuss A, et al. (eds): The Clinical Practice of Emergency Medicine. JB Lippincott, Philadelphia, 1991, pp 894–897.

Hunt M: Syncope. In Rosen P and Barkin RM (eds): Emergency Medicine: Concepts and Clinical Practice, ed 3. Mosby-Year Book, St. Louis, 1992, pp 1186–1199.

Wilson A: Syncope. In Tintinalli JE, Krome LR, and Ruiz E (eds): Emergency Medicine: A Comprehensive Study Guide, ed 2. McGraw-Hill, New York, 1988, pp 119–121.

Notes

CHAPTER 43

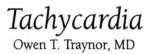

Tachycardia

Owen T. Traynor, MD

Presentation

The adult who has a heart rate in excess of 100 bpm is tachycardic. Tachycardia can be a physiologic response to stress; a compensatory mechanism for acute blood loss or hypoxia; or a sign of pathology, caused by heart disease, drugs, or an unknown mechanism. The clinical presentation of a patient with tachycardia depends on the heart rate, the duration of the tachycardia, the pumping effectiveness of the heart, the cardiovascular status of the patient, and the underlying health of the patient.

Immediate Concerns

- **What is the patient's hemodynamic status?** If the patient is hemodynamically unstable, immediate resuscitation is warranted, including oxygen administration, establishment of IV access, possibly IV medications, and synchronized cardioversion or defibrillation. If the tachycardia is a response to hypovolemia, fluid resuscitation and treatment for shock are necessary.

Important History

- **Is the patient symptomatic?** Tachycardias may lead to inadequate cardiac output resulting in the following common complaints: chest pain, dyspnea, fatigue, syncope, dizziness, or neurologic deficits. Chest pain may be either the result of an AMI, which may be causing the tachycardia, or the consequence of poor coronary perfusion secondary to the tachycardia. Asymptomatic patients require less aggressive immediate therapy.
- **Is the patient taking any medication?** Many medications, particularly sympathomimetic agents, aminophylline

derivatives, thyroid medications, and diuretics (reflex tachycardia secondary to hypovolemia) can cause tachycardias.

- **Is there a history of hyperthyroidism?** Excess thyroid hormones may cause an increased sensitivity to sympathetic nervous system hormones, thereby leading to tachycardias. Signs and symptoms of hyperthyroidism include heat intolerance, increased sweating, weight loss, insomnia, hyperkinetic movements, and tachycardias.
- **Does the patient have a previous history of heart disease?** Patients with valvular heart disease; prosthetic heart valves; cardiomyopathies; or pre-excitation syndromes, such as Wolff-Parkinson-White (WPW) syndrome, exhibit an increased incidence of tachycardia.
- **What events preceded the onset of the tachycardia?** Exercise, pain, emotional stress, fatigue, fever, dyspnea, and acute blood loss may cause tachycardias. Nicotine, alcohol, and caffeine may increase heart rate. The use of cocaine and other stimulants may also induce tachycardias.

Differential Diagnosis

SUPRAVENTRICULAR TACHYCARDIAS (SVT)

- *Sinus Tachycardia.* The sinus node rate is between 100 to 180 bpm, although it can be much faster with even moderate exertion. It is usually characterized by a gradual onset and a gradual recovery. Sinus tachycardia is a response to fever; hypotension; anemia; thyrotoxicosis; anxiety; exercise; pulmonary embolism; AMI; CHF; and drugs, such as sympathomimetics, alcohol, caffeine, and nicotine. Therapy should focus on the underlying etiology.
- *Atrial Flutter.* The atrial rate is between 250 to 350 bpm, with a ventricular rate between 80 to 175 bpm (conduction ratio may be 2:1, 4:1, or least commonly, 3:1). The presence of flutter (F) waves may be noted. Atrial flutter is an unstable rhythm, often spontaneously converting to atrial fibrillation or normal sinus rhythm. Chronic atrial flutter is usually associated with underlying heart disease: mitral and tricuspid valve stenosis, ischemic heart disease, and cardiomyopathies. Paroxysmal atrial flutter, however, can occur in patients without structural heart disease.
- *Atrial Fibrillation.* This rhythm is characterized by disor-

ganized, chaotic atrial activity, with P waves absent and
fibrillation waves present at a rate greater than 350 bpm.
Atrial fibrillation is a common arrhythmia, occurring in
1% of adults over 60 years of age. Incidence increases with
age. Most patients have underlying heart disease, such as
coronary artery disease (CAD), hypertensive heart disease,
CHF, or cardiomyopathy. Hyperthyroidism is an important
cause of new-onset atrial fibrillation. Patients with atrial
fibrillation have an increased risk of embolic events and
are often taking anticoagulants.

- *Atrial Tachycardias.* The atrial rate is greater than 100
  bpm but less than 150 bpm, as rates greater than this are
  usually considered to be paroxysmal supraventricular
  tachycardia (PSVT); P-wave morphology is different from
  sinus node P waves in atrial tachycardia. Unlike sinus
  tachycardia, which has a gradual onset, atrial tachycardia
  is characterized by a sudden onset, hence paroxsysmal. If
  heart block is present in patients taking digitalis preparations, consider digitalis toxicity.
- *Multifocal Atrial Tachycardia (MAT).* Atrial rates are usually from 100 to 130 bpm. There is a variation in P-wave
  morphology of at least three etiologies. The rhythm is irregular. This rhytm occurs most commonly in elderly patients with COPD or CHF; it may degenerate into atrial
  fibrillation.
- *Sick Sinus Syndrome.* A sinoatrial (SA) node abnormality
  that includes persistent spontaneous inappropriate sinus
  bradycardia, episodes of sinus arrest or sinus exit block, a
  combination of SA or atrioventricular (AV) node conduction anomalies, or alternating periods of paroxysmal atrial
  tachycardias with slow atrial and ventricular rhythms. This
  is also known as the bradycardia-tachycardia syndrome.
- *Junctional Tachycardias.* These tachycardias may result
  from increased automaticity or, more commonly, a re-en-
  trant phenomenon. They are characterized by a regular
  rhythm, normal QRS complexes, and P waves that may be
  absent, precede, or follow the QRS complex. The P waves
  may be positive, biphasic, or negative in ECG leads where
  normally positive. Where the P wave is positive, the PR
  interval is usually less than 0.12 second. Ventricular rates
  are usually from 130 to 180 bpm.
- *Pre-Excitation Syndrome.* A syndrome in which an atrial

or a ventricular impulse travels not only along the normal conduction system, but along an anomalous pathway through the myocardium, resulting in conduction of an impulse earlier than expected. WPW syndrome, where impulses are conducted along an accessory AV pathway, is the most common type of pre-excitation syndrome, with an incidence of 1.5 per 1000 persons. Two key characteristics of WPW syndrome are PR intervals less than 0.12 second during NSR and QRS complexes greater than 0.12 second, with slurred, slowly rising onset of the QRS complex (delta wave) in some ECG leads and usually a normal terminal QRS portion. Rapid ventricular rates are possible when impulses are conducted along the accessory pathway, bypassing the AV node. The most common ventricular rates are 150 to 250 bpm. The tachycardias usually occur with a sudden onset and a sudden termination. Atrial fibrillation is a particularly dangerous rhythm in these patients because very rapid ventricular rates are possible. Atrial fibrillation can lead to ventricular fibrillation in WPW patients. The accessory pathways can be mapped and then destroyed using high-frequency radio frequency energy at specialty centers.

VENTRICULAR TACHYCARDIA

Ventricular tachycardia (VT) is defined as three or more consecutive beats of ventricular origin in a row. The QRS complex is usually wide (greater than 0.12 second), and the ST and T waves are usually opposite in direction to the QRS deflection. VT arises distal to the bifurcation of the His bundle, in the conduction system, in the myocardium, or in both locations. The rate is usually from 70 to 250 bpm. VT may be paroxysmal or nonparoxysmal, multiform or monoform. It may be difficult at times to differentiate between VT and an SVT with aberrant conduction.

NOTE: Ventricular tachycardia is the most common cause of wide-QRS complex tachycardia.

POLYMORPHIC VENTRICULAR TACHYCARDIA

Also known as torsades de pointes, this is a VT variant characterized by a gradual fluctuation in amplitude and axis of the

QRS complex. It is generally found in the context of a prolonged QT interval in patients taking type IA antiarrhythmic agents such as procainamide, quinidine, and disopyramide. It also requires different treatment than conventional VT: overdrive transcutaneous pacing, IV magnesium sulfate, and possibly IV isoproterenol.

DIFFERENTIATION OF VENTRICULAR TACHYCARDIA VERSUS SUPRAVENTRICULAR TACHYCARDIA WITH ABERRANT CONDUCTION

Although it may be useful to distinguish between supraventricular and ventricular wide complex tachycardias (WCTs) as their therapeutic modalities differ, it is difficult to do so reliably in the prehospital environment.

Factors Favoring Ventricular Tachycardia

- QRS complexes have similar morphology to premature ventricular contractions (PVCs).
- Tachycardia was initiated by a PVC.
- Usually unresponsive to vagal maneuvers.
- Presence of AV dissociation.
- QRS complex greater than 0.14 second.
- Presence of fusion beats.
- History of CAD.

Factors Favoring Supraventricular Tachycardia With Aberrancy

- Similar morphology to previous baseline rhythm.
- Tachycardia may slow or break with vagal stimulation.
- Responsive to adenosine therapy.
- Tachycardia often initiated by a premature atrial contraction (PAC).

Key Physical Examination Findings

The physical examination is geared toward assessing the cardiovascular status of the patient and potential sources of sinus tachycardia.

- *Initial Assessment.* Look for signs of shock and blood loss.
- *Vital Signs.* Monitor blood pressure, pulse, respirations,

and temperature. Hypotension may be present. Tachypnea may be present, indicating hypoxia. Fever may be present, indicating infection and causing sinus tachycardia.

- *Lungs.* Listen for the presence of rales, which indicates CHF.
- *Heart.* Listen for gallops.
- *Abdomen.* Look for signs of acute abdomen, another etiology for sinus tachycardia.
- *Extremities.* Assess for pain secondary to injury, which may explain sinus tachycardia.
- *Mental Status.* Assess for signs of altered mental status. Inadequate perfusion can cause an altered mental status.

ECG

An important diagnostic tool that will help determine therapy.

Treatment Plan

Treatment options begin with the assessment of the patient's stability. Instability is characterized by an altered mental status, chest pain, dyspnea, hypotension, pulmonary edema, CHF, and AMI. The patient's instability must also be related to the patient's tachycardia.

- *Patient Assessment.* Provide frequent reassessment owing to the potential for a worsening of hemodynamic status and CHF. Cardiac monitoring is necessary. Be prepared—potential for cardiac arrest exists. Treat for an AMI if the tachycardia is occurring in the context of a myocardial infarction. Transport decisions need to be considered early in the treatment of unstable patients. Early contact with medical control physicians is recommended when there are diagnostic or therapeutic modality difficulties, as well as when permission is required to institute therapy.

STABLE TACHYCARDIAS

The approach to treating stable tachycardias may be divided into four distinct scenarios based on the patient's ECG findings.

- *Atrial Fibrillation or Flutter.* In general, little field treatment needs to be given in cases of artial fibrillation or flutter other than observation and supportive care. When there is hemodynamic instability or a rapid ventricular response, however, prehospital therapy should be considered. The primary goal of therapy is rate control, not abolishing the arrhythmia. Patients with stable artial fibrillation rarely convert to sinus rhythm after vagal maneuvers, verapamil, or adenosine. Care is directed in the manner outlined below.

- Administer O$_2$ and **provide ventilatory support** as needed
- Establish **IV access with 0.9% NaCl at a KVO rate**.
- Perform **vagal maneuvers**, such as the Valsalva maneuver. If the diagnosis of artial fibrillation is in question, increased vagal tone may make flutter waves more apparent. Carotid sinus massage should not be performed in patients with carotid bruits. If artial fibrillation or flutter persists, consider:

  Verapamil, 2 to 5 mg/kg IV. Do not use verapamil if the patient has a history of severe bradycardia, is hypotensive, is in CHF, or has acutely received IV beta blockers. Verapamil may be repeated at 5 to 10 mg/kg IV in 15 to 30 minutes if there is inadequate rate control.

  Diltiazem 0.25 mg/kg IV over 2 minutes. If insufficient response, may re-bolus in 15 minutes with 0.35 mg/kg IV. If effective, start diltiazem infusion at 5 to 15 mg/hour.

  Procainamide, 20 to 30 mg per minute IV until effective, or 17 mg/kg total has been given, or the width of the QRS complex increases by 50%.

- If verapamil or procainamide are ineffective, **consider beta blockers** to control ventricular rate, followed by synchronized cardioversion. Prehospital cardioversion should be avoided, if the transport time to the ED is short, unless the patient's hemodynamic status is poor or the patient is symptomatic. Consider sedation before cardioversion.
- **Transport to appropriate ED**. Continue to **reassess** the patient's ECG and hemodynamic status. Ensure patient comfort en route.

Paroxysmal Supraventricular Tachycardia

It can be difficult at times to distinguish between the various types of tachycardias, ventricular and supraventricular alike. Two general principles may help guide therapy: (1) treat unstable tachycardias with DC electrical therapy, and (2) if the tachycardia is a WCT, treat the patient as if in VT. General treatment guidelines for the treatment of PSVT follow:

- Administer O$_2$ and **provide ventilatory support** as needed.
- Establish **IV access with 0.9% NaCl at a KVO rate**.
- **Perform vagal maneuvers,** such as the Valsalva maneuver, if trained in their proper use. Carotid sinus massage should not be performed in patients with carotid bruits.
- If PSVT persists, administer **adenosine, 6 mg rapid IV bolus**. Adenosine may be repeated at 12 mg IV in 1 to 2 minutes if ineffective. Drug may be repeated a second time at same dosage.
- If PSVT persists, re-evaluate width of QRS complex.

Narrow Complex Tachycardia (With Normal or Elevated BP)

- Administer **verapamil, 2 to 5 mg/kg IV**. Do not use verapamil if patient has a history of severe bradycardia, is hypotensive, is in CHF, or has acutely received IV beta blockers. Verapamil may be repeated at 5 to 10 mg/kg IV in 15 to 30 minutes if PSVT persists.
- **Diltiazem 0.25 mg/kg IV over 2 minutes.** If insufficient response, may re-bolus in 15 minutes with 0.35 mg/kg IV. If effective, start diltiazem infusion at 5 to 15 mg/hour.
- Repeat vagal maneuvers between pharmacologic interventions.
- If adenosine or verapamil are ineffective, **consider beta blockers** to control ventricular rate, **followed by synchronized cardioversion**. Prehospital cardioversion should be avoided, if the transport time to the ED is short, unless the patient's hemodynamic status is poor or the patient is symptomatic. Consider sedation before cardioversion.
- **Transport to appropriate ED.** Continue to reassess the patient's ECG and hemodynamic status. Ensure patient comfort en route.

Narrow Complex Tachycardia (With Low or Unstable BP)

- **Synchronized cardioversion** at the following suggested initial energies: atrial flutter 50 J; PSVT 50 J; atrial fibrillation 100 J; polymorphic VT 200 J. Consider sedation before cardioversion. If patient's hemodynamic stability worsens and delays in synchronization occur, proceed to immediate unsynchronized cardioversion.

- If rhythm persists, **repeat synchronized cardioversion** using the following incremental dosage scheme: 100 J, 200 J, 300 J, 360 J.
- **Transport to appropriate ED.** Continue to reassess the patient's ECG and hemodynamic status. Ensure patient comfort en route.

Wide Complex Tachycardia

- Give **lidocaine, 1 to 1.5 mg/kg IV**.
- If WCT persists, give **procainamide, 20 to 30 mg per minute IV until effective**, or 17 mg/kg total has been given. If ineffective, or the width of the QRS complex increases by 50%.
- **Synchronized cardioversion** as in unstable patients. Consider sedation before cardioversion. Prehospital cardioversion should be avoided if the transport time to the ED is short, unless the patient's hemodynamic status is poor or the patient is symptomatic.
- **Transport to appropriate ED.** Continue to reassess the patient's ECG and hemodynamic status. Ensure patient comfort en route.

Wide Complex Tachycardia of Uncertain Type

Prehospital EMS providers should not attempt to use either clinical criteria or ECG criteria to distinguish between SVT with aberrant conduction and VT. The value of the treatment outweighs the prehospital differentiation of these dysrhythmias. General treatment guidelines follow.

- Administer O_2 and **provide ventilatory support** as needed
- Establish IV access with 0.9% NaCl at a KVO rate.
- Administer **lidocaine 1 to 1.5 mg/kg IV**. Lidocaine may be repeated at 0.5 to 0.75 mg/kg every 5 to 10 minutes until WCT resolves or 3 mg/kg total has been given.
- If WCT persists, administer **adenosine, 6 mg rapid IV bolus**. Adenosine may be repeated at 12 mg IV in 1 to 2 minutes if ineffective. Drug may be repeated a second time at the same dosage.
- If WCT persists, administer **procainamide, 20 to 30 mg/ min IV until effective** or 17 mg/kg total has been given, or the width of the QRS complex increases by 50%.

- If ineffective, consider **bretylium, 5 to 10 mg/kg IV** (diluted to 50 ml) over 8 to 10 minutes.
- If VT persists, perform **synchronized cardioversion** as in unstable patients. Consider sedation before cardioversion. Prehospital cardioversion should be avoided if the transport time to the ED is short, unless the patient's hemodynamic status is poor or the patient is symptomatic.
- **Transport to appropriate ED.** Continue to reassess the patient's ECG and hemodynamic status. Ensure patient comfort en route.

Ventricular Tachycardia

- Administer O_2 and **provide ventilatory support** as needed.
- Establish IV access with 0.9% NaCl at a KVO rate.
- Give **lidocaine, 1 to 1.5 mg/kg IV**. Lidocaine may be repeated at 0.5 to 0.75 mg/kg every 5 to 10 minutes until VT resolves or 3 mg/kg total has been given. If VT persists,
- Administer **procainamide, 20 to 30 mg/min IV until effective** or 17 mg/kg total has been given, or the width of the QRS complex increases by 50%.
- If ineffective, consider **bretylium, 5 to 10 mg/kg IV** (diluted to 50 ml) over 8 to 10 minutes.
- If VT persists, perform **synchronized cardioversion** as in unstable patients. Consider sedation before cardioversion. Prehospital cardioversion should be avoided if the transport time to the ED is short, unless the patient's hemodynamic status is poor or the patient is symptomatic.
- **Transport to appropriate ED.** Continue to reassess the patient's ECG and hemodynamic status. Ensure patient comfort en route.

Pre-Excitation Syndromes

Patients with WPW who exhibit stable regular narrow complex tachycardias should be treated as noted for stable PSVT above. Adenosine may be administered as the first-line drug, then verapamil (see note). If the tachycardia is an irregular wide complex tachycardia, atrial fibrillation or flutter may be present. Drugs that prolong the refractoriness of the accessory pathway, like procainamide, must be used to prevent ventricular fibrillation.

NOTE: Verapamil may be dangerous as it may increase the number of impulses conducted down the accessory pathways by prolonging the refractoriness of the AV node, thereby further increasing the heart rate.

Polymorphic Ventricular Tachycardia
(Torsades de Pointes)

Torsades de pointes requires different treatment than conventional VT—overdrive transcutaneous pacing (at a rate greater than the ventricular rate), IV magnesium sulfate (1 to 2 g IV over 1 to 2 minutes), and possibly IV isoproterenol (2 to 10 µg/min). Type IA antiarrhythmic agents such as procainamide and quinidine are contraindicated. If polymorphic VT is recurrent or sustained, defibrillation should be performed.

UNSTABLE TACHYCARDIAS
Ventricular Tachycardia

The unstable patient with VT requires emergent treatment. Unstable patients are defined as patients with an altered mental status, CP, dyspnea, hypotension (systolic BP less than 90 mm Hg), CHF, ischemia, or infarction. VT without a pulse should be treated as ventricular fibrillation.

- Administer O_2 and **provide ventilatory support** as needed.
- Establish **IV access with 0.9% NaCl at a KVO rate**.
- **Synchronized cardioversion at 100 J.** Consider sedation prior to cardioversion. If patient is hypotensive, unconscious, or in pulmonary edema, unsynchronized cardioversion should be performed to avoid delay associated with synchronization. A precordial thump may be employed before synchronized cardioversion in those patients who are not hypotensive, unconscious, or in pulmonary edema.
- If VT persists, **repeat synchronized cardioversion** using the following dosage scheme: 200 J, 300 J, 360 J.
- If recurrent, add **lidocaine** (1.0 to 1.5 mg/kg IV initially, repeated at 0.5 to 0.75 mg/kg every 5 to 10 minutes until VT resolves or 3 mg/kg total has been given) and **cardiovert again** at level which was previously successful. If lidocaine is not successful in converting the rhythm, use **procainamide** (20 to 30 mg per minute IV until VT resolves, or 17 mg/kg total has been given, or the width of the QRS complex increases by 50%) or bretylium (5 to 10 mg/kg IV over 8 to 10 minutes). If hypotension, pulmonary edema, or unconsciousness is present, **bretylium** should be used rather than procainamide. In other cases, lidocaine should be followed by procainamide and then bretylium.

- If VT resolves, give IV infusion of antiarrhythmic agent that has aided in its resolution—lidocaine, 2 to 4 mg per minute, procainamide, 1 to 4 mg per minute, or bretylium, 1 to 2 mg per minute.
- **Transport to appropriate ED.** Transport decisions need to be considered early in the treatment of unstable patients. Continue to reassess the patient's ECG and hemodynamic status. Ensure patient comfort en route.

Supraventricular Tachycardia

- Administer O_2 and **provide ventilatory support** as needed.
- Establish **IV access with 0.9% NaCl at a KVO rate**.
- Consider a trial of antiarrhythmic agents based on the arrhythmia (see previous discussion).
- Perform **synchronized cardioversion** at the following suggested initial energies: atrial flutter 50 J, PSVT 50 J, atrial fibrillation 100 J, polymorphic VT 200 J. Consider sedation prior to cardioversion. If patient's hemodynamic stability worsens and delays in synchronization occur, proceed to immediate unsynchronized cardioversion.
- If rhythm persists, **repeat synchronized cardioversion** using the following incremental dosage scheme: 100 J, 200 J, 300 J, 360 J.
- **Transport to appropriate ED.** Continue to reassess the patient's ECG and hemodynamic status. Ensure patient comfort en route.

  NOTE: If the ventricular rate is less than 150 bpm, immediate cardioversion is seldom needed.

Polymorphic Ventricular Tachycardia

Torsades de pointes requires different treatment than conventional VT, which includes **overdrive transcutaneous pacing** (at a rate greater than the ventricular rate), **IV magnesium sulfate** (1 to 2 g over 1 to 2 minutes), and possibly **IV isoproterenol** (2 to 10 µg/min.). Type IA antiarrhythmic agents such as procainamide and quinidine are contraindicated. If polymorphic VT is recurrent or sustained, **defibrillation** should be performed.

Bibliography

Brown KR and Jacobson K: Mastering Dysrhythmias: A Problem-Solving Guide. FA Davis, Philadelphia, 1988.

Essentials of ACLS. In Textbook of Advanced Cardiac Life Support, ed 3. American Heart Association, Dallas TX, 1994, pp 1-32 to 1-40.

Guidelines for Cardiopulmonary Resuscitation and Emergency Cardiac Care. JAMA 268:2222–2226, 1992.

Zipes DP: Specific Arrhythmias: Diagnosis and Treatment. In Braunwald E (ed): Heart Disease: A Textbook of Cardiovascular Medicine, ed 4. WB Saunders, Philadelphia, 1992, pp 667–693, 701–706.

Notes

CHAPTER 44

Vaginal Bleeding

Jonathan S. Rubens, MD, FACEP

Presentation

Vaginal bleeding is one of the most common gynecologic complaints in emergency medicine. Patients may present with a variety of signs and symptoms, including those of shock and passage of blood, clots, or tissue from the vagina.

Immediate Concerns

- **ABCs.** If the patient is exhibiting signs of shock, resuscitation should be initiated with oxygen, two large-bore IV lines, isotonic fluids, and possibly the use of the PASG.

Important History

- **Is the patient pregnant (gravid)?** Bleeding in pregnancy varies in cause depending on the trimester. Pregnant patients may bleed early on owing to implantation (fetal sac implants onto uterine wall), spontaneous abortion, or ectopic pregnancy or later in the pregnancy from placenta previa, abruption, or even uterine rupture. A history of pelvic inflammatory disease, ectopic pregnancy, tubal surgery, previous pelvic surgery, and induced abortions are important findings.
- **Last normal menstrual period?** Does current bleeding coincide with the expected cycle of menses?
- **Is there pain associated with the bleeding?** Cramping is common in menstruation and spontaneous abortion. Pain is often associated with ectopic pregnancy and abruptions. Painless blood can be seen in a patient with placenta previa.
- **What is the amount of bleeding?** This can often be quantified by number of pads used in a period.
- **Is the patient taking any medications?** Aspirin, warfarin

(Coumadin), and nonsteroidal anti-inflammatory agents may all contribute to bleeding.

- **What is the patient's other medical history?** Is there any history of malignancy or bleeding tendencies? Women who have undergone embryo transfer techniques and treatment for infertility are at increased risk for ectopic pregnancy.
- **Is there a history of trauma?** Examples include intercourse, sexual assault, or instrumentation (foreign objects).

Differential Diagnosis

THE PREGNANT PATIENT

- *Ectopic Pregnancy.* Any woman of childbearing age with vaginal bleeding should be considered ectopic until proven otherwise (with or without pain).
- *Hydatidiform Mole.* An abnormal development of the tissue which forms the placenta. Molar pregnancies occur in approximately 1 out of 1500 live births. The uterus is usually larger in relation to dates in the pregnancy cycle. Risk is 10 times greater in women older than 45 years of age.
- *Spontaneous Abortion.* Termination of pregnancy occurs before the 20th week of gestation. Approximately 15% to 20% of pregnancies end this way.
- *Placenta Previa.* A portion of the placenta overlies the cervical os (or opening), usually painless bright red blood.
- *Abruptio Placentae.* Painful separation of the placenta from its implantation site. Bleeding may or may not be present—it is sometimes contained within the uterus.
- *Uterine Rupture.* This grave complication occurs in 1 out of 2000 pregnancies, and results in high maternal and fetal mortality.

THE NONPREGNANT PATIENT

- *Normal Menses.*
- *Neoplasms.* These are of the uterus, ovaries, or cervix.
- *Ovarian Cysts.* These cysts result in hormonal disruption
- *Endometriosis.* Endometrial tissue develops outside of the uterus.
- *IUDs* (intrauterine devices).
- *Trauma.* Trauma results in disruption of the integrity of the vaginal or cervical anatomy

- *Infection.* A history of vaginal discharge, fever, and dyspareunia (painful intercourse) is usually present.
- Other systemic disease or coagulation disorders

Key Physical Examination Findings

- *Initial Assessment.* Monitor airway, breathing, and circulation. Look for signs of shock.
- *Vital Signs.* Include orthostatic blood pressures. Remember that pregnant patients may have up to one third greater blood volume, and thus may not show signs of shock as early as the nongravid patient.
- *Abdomen.* Is a gravid abdomen present? Tenderness, masses, rebound tenderness, and involuntary guarding should all be assessed. Listen for bowel sounds; attempt to gently palpate any uterine contractions.
- *Genital.* Inspect the external genitalia for amount of bleeding and the presence of any tissue. Do not perform any internal examination of the vaginal opening in the field.

Treatment Plan

- Continued vital sign assessment.

GENERAL TREATMENT GUIDELINES: HEMODYNAMICALLY UNSTABLE PATIENT

- Administer O_2 and **provide ventilatory support** as needed. Monitor O_2 saturation with pulse oximetry if available.
- Establish **two large-bore IV lines with 0.9% NaCl or LR**.
- **Position gravid patients on their left side** to avoid inferior vena cavae compression by the uterus and to increase venous return.
- Monitor ECG
- **Transport expeditiously to appropriate ED.** Do not needlessly delay transport—expedite transport. Ensure patient comfort en route.

GENERAL TREATMENT GUIDELINES: HEMODYNAMICALLY STABLE PATIENT

- **Transport to appropriate ED.** Ensure patient comfort en route.

Bibliography

Hochbaum S: Vaginal bleeding. In Rosen P and Barkin RM (eds): Emergency Medicine: Concepts and Clinical Practice, ed 2. CV Mosby, St. Louis, 1988, pp 1605–1611.

Pritchard JA, et al.: Williams Obstetrics, ed. 17. Appleton-Century-Crofts, New York, 1985.

Scott V: Complications of Pregnancy. In Rosen P and Barkin RM (eds): Emergency Medicine: Concepts and Clinical Practice, ed 2. CV Mosby, St. Louis, 1988, pp 1581–1589.

Notes

CHAPTER 45

Wheezing
Deepi Goyal, MD

Presentation

A wheeze is an abnormally high-pitched sound produced by breathing through partially obstructed or narrowed airways. It is more prominent during exhalation and is associated with a prolonged expiratory phase. The wheezing patient may present in many different ways. In fact, the patient may not even complain of wheezing. Quite often, the patient may present with complaints of shortness of breath, cough, or chest tightness. Wheezing patients are often apprehensive and distressed. Their shortness of breath may be so severe that they may not be able to speak in complete sentences. Oxygenation may be compromised to the point that there is a decrease in the patient's level of consciousness. These signs are clues that the patient needs immediate and aggressive therapy. In evaluating the wheezing patient, it is always important to remember the adage that "all that wheezes are not asthma" (or COPD).

Immediate Concerns

- **What is the patient's state of oxygenation? Are they cyanotic?** Can they talk? Patients that are clearly hypoxic may exhibit symptoms including a decreased level of consciousness and cyanosis. A note of caution: the hypoxic patient may not be cyanotic. Cyanosis occurs when 5 mg% of hemoglobin is unsaturated. Therefore, the severely anemic patient may not be able to produce cyanosis and yet be quite hypoxic. Hypoxic patients need immediate and aggressive therapy, including supplemental oxygen, inhaled bronchodilators, and possibly, intubation.

Important History

- **Is there a history of wheezing in the past?** Patients who have had episodes of wheezing in the past may know if they have a history of asthma, COPD, or other respiratory disorders. It is important to determine the average duration of prior attacks and the therapy that has been effective in terminating these acute attacks. Furthermore, knowledge of the patient's ventilatory capacity between attacks can help determine the patient's baseline level of functioning, which can help in assessing the patient's response to therapy. For instance, if a patient normally has a poor level of pulmonary function between attacks, the endpoint of therapy will be different from the patient with a normal level of function between attacks. Does the patient have a previous history of intubation?

- **Is the patient taking any medications?** Certain medications (eg, beta blockers) can acutely precipitate asthmatic attacks. Furthermore, the patient's medications, such as metered dose inhalers or cardiac medications, can provide clues to other medical problems and thus help to guide therapy.

- **Does the patient have any allergies?** A history of prior allergic reactions may indicate that the patient's symptoms are a manifestation of anaphylaxis.

Differential Diagnosis

- *Chronic Obstructive Pulmonary Disease.* Emphysema and chronic bronchitis account for a large percentage of EMS calls for shortness of breath. These patients will almost universally have a significant tobacco smoking history. Smoking leads to chronic damage to both the small and large airways, with most of the damage occurring in the large airways. These patients usually have a lowered baseline level of pulmonary function, as opposed to the patient with pure asthma who will return to a normal level of function between asthmatic attacks. Although emphysema and chronic bronchitis are categorized as entirely different entities, there is often a component of both disorders in the patient who presents with wheezing and shortness of breath. These patients often have a history of chronic cough, sputum production, and dyspnea on exertion. The classic case of a person with emphysema has the appearance of the "pink puffer," with rapid, shallow breathing through pursed lips, a thin body habitus with a barrel chest, and the use of accessory muscles of breathing. The classic case of a person with bronchitis has characteristics associated with the "blue bloater": they are cyanotic and overweight, with slow, deep, and labored breathing.

- *Asthma.* Asthma is characterized by a hypersensitivity of the tracheobronchial tree to a variety of stimuli, leading to bronchoconstriction, inflammation, and increased airway secretions.
- *Congestive Heart Failure.* This is often overlooked as a cause of wheezing, but wheezing may be the only sign of CHF. This diagnosis should be suspected in every middle-aged or older person who complains of wheezing, especially if there is also a history of heart disease.
- *Aspiration.* Persistent localized wheezing can suggest the diagnosis of foreign body aspiration, especially in individuals who may not protect their airways well. Foreign body aspiration, however, usually produces an obstruction of the upper airway and therefore is more likely to produce stridor than frank wheezing. Aspiration is more likely in young children and older, debilitated patients who cannot protect their airways.
- *Anaphylaxis.* Wheezing may be a manifestation of anaphylaxis, as histamine release and inflammation lead to narrowing of the airways. Usually, however, other clues are present to indicate an anaphylactic reaction, such as rash, edema, hypotension, and so forth.
- *Other Causes.* Pneumonia, pulmonary embolism, thoracic cage deformities, tuberculosis, and lung cancer are among the other causes of wheezing. Wheezing, however, is a less common manifestation of these disorders than those mentioned previously.

Key Physical Examination Findings

- *Initial Assessment.* Look for signs of shock or airway compromise. The use of accessory muscles to breathe or the inability to speak in complete sentences secondary to shortness of breath indicates that the patient's respiratory status is in jeopardy.
- *Vital Signs.* Monitor respirations and pulse. The respiratory rate is usually increased. Tachycardia is often prominent if cardiac output must be increased to compensate for decreased oxygenation.

- *Peak Expiratory Flow Rate.* Measure peak expiratory flow rate (PEFR). The PEFR provides the only objective measurement of the degree of airway obstruction and can be used to follow the patient's progress. It does depend on the patient's technique and efforts; therefore, the patient must be coached in its use and encouraged to give their best effort.
- *Neck.* Look for distended neck veins as an indicator for CHF or possible pulmonary embolism.
- *Chest.* Listen to the nature and character of the breath sounds. Beware, you may be fooled into a sense of security by a previously noisy chest that becomes quiet. Often this is a sign of impending doom as the patient becomes fatigued and cannot generate enough airflow to create wheezes. This is an indication that the patient is rapidly deteriorating and that steps should be taken immediately to prevent loss of the airway.
- *Accessory Muscles.* The use of the neck muscles and chest wall muscles are a sign that the work of breathing is too great for the diaphragm alone. Abdominal breathing is an even later sign, which indicates that the patient is beginning to tire. The energy required to breathe in this manner is great, and once fatigue sets in, the patient will no longer be able to compensate for the extra airway resistance.
- *Extremities.* Check for signs of peripheral edema. Peripheral edema is a sign of heart disease and should make you suspicious that the patient's wheezing may be due to CHF. Right heart failure is common in advanced lung disease (cor pulmonale). Clubbing of the fingers is an indication of longstanding hypoxia.

Treatment Plan

- *Patient Assessment.* Reassess the patient frequently for both response to therapy and for signs of further deterioration. The patient may need assisted ventilations with a bag-valve-mask or even require intubation. The fatigued-appearing patient warrants early intervention.
- Administer O_2 either via nasal cannula, face mask, or bag-valve-mask, depending on the patient's degree of respiratory compromise. A pulse oximeter may be very useful in determining the patient's O_2 saturation.

- Establish **IV access**, as it may be necessary for the administration of medications.
- *Medications.* For the treatment of asthma or COPD, give nebulized beta agonists, such as albuterol or metaproterenol sulfate (Alupent) back to back until the patient's status improves. Steroids are not used often in the field as their benefits take several hours to manifest themselves and they may actually worsen some conditions that may mimic asthma. If there is evidence of CHF, sublingual nitroglycerin, furosimide (Lasix), and morphine may be indicated. The following agents are most commonly used to treat bronchospasm:

  Albuterol, 2.5 mg in 3 ml 0.9% NaCl via nebulizer (pediatric dose: age younger than 12 years, one half of the adult dose (1.25 mg); age older than 12 years, use full adult dosing). Dose may be repeated every 6 hours; however, in cases of severe bronchospasm it may be given as frequently as back to back. Other beta agonists such as metaproterenol, isoproterenol, or isoetharine (Bronkohsol) may be considered.

  NOTE: More frequent dosing may result in a greater incidence of side effects.

  Epinephrine (1:1000), 0.3 to 0.5 mg SC injection (pediatric dose: 0.01 mg/kg, not to exceed 0.5 mg per dose). Dose may be repeated every 20 minutes.

  Aminophylline loading dose 5 to 6 mg/kg IV infusion over 20 to 30 minutes (pediatric dose: 6 mg/kg IV infusion over 20 to 30 minutes). This dosage may be used in patients who are not currently using aminophylline or theophylline. For patients using a theophylline or aminophylline agent, this loading dose should be reduced by one half (2.5 to 3.0 mg/kg).

- **Transport expeditiously to an appropriate ED.** Do not delay patient transport needlessly—expedite transport. A delay in transport may hinder further diagnostic and therapeutic maneuvers. Ensure patient comfort en route.

Bibliography

Cooper KR: Wheezing. In Glauser FL (ed): Signs and Symptoms in Pulmonary Medicine. JB Lippincott, Philadelphia, 1983, pp 43–52.

Fanta CH: Symptoms and Signs of Respiratory Disorders. In May HL, Aghababian RV, and Fleisher GR (eds): Emergency Medicine, ed 2. Little, Brown & Co, Boston, 1992, pp 115–118.

Montenegro HD and Cherniak NS: Chronic Obstructive Pulmonary Disease. In Callaham ML (ed): Current Practice of Emergency Medicine, ed 2. B.C. Decker, Philadelphia, 1991, pp 407–409.

Tokarski GF and Nowak RM: Adult Asthma. In Callaham ML (ed): Current Practice of Emergency Medicine, ed 2: B.C. Decker, Philadelphia, 1991, pp 402–407.

Vargas J: Chronic Obstructive Pulmonary Disease. In Schwartz GR (ed): Principles and Practice of Emergency Medicine, ed 3. Lea and Febiger, Philadelphia, 1992, pp 1476–1482.

Notes

SECTION II

*Special
Situations*

CHAPTER 46

Advance Directives for Health Care

Thomas J. Rahilly, MS, EMT-CC

In the increasingly complex world of medicine, it is becoming more common for individual states to allow its residents to make informed decisions regarding their health care in advance of the need to do so. The need to make such decisions can be the result of a current serious illness or injury with a poor prognosis for recovery. In this case, the individual may assign their medical treatment decision-making authority to someone they trust. Advance directives may also be written by those who prefer to have their treatment decisions made by someone they trust, should they suffer a catastrophic illness or injury at some time in the future.

There are three main types of advance directives: do not resuscitate (DNR) orders, living wills, and health care proxies. Although not all states have approved legislation allowing these documents, they are becoming more prevalent. It can be expected that prehospital healthcare providers will begin to encounter these directives in the near future.

Do Not Resuscitate Order

A DNR order, which requires that resuscitative measures not be instituted when the patient expires, is issued by a physician at the request of the patient or by the patient's legally authorized representative. The DNR order is a written directive that must be signed by the attending physician and, in most states, honored by the EMS providers if they do not have a valid reason to disregard it. A few states have developed standardized DNR forms as well as DNR bracelets. These items must clearly identify the individual patient and must not have exceeded the expiration date if applicable.

Do not resuscitate orders are not generally considered legal authority for withholding other medical treatment, such as the administration of oxygen and other life-sustaining measures. In the absence of a valid form of documentation indicating that the patient has specifically requested not to be resuscitated, the EMS provider must follow the standard of care as stated in statute and/or provided by medical control policies through prehospital protocols.

Living Wills

A living will is a legal document that adults may, while in a competent state of mind, use to express their wishes regarding their future health care. The living will can be used to stipulate their desire for certain life-sustaining medical treatments. In many cases, however, the persons who authorize a living will want to make clear their objection to unwanted medical interventions while they still have the capacity for such decisions. The living will is most often intended to apply to situations where the person would suffer an illness or injury that results in a terminal condition accompanied by a permanent state of unconsciousness. It could also apply to those situations where the person could maintain consciousness, but damage to the brain would be so severe that an expression of wishes regarding treatment cannot be made.

Health Care Proxy

A healthcare proxy is another mechanism whereby persons are able to decide what health care they will receive during a period in which they are incapacitated. By appointing a health-care proxy (in writing), a person transfers the authority for informed consent to another person who has the best interests of the patient in mind. Healthcare providers will often look to family members for guidance when a person is too sick to make an informed decision about their health. But family members are not usually permitted to withhold or stop treatment. The line of authority may be complete or specific to a certain treatment that is to be administered or withheld. The healthcare proxy may receive detailed instructions to be followed in the event of a temporary loss of decision-making ability, such as during surgery. Unlike a living will, a healthcare proxy agreement does not require that all of the decisions be made in advance. Unless otherwise specified, the healthcare proxy may interpret the medical circumstances surrounding a particular healthcare situation and make decisions accordingly. In other words, the proxy may make decisions as the patient's condition either improves or deteriorates.

As is the case with most healthcare issues, there is no universal acceptance of the healthcare proxy as a legal document in the prehospital EMS environment. Each provider must be familiar with all of the regulations associated with not only advance directives, but also each of the medicolegal requirements of their states and local jurisdictions.

Notes

CHAPTER 47

Critical Incident Stress
Thomas J. Rahilly, MS, EMT-CC

The providers of emergency services are not born psychologically iron-clad human beings who can walk among the worst events of society and have their psyches remain intact forever. In addition, there is no reason to believe that the way to condition the human spirit to adversity is to constantly expose a person to human tragedy, suffering, and death. To the credit of the many healthcare professionals who have taken an interest in the stress experienced by the providers of emergency services, the psychological well-being of the EMS provider is being recognized and addressed.

Stress has finally become a recognized problem in the American workplace and has found a niche in the field of occupational medicine. We are bombarded with seemingly never-ending tales of work-related events that have pushed employees to vent their frustrations through overt acts of violent behavior. Of course, these events are only the most severe manifestations of stress in the workplace, and it can be safely stated that they represent only a fraction of the real problem. The occupational stress of EMS workers is more covert and is often exhibited by changes in personality, substance abuse, failures within the family setting, and a premature departure from EMS.

The stress experienced by the emergency responder has the potential to be managed effectively. As with the other areas of personal health and safety, stress management is a shared responsibility between the providers of service and their employers. The management of the day-to-day stressors affecting the emergency medical provider can be accomplished by many of the same methods used for other occupations. Although often considered a special breed of person, EMS providers are still part of mainstream society and are subject to the same environmental and psychological stressors as their friends and neighbors. When it comes to job-related stress, however, there is a marked difference between the emergency service provider and all others. This special classification of stress, caused by a critical incident, requires a special type of mental health care. That care is most appropriately provided by professionals trained in critical incident stress management.

A moderate amount of stress can be helpful and productive for the person experiencing it. The reactions to stress are usually comparable to the level of stress. That is, a situation that produces a mild amount of stress will most likely result in a mild reaction. But as the level of stress rises, there will generally be a corresponding increase in the intensity of the response. Fortunately, most people exhibit a variety of signs and symptoms associated with stress of high intensity. It is essential that emergency service providers learn to recognize these warnings signs, in both themselves and their coworkers. It is equally important that there be a mechanism to provide relief from this stress. Through counseling and treatment, help must be made available to the providers so that they may recover their mental health as soon as possible.

Critical Incidents

It would be helpful to identify those incidents that have the potential to cause an inordinate amount of stress. They do not occur everyday in each community, and it is possible that an EMS provider may complete an entire career without ever experiencing a critical incident. For the most part, critical incidents are unpredictable and give no early warning signs. Among those that can be classified as critical incidents are an on-the-job death or serious injury to an emergency worker, treating a seriously ill or injured loved one or friend, the suicide of a fellow worker, a disaster or multi-casualty incident, death or severe illness or injury involving a child, and death or severe injury to a civilian as the result of an emergency response.

It should be noted that the definition of a critical incident is open-ended. That which is critical to one responder may not be to another. Studies have shown that an overwhelming majority of emergency workers have experienced an acute stress reaction after one of the situations mentioned previously. Therefore, if an incident produces stress in one EMS provider, the others present at the scene will probably feel at least some amount of stress also. Do not forget to consider the support personnel associated with the event such as supervisors and dispatchers.

Indicators of Critical Incident Stress

Critical incident stress exists when the stressors of an event overcome the coping mechanisms of the individual. This level of stress can also be produced by the cumulative effects of a series of other, less taxing incidents. It can also occur as the result of job-related stressors in combination with the environmental and psychological stressors experienced at home and in other non–work-related situations. In each of these situations, the indicators of stress will be physical as well as emotional in nature. Usually a variety of indicators are present at one time, and they can reveal themselves in any combination.

The most commonly reported physical abnormality is sleep disturbance. Some people who suffer from the effects of high-level stress will have dreams that are upsetting or wake them during the sleep cycle. Other physical signs should be quite familiar to the EMS provider. These include chest pain, difficulty breathing, nausea and vomiting, elevated blood pressure, and a general feeling of fatigue or even exhaustion. Any noticeable change in the provider's physical condition may be related to an inability to cope with the amount of stress to which they have been subjected. These signs are the body's ways of telling the individual that something is wrong and there is a need to obtain a medical evaluation and follow-up care.

The emotional signs of critical incident stress may be somewhat more difficult for the person under stress to recognize. These changes are closely associated with those in behavior and cognitive reasoning ability. All of the signs are too numerous to list in this section, and further readings are provided in the references at the end of the chapter. However, those that are most serious and that pose the greatest danger to the provider and patient include emotional states of panic or shock that may result in a loss of control or an inappropriate response to a particular stimulus. Overreactions to an otherwise stable situation may place the emergency workers and the patients in a compromised position and produce an unwanted outcome. It is possible for those with untreated stress disorders to "lose their edge" and become less sensitive to their surroundings. This can bring about delayed, inappropriate, or incorrect decisions that are contrary to accepted protocols and procedures. Left uncorrected, these actions place everyone at the emergency scene at risk for injury or even death.

Too often, EMS providers attempt to rationalize these changes in their physical or mental health brought on by excessive stress. Denial is just another of the factors influencing the providers reaction to the stress condition. Emergency service workers often develop a "macho" attitude that inhibits their ability to realize that they could possibly be suffering from something as abstract as stress. This is why it is so important for the entire "family" of emergency service providers to understand the pattern of behavioral changes that indicate one of their own is in trouble. This includes coworkers, supervisors, and significant others who are most able to note the changes that may not be as obvious to the casual observer or the individuals themselves.

Be Proactive

To be effective, stress management programs must be in place before the need for them arises. There are those areas of the country that are fortunate enough to have sufficient resources for programs staffed by current or former emergency providers. These programs are usually more effective at encouraging responders to view stress management as a form of help and not as an occupational stigma that singles them out as someone who "can't take it." There are also many programs that take advantage of the mental health professionals that serve the community at large. Critical incident stress debriefing teams are often a combination of these two resources and have proven their worth repeatedly.

Regardless of the provider of the service, stress management programs will be of little assistance if the EMS provider is reluctant to accept this form of help. Continuing education programs are an excellent forum for providing information on job-related stress and its management. If providers know in advance that their reaction to the events of a highly stressful vocation or avocation is not abnormal, they will be more willing to seek and accept the benefits that can come from participation in occupational health and safety programs.

Bibliography

Federal Emergency Management Agency, United States Fire Administration: Developing Stress Management Programs for Emergency Medical Services, USFA, Washington, DC, 1991.

Mitchell JT and Bray GP: Emergency Services Stress. Prentice-Hall, Englewood Cliffs, NJ, 1990.

Notes

CHAPTER 48

Exposure to Infectious Diseases

Thomas J. Rahilly, MS, EMT-CC

For many years the dangers associated with responding to emergencies were considered occupational hazards that came with the job. As federal and state labor departments continued to enact legislation to make the American workplace safer, the emergency service providers were, for the most part, left to work in an increasingly dangerous work environment without any regulation. To make matters worse, the emergency workers seemed to accept this as part of their working conditions. There was a certain mystique surrounding the life of the providers of emergency services. Most of these individuals could hardly think of the communities they served as workplaces, especially the volunteer providers.

It was not until the early 1980s that any concerted effort was made to improve the health and safety of emergency service responders. The National Fire Protection Association (NFPA) along with the US Fire Administration began to study the deplorable injury and death statistics of the fire service. It became apparent that if the firefighters of this country, and indeed all emergency service providers, were going to have a safer work environment, it would have to be brought about by legislation and regulation.

In 1970, Congress authorized the establishment of the Occupational Safety and Health Administration (OSHA). Assigned to the US Department of Labor, OSHA began promulgating standards designed to reduce injury and death in the workplace. Among the hazards identified as potentially harmful to healthcare workers, in particular, was communicable infectious disease. Although almost every hospital in the country was practicing some form of infection control, there was no uniform standard used by the healthcare industry. OSHA began the process of standardizing infection control by issuing a document entitled "Advance Notice of Proposed Rulemaking for Bloodborne Pathogens" on November 27, 1987. From this date on, many other agencies, organizations, and individuals began to address the problem in a variety of ways. OSHA completed their rulemaking process when, on December 6, 1991, it issued Final Rule 29 CFR 1910.1030, Occupational Exposure to Bloodborne Pathogens. The standard became effective March 6, 1992. The standard for airborne pathogens will be in effect when this book is published.

The exposure to disease has always been a hazard to humans. There have been a number of devastating diseases over the course of time that have been carefully recorded by historians. As the 20th century comes to an end, there are several diseases, both airborne and bloodborne, that may be included in the worst ever contracted by man. Hepatitis B virus, human immunodeficiency virus, and tuberculosis are serious threats to the health of the general population and especially that of healthcare workers.

Prehospital emergency medical service (EMS) providers comprise a segment of the healthcare field that are especially susceptible to acquiring an occupational exposure to disease. The prehospital area is more dangerous than that of other healthcare work environments because the worker has little, if any, control over the workplace where the health care is delivered. EMS workers often find themselves in unfamiliar surroundings that were never specifically meant to be places where health care was delivered. Motor vehicle and industrial accident sites as well as the homes, offices, and even the streets where people experience events that lead to the need for emergency medical assistance all pose a danger for the emergency medical technician. Unlike other areas where emergency medical care takes place, such as the emergency departments of hospitals, there is usually limited or no control of environmental conditions such as light, temperature, and the engineering controls that may reduce the potential exposure to communicable disease.

Having read the previous paragraph, you may feel that the acquisition of a communicable disease is only a matter of time. This, however, is not true. By implementing a comprehensive infection control program, EMS and first responder agencies can greatly improve the chances that their employees (including volunteers) can remain safe in their workplace. The establishment of an effective health maintenance system, the development of an objective-based training program, and the routine use of appropriate personal protective equipment can provide a high level of protection for the EMS worker. Although the potential for infection will always be present, the risk of becoming occupationally exposed to a communicable disease can be minimized.

Governmental agencies such as OSHA and state departments of labor require employers in the broad spectrum known as the "healthcare industry" to develop and maintain an exposure control plan for the protection of its employees. Most of these agencies—including OSHA—specify a plan that protects against bloodborne pathogens. The components of an effective plan, however, will provide protection from all pathogens. At a minimum, such a plan will include policies for:

- Health maintenance
- Personal protective equipment
- Incident operations and recovery
- Postexposure
- Equipment disinfection and storage

To prevent the spread of infection in the prehospital field, EMS providers must develop a proactive attitude. The procedures needed to reduce the risk of acquiring an infectious disease are known as body substance isolation (BSI). Those who practice BSI consider the blood, body fluids, and tissues of all patients to be infectious. This differs from the "universal precautions" infection control strategy used by most hospitals, which considers only blood and *certain* body fluids to be potentially infectious. Universal precautions were designed for the controlled environment of a healthcare facility and will not provide the level of protection afforded by BSI. BSI requires those emergency service personnel who have the potential to come in contact with a patient to place a barrier between themselves and the potentially infectious materials found at every emergency medical incident. By using barrier protection, or personal protective equipment, the responders isolate their skin and mucous membranes from contact with the potentially infectious materials. The only exceptions to using of barrier protection are when the use of personal protective equipment interferes with the proper delivery of healthcare or when such equipment poses a significant risk to the personal safety of the responder or a coworker. These cases are considered extraordinary situations and the decision not to use personal protection rests solely with the emergency service providers, not their employers.

At a minimum, BSI requires the use of disposable gloves. They should be donned prior to any patient contact, worn until all patient care and cleanup activities are complete, and disposed of according to the response agency's written policy. There must also be written policies that indicate when masks, protective eyewear, gowns, and other forms of personal protection must be worn. Training programs that inform emergency providers about the use of these devices must be included in the agency's exposure control plan.

All emergency service providers are at risk for acquiring an infectious disease while providing healthcare. They may, however, provide a high degree of personal protection by maintaining their health, practicing BSI, and ensuring that their patient care equipment and transport vehicles are kept free from potentially infectious materials.

Bibliography

National Association of Emergency Medical Technicians: NAEMT Emergency Management Committee's Report on Infection and Infection Control. NAEMT, Kansas City, MO, 1987.

National Fire Protection Association: NFPA 1581: Standard on Fire Department Infection Control Program. NFPA, Quincy, MA,1990.

US Fire Administration: Infection Control for Emergency Response Personnel: The Supervisor's Role. USFA, National Fire Academy, Emmitsburg, MD, September, 1992.

West K: Infectious Disease Handbook for Emergency Care Personnel. JB Lippincott, Philadelphia, 1987.

Notes

CHAPTER 49

The Fire Scene

Thomas J. Rahilly, MS, EMT-CC

In many communities, the fire department is also the provider of emergency medical services. This means that when responding to a fire call, the ambulance personnel are under the direct control of the chief fire officer and are fully integrated into the department's response plan. The ambulance usually accompanies the fire apparatus. Firefighter/emergency medical technicians (EMTs), or other fire-medic personnel, perform specific tasks on the fire scene that are delineated in the fire department's standard operating procedures. Not all emergency medical services (EMS), however, are provided by the fire service. In fact, there are a great many areas where the provider of EMS may serve a region that is protected by several different fire departments. Because a chance exists that there may either be an injured person at the fire scene as a result of the fire or that one of the firefighters could be injured during the firefighting operation, ambulances are generally dispatched to the scene of a fire. It is, therefore, imperative that EMS responders know exactly what their responsibilities are at the scene of a fire.

Over the past several years, a massive national effort has been underway to organize more effectively the response of the emergency services. For the most part, the fire service has been the leader in a move to establish a system whereby the scene of an emergency is managed in a coordinated manner. The incident command system (ICS), when properly implemented, assigns areas of responsibility according to the task being performed. These responsibilities are assigned to sectors with an officer in charge who reports to a single incident commander. The desired effect of this system is to reduce the amount of "freelancing" by the various agencies that may become involved during a fire or other multiagency response. ICS provides more efficient use of resources, reduces personal risk, and improves on-scene communication.

All EMS responders, whether fire or third service, must report to the incident commander on arrival at the scene of a fire or other emergency where the chief fire officer has been placed in charge. In communities where there is an integrated approach to emergency management, each response organization has knowledge of its specific responsibility within the system. The ICS identifies EMS as a separate sector, and an officer, preferably from EMS will be assigned as the sector commander. Under this system all emergency medical providers must report to the sector commander on arrival at the emergency scene. From this point, personnel can be assigned to activities in the order of highest priority. There may be a need for the treatment of fire victims and firefighters, or EMS responders may be needed to staff the rehabilitation sector, where emergency workers are evaluated and monitored for any negative physiologic effects resulting from the operation.

In the event a community has not implemented an emergency incident management system, or if the ambulance arrives before the fire department, EMS personnel should not undertake firefighting operations on their own. This includes the entering of structures that are on fire or those that appear to be emitting smoke. Untrained or poorly equipped persons who attempt to gain entry to a fire building not only risk personal injury to themselves, they place an added burden on firefighters who now must consider them to be potential victims. This may actually delay the rescue of the building's occupants. Additionally, the EMS responders will be needed to treat any victims who are rescued from the building. If they become injured themselves, they only add to the problem at hand.

It is not uncommon for an ambulance to come on a structure that is on fire or arrive before the firefighters. The EMS responders first action must be to notify the fire department. Do not rely on reports at the scene that the fire department has already been called. Advise the EMS dispatcher to make a separate notification. The EMS responders next action should be to alert the occupants of the building from a position of personal safety. The use of the ambulance public address system and siren are a particularly effective means of accomplishing this. Once again, without the proper training and personal protective equipment, EMS personnel should not enter a burning building.

Bibliography

International Fire Training Association: Essentials of Firefighting. Stillwater, OK, International Fire Training Association, 1992.
National Fire Protection Association: NFPA 1500: Standard for Fire Fighter Health and Safety, Batterymarch Park, MA, NFPA, 1992.

Notes

CHAPTER 50

The Hazardous Materials Incident

Thomas J. Rahilly, MS, EMT-CC

Everyday millions of pounds of hazardous materials are produced, transported, stored, and used worldwide to support modern technology. Considering the number of industries that are using substances that are potentially harmful to humans and the environment, there are surprisingly few accidents. But they do occur and will continue to place workers and the public in danger. As is the case in just about every other emergency incident, an emergency medical service (EMS) response will be necessary either to help mitigate the problem or provide support services to those who must confine and control the situation.

When called to the scene of a hazardous materials (hazmat) incident, emergency service workers must take a more conservative approach to the operation than they would at another type of incident. The danger to the responders are great, and many of them are not very obvious. Hazardous material incidents should not be considered routine, as the use of day-to-day procedures can result in longer exposure for the victims and contamination of ambulance and emergency department personnel and equipment. The Occupational Safety and Health Administration (OSHA) requires all emergency service personnel who respond to emergencies as first responders to complete a hazardous materials awareness training course. This course is the first step in recognizing the inherent dangers associated with hazardous materials incident response. It does not, however, prepare the emergency worker to mitigate the problem or to treat victims associated with these emergencies.

The Incident Command System

Any emergency response organization that may be called to the scene of a hazardous materials incident should have an operational plan that has been developed in cooperation with the other agencies that will also be on the scene. The use of the incident command system (ICS) will help to ensure a coordinated approach to a situation that is as dangerous to the responders as it is to the victims. Responding EMS units should report to the incident commander and follow the directions of the command post.

An effective hazardous materials operation managed by ICS will have zones established to identify the areas that pose a danger to victims of the incident as well as to the emergency responders. The "hot zone" is the area that actually contains the material that has caused the event. Depending on the material involved and the atmospheric conditions present or expected, this zone will vary in size. No responders may enter this area unless they are expressly ordered to do so by the command post, and then, only if they are currently certified to work there. Activity in the hot zone requires special equipment and training. Independent actions by unauthorized persons may result in injury or death and will, most often, endanger the safety of the other emergency responders.

The "warm zone" is that area immediately surrounding the hot zone. This is where such activities as patient and hazardous materials technician decontamination is accomplished. Once again, if responders are not adequately trained and protected, entry to this zone is restricted. Perimeter identification and control are essential to ensure that unwary responders do not inadvertently enter a dangerous area of the incident.

The "cold zone" is established well beyond the area of potential danger. It is here that all of the support functions, such as the provision of emergency medical services, occurs. The "cold zone" contains the command post, EMS sector, and staging areas for additional resources. Incoming EMS units should receive direction from the command post before their arrival whenever possible. Preplanning and multiagency training drills help to avoid the confusion associated with multiagency emergency response when these agencies do not normally work with each other on a day-to-day basis.

The Emergency Medical Services Sector

The EMS, or medical, sector of the ICS has several important functions. Depending on the other resources available, they may include medical surveillance of the hazardous materials response team, the decontamination of victims, and their treatment and transport to an appropriate medical facility. Rarely will EMS providers be part of the hazardous materials team, which is responsible for rescuing victims or controlling the release of the material. A well-designed hazardous materials plan will assign the following responsibilities to the EMS sector:

- *Medical Surveillance of the Hazardous Materials Team.* Members of the hazardous materials team are frequently placed under severe physical stress due to the effects of the personal protection equipment that must be used to protect them from the hazardous materials present. EMS personnel should be present to establish baseline vital signs of the team before the commencement of their operations. All members of the team should be monitored after the completion of their duties to ensure that they have not been adversely affected by either the stress of the incident or the hazardous materials themselves. Complete documentation is essential for the protection of the team's future health benefits.

- *Decontamination of Patients.* Although many hazardous materials response teams are trained and equipped to handle this task, there may be a need in certain jurisdictions for the EMS sector to assume this responsibility. When developing the overall response plan, the emergency management staff must determine which agency will be given the resources and training to properly perform patient decontamination. There are hazardous materials plans that identify decontamination as a separate sector. Regardless of which agency or organization is charged with the responsibility of decontaminating patients exposed to hazardous substances, proper training and equipment are necessary if the decontamination process is to be successful. During decontamination, victims should be decontaminated in the "warm zone."

- *Treatment of Patients.* After each patient has been decontaminated, they must receive a thorough evaluation and treatment according to the presenting problem, with consideration given to the substance involved. Before any patient contact, EMS personnel should don the appropriate personal protective equipment. Use extreme caution during patient care as incomplete decontamination may result in personal injury to the caregiver.

Because most chemical emergencies will adversely affect the respiratory system of those victims exposed, basic life support is a priority. Immediate attention must be given to protecting the airway with ventilatory assistance as appropriate. Information about the treatment of specific injuries from substances identified by the hazardous materials technicians may be found in the US Department of Transportation (DOT) *Hazardous Materials Response Guidebook*. This reference is updated periodically and often contains the method for neutralizing the substance. All EMS vehicles should have a copy of the DOT guidebook, which is available from the US Government Printing Office.

Whenever possible, labels used to identify the material should be brought to the emergency department to assist the physician in treating the patient. If material safety data sheets (MSDS) are available, copies of these documents will also be useful in the evaluation and treatment of the patient. Because all entities that use or store hazardous materials must disclose their use to the agency responsible for hazardous materials, it might prove helpful to provide the medical facility with copies of the disclosure documents before an emergency.

- *Transport of Patients.* After treatment and packaging of the patients is complete, they should be transported to the closest appropriate medical facility. Before placing a patient who has been exposed to hazardous materials in the ambulance, it may be necessary to remove nonessential equipment and supplies to keep them from potential contamination. In addition, it may be prudent to drape the inside of the patient compartment with a plastic sheet to help protect the interior of the ambulance. Seal off the opening to the driver's compartment as well if there is such an opening.

Because not all medical facilities are staffed with appropriately trained personnel or equipped to handle victims of a hazardous materials incident, preplanning is essential to a successful outcome for the victims. Medical facilities identified as prepared and willing to receive patients exposed to hazardous materials must be included in the planning process and involved in training drills to increase the likelihood that they will maintain a high level of readiness. Notification from the command post will help the medical facility prepare itself and its personnel for the arrival of a patient that may pose a danger to the other people in the facility.

The nature of emergency response is becoming more complex and, if not adequately planned, may be cause for injury or death to those called on to control the incident. EMS providers must be prepared to assume their role in the overall response to hazardous materials incidents. Training, personal protective equipment, and most of all, self-discipline, are the fundamental components of a plan that will help to ensure that the rescuers will not become victims themselves.

Bibliography

Cashman JR: Hazardous Materials Emergencies: Response and Control, ed 2. Lancaster, PA, 1988.

Stutz DR, Ricks RS, and Olsen MF: Hazardous Materials Injuries. Bradford Communication, Greenbelt, MD, 1982.

Notes

CHAPTER 51

Interpreting the 12-Lead Electrocardiogram

David R. Adamovich, EdD, FACSM, EMT-P

A September 1993 emergency medical services journal ran an advertisement for a 12-lead electrocardiograph defibrillator with computerized interpretation. This is an example of the state-of-the-art in paramedicine. The idea of viewing standard lead II for rhythm (ie, normal sinus, atrial fibrillation, ventricular tachycardia) will soon be something of the past. With the advancement of ECG from a single-lead to the full-component 12-lead system, the level of prehospital emergency medical services (EMS) training and expertise is about to take another major step forward into the realm of technologic sophistication.

The format of this book calls for you to make a differential diagnosis based on answers to a series of thought-provoking questions related to a specific disorder. Essential to making the correct differential diagnosis is the ability to sort out this information and move through a hypothetical algorithm ultimately arriving at the most likely conclusion. The 12-lead ECG processes information in much the same way. The use of the 12-lead ECG enables you to view the larger picture by piecing together many more pieces of the puzzle, that is, 12 pieces versus the one obtained with conventional systems. Analysis of lead II allows for an occasional peek at the changes associated with an acute myocardial infarction (AMI). Adding the full complement of 12-leads permits a view of the entire myocardium: posterior, high lateral, low lateral, anterior, and septal views as well.

You should recognize the ECG for precisely what it is—a presentation of the electrophysiologic events of depolarization and repolarization. The best way to convey this message is to take a look at what happens electromechanical dissociation, a form of pulseless electrical activity (PEA). In EMD, a patient presents with what appears to be a normal-looking ECG image (ie, the normal looking PQRST at a normal RR interval), but no pulse.

With the addition of the 12-lead ECG you can add the full component of ECG interpretation to your diagnostic ability.

The 12-lead ECG uses 10 electrodes compared with the 4 used in conventional telemetry systems. Thus, in the three-lead telemetric system, standard leads I, II, and III, the electrodes placed at the right arm (shoulder), left arm, and left leg (hip) positions, enter the configuration process. (As a matter of academic interest, the axis component of a 12-lead ECG is slightly modified when the electrodes are placed at the shoulders and hips versus the standard position of wrists and ankles. This may be compensated for by placing the left arm electrode on the posterior of the trunk in a position comparable to that of its previous position on the anterior of the trunk.) The electrode placed on the right leg (hip) is for grounding purposes only. In 12-lead ECG nine electrodes enter the configuration process, and the right leg electrode is for grounding only.

The 12-lead configuration consists of three lead sets:
- Three bipolar: I, II, III (three leads with one negative and one positive electrode location)
- Three augmented unipolar: aVR, aVL, aVF (three leads with one positive electrode location)
- Six unipolar or precordial: V^1, V^2, V^3, V^4, V^5, V^6 (six leads with one positive electrode location)

Conventional single-lead telemetry focuses on standard lead II. This allows for visualization of leads I and III in the ambulance. Transmission of I and III is usually not permitted, however.

To best understand the differences between each of the lead sets, it is easiest to consider the examiner's view as though you are looking at the heart from the direction of the positive electrode. Thus, in leads I, II, and III you are viewing the heart from the left shoulder, left hip, and right shoulder, respectively. The difference between the last two views is that although they both look at the heart from the left hip, one looks toward the right shoulder and the other toward the left shoulder. The three augmented unipolar and six precordial leads act as "eyeballs" looking at the heart from the extremities, moving across the chest from precordial positions V^1 through V^6; moving laterally around the left ventricle.

Some key points to help you begin on the right foot:
- Always look in lead aVR. It should always be positioned downward (negative). If it is not, check for an error in limb

lead placement (ie, transposition of either the arm or leg electrode wire to the electrode). Lead aVR may appear upright (positive) in a patient with dextrocardia—a heart on the right side of their chest; but this is extremely rare and the patient usually knows about it.

- Check the calibration. It should always be at 1 mV/cm. The only reasons to change calibration to either 1/2 or 2X would be if precordial voltage is too high (eg, left ventricular hypertrophy) or too low (eg, in emphysema).

There are many ways of approaching 12-lead interpretation, perhaps as many ways as there are textbooks on the topic. Most anyone familiar with 12-lead interpretation will tell you they see "everything in one glance." They must, however, have started somewhere—one step at a time. One of the easiest ways to do that is to break interpretation into separate components. An example is to gather data or each of the following components:

- Rate
- Rhythm
- Axis
- Hypertrophy
- Infarction
- Electrolyte abnormalities

Once all the information is gathered, it is time to draw a conclusion, that is, to make a value judgment based on the available data. Thus, the differential diagnosis can be arrived at with the highest level of confidence.

Whereas axis, hypertrophy, and electrolyte abnormalities are of value in 12-lead interpretation, the most important aspects of field interpretation should focus on:

> rate—both atrial and ventricular as they can be
> different
>
> rhythm—there are 14 possible rhythms to identify
> infarction—acute versus healed

Rate does not usually have to be calculated because most ECG machines have a rate meter. On the other hand, rate may be calculated very accurately using the 300, 150, 100, 75, 60, 50 method. To calculate ventricular rate, start with any R wave (use the P wave for atrial rate) on a dark line (one of every five is dark) and begin counting dark lines until the next R wave is encountered. For example, if the next R wave falls on the 4th dark line, the ventricular rate equals 75 bpm. Complexes falling between dark lines are a simple matter of interpolation. For example, the complex determining rate that falls between dark lines identifying 150 and 100 would be evaluated in units of 10 as the difference between 150 and 100 equals 50. Fifty divided by the 5 boxes between dark lines is 10 beats per unit or line. Between 100 and 75, each line equals 5 bpm; between 75 and 60, each line equals 3 bpm.

To identify the inherent rhythm follow these steps: (1) evaluate the atrial and ventricular rates, (2) evaluate the P wave configuration in lead II, (3) establish the relationship between the number of P waves to the number of QRS complexes (ie, 1:1, 2:1, etc.), and (4) evaluate the configuration of the QRS complex. Table 51–1 identifies 14 inherent rhythms distinguishable from each other by four independent criteria: rate, P wave, P to QRS ratio, and QRS complex. For example, an atrial rate of 300 bpm with a ventricular rate of 60 bpm, showing upright P waves in lead II and having a normal width QRS complex, identifies atrial flutter. Each inherent rhythm possesses only one of all four criteria. Exceptions do exist where different ECG abnormalities appear identical on a rhythm strip (eg, supraventricular tachycardia mimicking ventricular tachycardia). This rarely becomes an issue except when incorrect differential diagnosis and subsequent pharmacologic intervention alter outcome.

Infarction is evaluated as either acute or healed. For the purpose of field interpretation an AMI may manifest either ST elevation or depression—in most cases elevation. Depression by itself is seen in angina. During an AMI, ST depression may be seen in those leads that are opposite to the site of the infarct (eg, in the inferior leads during an acute anterior wall myocardial infarction).

For the purpose of prehospital interpretation, the two major areas to search for ST elevation, the hallmark of an AMI, are in the inferior leads II, III, and aVF, and in the anteroseptal leads V^1 through V^3. It is these locations where most MIs occur. A healed MI, on the other hand, presents with scarred myocardium, causing "significant" Q waves in the same locations as previously described. A significant Q wave is defined as greater than 0.04 second (1 mm) or exceeding 25% of the total QRS complex, that is, if the Q wave exceeds 3 mm (0.03 mV) of a QRS complex with a total amplitude of 10 mm (1 mV).

Table 53-1. Characteristics of Selected Cardiac Arrhythmias

Rhythm	Atrial Rate	Ventricular Rate	P Wave in Lead II	P to QRS Ratio	QRS Morphology
Sinus bradycardia	<60	Equal	Upright	1 to 1	Normal width
Normal sinus rhythm	60–100	Equal	Upright	1 to 1	Normal width
Sinus tachycardia	>100	Equal	Upright	1 to 1	Normal width
Atrial tachycardia	120–150	Equal	Usually upright	1 to 1	Normal width
Atrial flutter	250–350	60–120*	Upright and spiked	4 or more:1	Normal width
Atrial fibrillation	>350	60–120*	Upright and irregular	Indeterminable	Normal width
Nodal rhythm†	40–60	Equal	Missing/downward	1 to 1 (if present)	Normal width
Accelerated nodal rhythm	60–100	Equal	Missing/downward	1 to 1 (if present)	Normal width
Nodal tachycardia	>100	Equal	Missing/downward	1 to 1 (if present)	Normal width
Ventricular rhythm†	xxx	<50	Missing	xxx	Wide/aberrant
Accelerated ventricular rhythm	xxx	50–1000	Missing	xxx	Wide/aberrant
Ventricular tachycardia	xxx	100–200	Missing	xxx	Wide/aberrant
Ventricular flutter	xxx	200–300	Missing	xxx	Wide/aberrant
Ventricular fibrillation	xxx	150–300	Missing	xxx	Wide/aberrant

* These values are approximate and show that a varying ventricular response is not unusual. In the case of atrial flutter, a fixed ventricular response is most frequent. In the case of atrial fibrillation, on the other hand, a varying ventricular response is both classic and a hallmark sign.

† These are the "truly" inherent rhythms occurring within the specialized conductive system of the heart. Atrial and ventricular rhythms such as tachycardia, flutter, and fibrillation are not "true" rhythms as they occur outside the normal conductive system.

Bibliography

Adamovich DR: The Heart: Fundamentals of Electrocardiography, Exercise Physiology and Exercise Stress Testing. Sports Medicine Books, East Moriches, NY, 1984.

Owen SG: Electrocardiography: A Programmed Text. Little, Brown & Co, Boston, 1973.

Rowlands DJ: Electrocardiography Pocket Book. Kluwer Academic Publishers, Norwell, MA, 1993.

Notes

CHAPTER 52

Multiple Casualty Incidents

John Fitzwilliam, BS, BA, EMT-CC

Statistics show that most advanced EMT experiences with multicasualty incidents (MCIs) are limited to motor vehicle accidents involving less than a dozen persons. Most paramedics spend their entire career without ever confronting a mass casualty disaster situation. Nevertheless, all paramedics and EMTs should be highly skilled in handling MCIs because of the potential for great loss of life. There are numerous definitions of an MCI. As a practical matter, we should understand that when the number of patients exceeds the number of rescuers, we must go into an MCI operations mode. Leadership, triage, rapid scene control, and intelligent resource utilization are the key elements to effective management of these situations.

Incident Command System (ICS)

Under the incident command system (ICS), one person, the incident commander (IC) is responsible for the overall management of the MCI. The IC delegates job assignments (sectorization) to the treatment sector, extrication (rescue) sector, staging sector, triage sector, supply sector or any other sectors, needed at a particular operation. Note that here a sector is a function, not necessarily a geographic location. The sector officer is the supervisor for that particular function. On-scene communications between sectors should occur primarily through sector officers, not through providers. This allows command personnel to have "the big picture," and to use their resources more efficiently. Personnel assigned to a specific task report to only one supervisor. ICS vastly improves efficiency and supervision. Its scope can be narrowed or expanded as needed for each MCI. Using ICS on a routine basis every day is good training. Different colored vests should be used to identify sector officers whenever possible.

Early On-Scene Operations

The first ambulance on the scene becomes the initial medical aid station, supply pool, and communications center. Do not let this ambulance drive off with the first victim. You will be stranded without any resources in the middle of chaos. These first arriving personnel will be the medical sector officers until relieved by later arriving officers. Their initial responsibilities include:

- Confirmation of the location
- Assessment of scene safety
- Sizing up the scene
- Establishing communications
- Triage
- Designation of a staging area and a central patient collection area
- Implementation of the ICS
- Implementation of the local MCI protocol

TRIAGE

Triage is the sorting of patients into categories based on the severity of their injuries and their potential for survival. The most medically experienced person should do the triaging. Most systems sort patients into three groups:

- Critical (RED)—Those who need immediate care or transportation;
- Serious (YELLOW)—Those who are urgent, but can wait up to 1 hour;
- Delayed (GREEN)—Those who are non-urgent and can wait over 1 hour. Deceased patients or those not expected to survive are often included in this last group.

Triage is an ongoing process, because patient conditions can change. Emergency medical personnel must try to do the most good for the most victims. A popular triage system is called "START" (simple triage and rapid treatment).

- On arrival at an MCI, tell anyone who can walk to move to a designated area. This immediately places them in a "delayed" category until triaged later.
- Now go to those patients left behind. Check their ventila-

tion. If no ventilations are present, position airway once. If still no ventilation, this patient is dead.
- If ventilation is present at rates over 30 breaths per minute, this patient is an immediate priority.
- If rate is less than 30 per minute, assess capillary refill. If capillary refill exceeds 2 seconds, this patient is an immediate priority.
- If capillary refill is less than 2 seconds (normal), proceed to assess mental status. If patient can follow simple commands, this patient is a delayed priority.
- If this patient cannot follow simple commands, this patient is categorized as an immediate priority.
- While triaging patients, do not start treatment. The only exceptions would be to attempt to open the airway once or put a pressure bandage on severely bleeding patients. Cardiopulmonary resuscitation (CPR) is not started during field triage.

The first arriving EMT or paramedic starts triage, not treatment. The use of triage tags is strongly recommended to provide an at-a-glance assessment of the patient's triage category, to speed documentation of medical care, and to track the condition and disposition of each patient at the scene.

STAGING AREA

The staging area should have good access and exit routes. Have police control traffic as soon as possible. Drivers should stay with ambulances (or at least have keys available). The staging area should be away from the actual incident but near enough to respond rapidly.

CENTRAL PATIENT COLLECTION POINT

The central patient collection point (often called the medical aid station or treatment sector) is a location where all triaged patients are taken for continuing care and to await disposition. It should be located close enough to the incident site to offer rapid care, yet far enough to offer protection from fire, smoke, explosion, hazardous material run-off, toxic fumes, leaking fire hoselines, vehicle exhaust, and so forth. It should be an area large enough to handle the anticipated number of casualties and then some. Consider uphill and upwind positioning, or place a fire engine between you and the threat. It is generally better to establish only one treatment area.

The most efficient means of moving patients is via backboards. Use non–EMS-trained personnel for patient transfer roles as much as possible. Use of a central patient collection point permits maximum utilization of rescuers and resources on hand. These EMS providers can function as a team and gain scene control rapidly. Whenever possible, advanced life support (ALS) trained personnel should perform ALS tasks; they should not be litter carriers or drivers.

The use of physicians at an MCI site is controversial. Many believe that doctors should stay at the hospital where they are more useful. Others say that on-scene physicians are valuable for making difficult triage decisions or performing advanced procedures on trapped victims.

Contact your Medical Control Communications Center (MEDCOM) early. This will allow local hospitals time to implement their MCI plans to be ready for the delivery of patients. MEDCOM contact with the scene, other than patient-specific on-line medical direction, should be through the medical sector commander only. Have MEDCOM determine individual hospital availability and treatment capability.

Do not overload the nearest hospital. This only moves the disaster from the field to the hospital. The patient's condition or chief complaint should be transmitted to MEDCOM for appropriate hospital destination assignments. Individual ambulances should not use the radio to contact MEDCOM during an MCI except for on-line medical direction.

ON-SCENE COMMUNICATIONS

Effectively managing communications at an MCI can be challenging. The radio communications system can easily be overwhelmed. The best communication on scene is "face-to-face." Do not hesitate to use messengers. The IC should have access to a portable radio from each agency at the MCI (if not, consider parking a fire chief's car, police car, ambulance, and so forth. together for coordinated radio coverage). Use plain English, not radio codes. Interjurisdictional operations make the use of codes confusing and, at times, dangerous. An MCI is not the time to experience mistaken messages.

Prevent open microphones at scene by placing the microphone

in its proper holder. Some people drop the microphone on a car seat or inadvertently depress the "push to talk" switch. One open microphone causes enormous frustration at the MCI. Proper radio procedure and frequency coordination is critical. Try to establish separate channels for administration, scene-to-hospital contact, and so forth. There should be no unnecessary transmissions; only talk when you have something important to say. In rural areas, consider involving amateur radio (ham) clubs in providing state-of-the-art communications assistance.

Hints For Increased Effectiveness

- Use red, yellow, or green plastic tarps, flags, or tape to indicate the treatment area.
- Have stocked disaster boxes available for rapid transport to scene. These can also be colored coded to indicate ALS or basic life support (BLS) supplies.
- Have a stockpile of backboards for MCIs. Take a 4×8 piece of 3/4-inch plywood. You can make two 2×6-inch boards and one 2×4-inch board (child) from each piece. You can have three boards if you make them 16 inches wide. Keep 25 or more at various locations with cravats.
- Have available some portable oxygen manifolds, a box of non-rebreather masks, and a large oxygen tank to treat the many patients requiring oxygen.
- Use worksheets to write everything down.
- Bring extra pencils, triage tags, writing paper, grease pencils, and portable radio batteries.
- Have colored sector officer vests widely available at any hour.
- Remove injured or emotionally distraught EMS providers and rescue workers from the scene immediately. The other EMS providers will not remain focused on their tasks if a fellow worker is suffering. It is also better for scene morale and control to remove injured children and hysterical persons as soon as possible.
- Have plans to protect patients from inclement weather. You might be able to move patients indoors to schools, shopping malls, barns, airplane hangars, or other structures. You can also bring shelter to the scene in the form of school buses, moving vans, or tractor trailer trucks.
- Have plans in place for situations in which there are not

sufficient ambulances available. Consider transporting via school bus. Place the wooden backboards over the seat tops and secure in place with cravats. Place several EMTs or paramedics on board with standard portable ambulance equipment and proceed to the hospital with police escort.

- Make arrangements to supply local maps to incoming units. Keep a resource book and the local Yellow Pages phone directory on hand to use as needed. If all else fails, do you have a quarter to make a phone call?

In conclusion, remember the six Ts of MCI operation:

- **Take charge**
- **Triage**
- **Treat**
- **Transport**
- **Terminate** (field and hospital emergency operation)
- **Talk** (critical incident stress debriefings)

When people are accustomed to following a procedure, that procedure becomes a habit. EMS personnel must develop good habits to successfully handle MCIs.

Bibliography

Auf der Heide E: Disaster Response: Preparation and Coordination. CV Mosby, St. Louis, 1989.

Butman AM: Responding to the Mass Casualty Incident: A Guide for EMS Personnel. Emergency Training, Westport, CT, 1981.

Notes

CHAPTER 53

Psychiatric Emergencies

Alan Cooper, MA, EMT-P
Owen T. Traynor, MD

Patients with a history of psychiatric illness can pose a challenge to the paramedics who have been called on to care for them. It is easy for the paramedic to focus on the abnormal behavior and fail to consider medical illness as a cause or exacerbation of underlying psychiatric illness. Some studies of inpatient and outpatient psychiatric patients have shown that between 5% and 30% of these patients have undiagnosed medical illness. Studies of patients who have been referred for emergency psychiatric evaluations have shown that between 3.5% and 16% also have undiagnosed medical illness. It is important, then, for the paramedic to develop a strategy for evaluating and caring for these patients.

The prehospital strategy involves these components: first, consider the safety of the patient, bystanders, and EMS workers; second, investigate and treat potential medical emergencies that may result in abnormal mental status or behavior; third, safely transport these patients to the appropriate emergency department (ED) for further evaluation and treatment; and finally, institute the appropriate procedures to forcibly retain the patient when indicated.

Safety is, of course, of paramount importance. Patients who are agitated, anxious, confused, or severely depressed may take actions that may be dangerous to themselves and others. A previous history of violent behavior may indicate a higher risk of future violent behavior. However, there is no good way to reliably predict someone's behavior. Clues to potential violent behavior include aggressive language and threats of violence. Steps should be taken, therefore, to minimize dangerous behavior. Knowledge of the dispatch information may alert you to a potentially dangerous situation awaiting at the scene. Police help should be actively sought when indicated. The police should help clear the patient of weapons. The area should be cleared of all nonessential people. Patients should be approached slowly,

311

in a non-threatening, compassionate manner. The goal is to keep the situation from escalating. You should position yourself near the room exit, so that a hasty exit may be made if necessary. The patient should be told that you are concerned about their safety and that you will provide a safe environment. If the patient appears dangerous and will not voluntarily consent to evaluation, treatment, and transport, physical or chemical restraint may be necessary. Local guidelines should be followed. Sometimes, a show of force, that is, the presence of several emergency personnel, may be all that is required to convince the patient to cooperate. Physical or chemical restraints should be a last resort and should be attempted only by those trained in their use.

Potential medical causes of abnormal behavior or altered mental status should be sought. These include hypoxia, hypovolemia, hypoglycemia, hypertensive encephalopathy, intoxication, poisoning, withdrawal syndrome, CNS infection, CNS trauma, intracranial hemorrhage, seizure disorder, and liver and renal failure. A thorough medical history, including a complete list of medications, both prescription and nonprescription medications, as well as a substance abuse history, should be obtained.

Although there are many psychiatric diagnoses, you should have familiarity with the following major psychiatric disorders: mood disorders, schizophrenic and delusional disorders, and anxiety disorders. The mood disorders, including major depression and bipolar or manic-depression, are the most prevalent psychiatric disorders, affecting up to 15% of the general population at some time in their lives. Major depression is defined as a persistent dysphoric or sad mood with loss of interest in normal activities, poor appetite, and sleep disturbances. The most significant complication of major depression is suicide. Suicide is the sixth leading cause of death in the United States. Therefore, it is recommended that depressed patients be evaluated for suicide risk.

Bipolar disorder, also known as manic-depressive disorder, is characterized by episodes of mania. These patients, when manic, may be euphoric, extremely energetic, and require little sleep. They frequently develop unrealistic plans, believe they possess special powers and abilities, often demonstrate poor judgment in spending money, and engage in promiscuous sexual behavior. This episodic disorder is characterized by periods of major depression. Complications include marital and occupational problems, substance abuse, and suicide.

Schizophrenia and delusional disorders are characterized by psychotic thinking, that is, difficulty in reality testing. These patients may have delusions and hallucinations. Delusions are fixed false beliefs. These beliefs will not be changed by facts to the contrary. Common delusions are paranoia and delusions of grandeur; that is, that the patient believes he or she has special powers or abilities.

Hallucinations are false perceptions; for example, the patient sees things that are not there or hears things others can not hear. In addition to auditory and visual hallucinations, the patient may have olfactory (smell), tactile, or gustatory (taste) hallucinations. Schizophrenia accounts for approximately one quarter of admissions to psychiatric hospitals. It is characterized by a gradual deterioration in functioning, delusions, hallucinations, and social withdrawal.

The anxiety disorders are characterized by fears, anxiety, apprehension, and increased sympathetic nervous system tone out of proportion to any real danger. The anxiety disorders include panic attacks, generalized anxiety disorder, phobias, and posttraumatic stress disorder.

Successful management of the psychiatric patient can be accomplished by following these suggestions:

- Look for and treat any possible medical causes before concluding that the patient's behavior is caused by a psychiatric illness.
- Demonstrate caring, compassion, and respect for the patient.
- Help protect the patient's privacy at the scene.
- Ensure the patient's safety.
- Approach the patient slowly and purposefully.
- Avoid any threatening actions.
- Do not talk down to the patient.
- Never lie to the patient or go along with their delusions.
- Use tact and firmness to persuade them to go to the hospital.

Bibliography

Coffman JA and Rund DA: Behavioral Disorders: Emergency Assessment and Stabilization. In Tintinalli JE, et al (eds): Emergency Medicine: A Comprehensive Study Guide, ed 3. McGraw-Hill, New York, 1992, pp 1074–1079.

Dubin WR: Disturbed Behavior: Functional and Organic Illnesses. In Harwood-Nuss A, et al.(eds): The Clinical Practice of Emergency Medicine. JB Lippincott, Philadelphia, 1991, pp 1157–1159.

Hockberger RS: Depression and Suicide. In Harwood-Nuss A, et al. (eds): The Clinical Practice of Emergency Medicine. JB Lippincott Philadelphia, 1991, pp 1159–1161.

Olson SC and Rund DA: Behavioral Disorders: Clinical Features. In Tintinalli JE, et al. (eds): Emergency Medicine: A Comprehensive Study Guide, ed 3. McGraw-Hill, New York, 1992, pp 1067–1073.

Shiener GA: The Agitated Acutely Psychotic, or Violent Patient. In Harwood-Nuss A, et al. (eds): The Clinical Practice of Emergency Medicine. JB Lippincott, Philadelphia, 1991, pp 1162–1164.

Notes

CHAPTER 54

The Pediatric Approach
Kemedy K. McQuillen, MD

The evaluation of the pediatric patient can be especially challenging because they differ significantly from adults in emotional development and physiologic function. In addition to being unable to communicate at a level that the adult caregiver can understand, they can be caught in a situation that they find terrifying, thereby limiting communication. What follows are general guidelines to approaching a pediatric patient in order to alleviate their fears while elucidating as much information as possible. Also included are signs and symptoms that are unique to children, which may give you important diagnostic information.

Approach

These guidelines apply to children who are aware of their surroundings. Children who are obtunded or rapidly deteriorating should be treated expeditiously to facilitate advanced care at an institution that can properly care for them .

General Guidelines

Remember that fear is often the limiting factor in the examination of a child. By keeping them comfortable, you will be able to clarify the situation more rapidly. Watch the child from a distance before approaching: Does the child smile? Does the child play? Whenever possible, allow the child to sit with or next to the parents. Because the child is more likely to talk to the guardian, have the guardian ask the questions. Start simple: what's the child's name; how old is the child; does the child go to school. If the child has a stuffed animal, do each part of the examination on the toy before you do it to the child. Most important, be honest and explain everything before you do it. If something is going to hurt, say so. Offer choices, and make the examination a game. "Do you want me to listen to your heart first, or your lungs first?" Do not ask to do something you have to do. If the child says "no," then you are stuck.

It may also be helpful to allow the child to touch the items you are going to use to examine or treat him or her if safe to do so. By permitting a child to hold the stethoscope for a few seconds, you may allay the fear that this is something that will hurt. It is also good practice to warm a cold stethoscope before placing it on the child's body.

Vital Signs

- Blood pressure is "a big hug on the arm." For kids older than two years of age, the normal systolic blood pressure is approximately 90 mm Hg plus 2 times the age in years, with a lower limit of 70 mm Hg plus 2 times the age in years.
- Temperature taking can be done by parents.
- Respiratory rate checks can usually be done visually from a distance.
  - Respiratory rate decreases with age: newborn, approximately 40, 1-year-old patient approximately 24 breaths per minute, 18-year-old patient approximately 18 breaths per minute.
  - Tachypnea is often the first sign of respiratory distress but can also be present with fever or anxiety.
- Heart rate decreases with age: infants approximately 120 to 150 bpm; toddlers approximately 100 to 120 bpm; school-aged approximately 90 to 100 bpm; teenagers approximately 70 to 90 bpm.
  - In general, heart rate increases in the earliest stages of shock, but in neonates the first response to hypoxia is bradycardia.
  - Tachypnea can also result from fever, anxiety, and excitement.

HEENT

- Offer a choice: "Should I look in your mouth or your eyes first?"
- Use keys or a toy (bears are the most popular) to track eye movement.
- To check for neck pain, or rigidity or, as it can be explained, a "tickle on the neck."

- In infants, check the fontanel (soft spot). Is it bulging or sunken?
  - Bulging fontanels may indicate rising intracranial pressure from various causes, such as head injury, meningitis, or hydrocephalus, or it may just be caused by crying.

Lungs

- Have mom or dad lift up or take off the child's shirt to watch respirations.
  - Does the child have retractions (intercostal, sternal, or supraclavicular)?
  - Does the child have paradoxical movement of the abdomen with respirations?
  - Is the child using accessory muscles? sitting forward? drooling?
- Let the child place the stethoscope on the chest, and listen for everything (heart rate, breath sounds, bowel sounds) wherever it lands.
  - Are breath sounds reduced or unequal?
  - Is there wheezing, stridor, or a prolonged expiratory phase?
  - Is the child grunting?
  - Have the child blow out a penlight to get good expirations.

Cardiac

- Distract child with a toy or medical instrument, or allow a baby to suck on a pacifier to get a quiet examination.
- Let the child listen to mom's heart before you listen to the child's.
- Tickle the feet or hands to evaluate temperature and capillary refill.
- Mucous membranes and nailbeds are good places to check for cyanosis.
  - Acrocyanosis (cyanosis of the hands and or feet) is normal in a newborn, and cutis mamorata (mottling of the legs) is normal in an infant.

Abdomen

- Use the stethoscope to push on the abdomen while listening.
- Tell the child you push on the belly to see if he or she is hungry.
- If the child is ticklish, have them place a hand on top of yours and do the pushing (while you do the feeling) to squelch the laughter and allow for a better examination.

Neurologic Examination

- Does the child recognize mom or dad?
  - By 2 months of age a child should be able to focus on parent's face
- Observe for confusion, lethargy, and agitation, which suggests a subacute hypoperfusion.
- Hold or have the parents hold the child to evaluate muscle tone.
  - Decreased muscle tone, convulsions, or pupillary dilatation suggest acute hypoperfusion.
- Watch the child play with parent to evaluate strength.
- Check with the parents to determine the child's baseline movements, gait, or truck before assuming the child is ataxic; the child may be just learning to walk or sit.
- Gently tickle the child to evaluate sensation.
- If a parent or guardian says the child is just not right, believe them—they know the child best.

Skin

- Ask the parents to direct you to any new rashes or discolorations.

These are just, suggestions. Good common sense and a certain degree of patience will carry you through even the most difficult evaluation.

For further information regarding emergent evaluation and treatment of children contact the American Heart Association for training in pediatric advance life support (PALS) or the American College of Emergency Physicians for its course in advanced pediatric life support (APLS).

Notes

CHAPTER 55

Pediatric Resuscitation
Owen T. Traynor, MD

Presentation

The paramedic must be expert in recognizing the pediatric patient who has significant illness—due to either traumatic or medical causes. Recall that pediatric patients have little reserve; that is, they may be able to compensate for the illness for a time, only to decompensate suddenly rather than gradually as adult patients. The principles of resuscitation, however, are the same in the pediatric patient as in the adult. Assessment of the airway, breathing, and circulation is key. In general, a cardiac etiology for cardiac arrest is not as common in children as in adults. For example, most pediatric cardiac arrests with a medical basis have a respiratory etiology. Therefore, attention to the airway may prevent cardiac arrest.

Immediate Concerns

- **Does the patient have an altered mental status?** An altered mental status may indicate evidence of head injury, respiratory distress or failure, inadequate perfusion, infection, a toxic ingestion, or a metabolic illness. Apply high-concentration oxygen and protect the cervical spine as indicated.
- **Is the airway endangered?** The airway of the pediatric patient is smaller than the adult's and therefore more vulnerable to obstruction. The tongue is also proportionately larger and may obstruct the airway of the pediatric patient with an altered mental status. The infant also is an obligate nasal breather, and even mild obstruction of the nasopharynx can cause an increased respiratory effort. Recall that there are medical causes of airway compromise (eg, epiglottitis and croup) and these will be worsened by examination of the airway. If a foreign body obstruction is suspected, begin the obstructed airway procedure.

- **Is there evidence of respiratory compromise?** Look for grunting, retractions, an altered mental status, tachypnea, stridor, wheezing, coughing, cyanosis, tripod positioning, cyanosis, poor respiratory effort, and a failure to feed in the infant. Apply high-concentration oxygen and be prepared to ventilate the patient.
- **Is the patient in shock?** The number one cause of death in children older than 1 year of age in the United States is trauma. In many of these cases, hypovolemia is the cause. Given the smaller blood volume of the pediatric patient, a loss of even a small amount of blood results in hypovolemic shock. The prehospital provider must recognize the signs and symptoms of early shock: delayed capillary refill, pallor, diaphoresis, tachycardia, tachypnea, decreased urine output, and poor feeding in the infant. Oxygen administration, fluid resuscitation, and expeditious transport are key components in the care of the patient in shock.
- **Has a cardiac arrest been caused by trauma or blood loss?** It is important to determine if this event is primarily cardiac or if it is the result of traumatic injuries. The management of traumatic arrest differs from a primary cardiac event. Arrests caused by blood loss or secondary to trauma generally require fluid resuscitation and surgical intervention (see Chapter 28, Multitrauma). An additional concern is hypothermia. The management of a hypothermic patient also differs (see Chapter 26, Hypothermia).
- **Is CPR indicated?** CPR is indicated for all apneic and pulseless patients without contraindications. Contraindications include obvious life-threatening injury, the presence of rigor mortis or extreme areas of dependent lividity, and a legal living will or DNR order that expresses the patient's wishes that CPR not be performed.

Important History

- **Is there a history of congenital disease?** Congenital heart disease occurs in up to 1% of births. Although most of these defects are non-life-threatening, some may have serious consequences. The most common defects involve the heart valves, the myocardium, or the major blood vessels. One way to classify these defects is to identify them as either cyanotic congenital heart defects or noncyanotic congenital heart defects. The child with a cyanotic congenital heart defect has less reserve than a normal child and therefore can become quite sick with illnesses that are considered mild or moderate in severity in healthy children.

- **Is the child taking any medications?** Most children will not be taking any medications; however, any medications taken may provide clues to past medical history or the possibility of medication side effects.

Differential Diagnosis

After accomplishing the initial treatment priorities, it is important to determine the patient's rhythm and perfusion status. While evaluating the electrocardiogram (ECG), assess for pulses. Always remember to treat the patient, not the monitor. If there is a change in the patient's rhythm, assess for the return of a pulse. A variety of rhythms may be present. It is important that you have the ability to interpret ECGs rapidly. This ability, combined with knowledge of the American Heart Association algorithms, will allow you to make a diagnosis and follow the correct treatment plan.

Key Physical Examination Findings

- *Initial Assessment.* Quickly check for unresponsiveness, a patent airway, adequate respirations, pulses, significant bleeding, and evidence of neurologic or spinal injury.
- *General Appearance.* Observe the patient for signs of dyspnea at rest. Effort and rate of breathing should be noted. Look for grunting, tracheal tugging, and use of accessory respiratory muscles.
- *Vital Signs.* Assess vital signs. There is a wide variability in vital signs based on the child's age. It is wise to carry a chart of pediatric vital signs.
- *Skin.* Is there pallor, flushing, cyanosis, or diaphoresis? The presence of a rash might indicate such causes as an allergic reaction or a specific infectious process.
- *HEENT.* Inspect the nose and mouth for clues to the presence of nasal discharge or bleeding. **NOTE:** If croup or epiglottitis is suspected, do not look into the mouth or do anything that may agitate the child and possibly cause complete airway obstruction.

- *Neck.* Assess for stridor as well as cough, which may be suggestive of a foreign body or of croup. Note the position of the trachea: is it midline or shifted, the latter suggesting a mass lesion or pneumothorax? Are the neck veins distended? This may suggest heart failure. Is the voice hoarse?
- *Chest.* Observe for any evidence of trauma, bruising, or asymmetric movement of the chest wall. Retractions of the sternum and intercostal areas give evidence of the work of breathing. Dullness to percussion or adventitious breath sounds—rales, rhonchi, wheezes, or rubs, may give clues to diagnosis. In addition, asymmetric sounds may point to areas of decreased ventilation.
- *Heart.* Listen for murmurs and extra heart sounds. These are often difficult to hear in the field, but can be evidence of underlying heart disease.
- *Abdomen.* Assess for tenderness, guarding, distention, contusions.
- *Extremities.* Assess for evidence of trauma, edema, capillary refill, and peripheral pulses.
- *Neurologic Examination.* Assess mental status, pupillary responses, interaction with parents and the environment, movement of all extremities, and sensation.

Treatment Plan

- *Patient Assessment.* It is important to remember to frequently reassess the patient. Any change in the patient's perfusion status or rhythm will require you to change algorithms/treatment. Remember: always treat the patient, not the monitor.
- *The Algorithmic Approach.* The American Heart Association (AHA) algorithms make a number of assumptions regarding the patient's status; the condition in the algorithm persists, the patient remains apneic and pulseless, and compressions and ventilations are continued throughout. The use of algorithms is to aid in treating the patient; however, they cannot replace clinical judgment. This section will focus on the specific pediatric resuscitation situations.
- *Neonatal Resuscitation.* The resuscitation of most newborns will require:
  - **Suctioning** of the airway using a bulb syringe. Be alert for the presence of thick meconium in the newborn's

airway. Meconium is a greenish fluid that results from fetal bowel movements in utero. Thick meconium must be evacuated from the airway to prevent meconium aspiration. More than half of infants with meconium in the airway will aspirate. One fifth of these neonates will develop complications including aspiration pneumonia, respiratory distress, and pneumothorax. If thick meconium is present, the hypopharynx must be suctioned once the head has delivered. Endotracheal intubation may be necessary, with the endotracheal tube attached directly to the mechanical suction unit. Withdraw the ET tube as you suction. Repeat this procedure again. Thin, watery meconium does not require endotracheal resuscitation.

○ Gentle **stimulation.**

○ **Maintain** their body **temperature.**

○ **Assess** the **respiratory effort, heart rate, color,** and **Apgar** score follows the initial interventions.

○ **Ventilate** with a bag-valve-mask and high concentration oxygen if respiratory effort is poor or absent, or if the heart rate is less than 100 bpm.

○ Begin **chest compressions** for a heart rate less than 60 bpm, or if the rate is between 60 and 80 bpm and not increasing after 30 seconds of ventilation with 100% oxygen.

○ Administer **high concentration oxygen** if there is central cyanosis despite a heart rate greater than 100 bpm and adequate ventilations. Cyanosis of the extremities need not be treated during the first few minutes of life—it is usually caused by sluggish circulation in the periphery.

○ The **Apgar** score should be noted at 1 minute and 5 minutes after delivery. Resuscitation efforts should not be delayed to record the Apgar score.

Sign	0	1	2
Heart rate	Absent	Slow (<100 bpm)	Fast (>100 bpm)
Respirations	Absent	Slow, irregular	Good, crying
Muscle tone	Limp	Some flexion	Active motion
Reflex irritability	No response	Grimace	Cough or sneeze
Color	Pale or central cyanosis	Peripheral cyanosis	Completely pink

- ○ **Endotracheal intubation** is indicated if bag-valve-mask ventilation is not effective; endotracheal suctioning is required for thick meconium or prolonged ventilation is required.
- ○ The use of **medications and fluids** should wait until adequate ventilations and CPR have been performed for 30 seconds, because the hypoxia is the most likely cause of the cardiac dysfunction. Venous access may be difficult and therefore transport should be initiated early. Use 0.9% NaCl or lactated Ringer's solution at 10 ml/kg over 5 to 10 minutes in the hypovolemic neonate. Monitor the ECG and follow the AHA treatment guidelines that follow.
- **Bradycardia Algorithm**
  - ○ Monitor **ABCs.**
  - ○ Secure the **airway.**
  - ○ Administer **100% oxygen, and ventilate** with a bag-valve-mask **if necessary**
  - ○ Establish intravenous or intraosseous access with 0.9% NaCl or lactated Ringer's solution.
  - ○ Assess **vital signs.**
  - ○ If there is **no evidence of cardiorespiratory instability** (poor perfusion, hypotension, or respiratory distress), continue to **observe** the patient and **transport** to the appropriate emergency department (ED).
  - ○ If there is cardiorespiratory compromise, reassess heart rate: If **heart rate is less than 80 bpm in the infant or less than 60 bpm in a child**, despite adequate oxygenation and ventilation, begin **CPR.**
  - ○ Administer **epinephrine 0.01 mg/kg (1:10,000) via IV/IO**, or **0.1 mg/kg (1:1000) via ET.** Repeat as needed every 3 to 5 minutes at the same dose.
  - ○ Administer **atropine, 0.02 mg/kg via IV/IO/ET.** Minimum dose 0.1 mg; maximum single dose 0.5 mg for a child, 1.0 mg for an adolescent. Dose may be repeated once in 3 to 5 minutes.
  - ○ Consider transport to the appropriate ED.
  - ○ If asystole develops continue CPR and administer **epinephrine** at the previous dose for the first dose and, for subsequent doses, at **0.1 mg/kg (1:1000) via IV/IO/ET.** Repeating every 3 to 5 minutes. **NOTE:** IV/IO doses at up to 0.2 mg/kg may be effective.
- **Cardiac Arrest General Algorithm**
  - ○ Determine pulselessness and begin **CPR.**

- ○ **Confirm ECG rhythm** in more than one lead.
- ○ Follow the appropriate treatment guideline—ventricular fibrillation (VF)/pulseless ventricular tachycardia (VT), pulseless electrical activity, or asystole.
- **Ventricular Fibrillation/Pulseless Ventricular Tachycardia**
  - ○ Continue **CPR.**
  - ○ Secure the **airway.**
  - ○ **Hyperventilate** with 100% oxygen.
  - ○ **Establish IV or IO access** with 0.9% NaCl or lactated Ringer's solution, but do not delay defibrillation.
  - ○ **Defibrillate** up to 3 times, if indicated, at **2 J/kg, 4 J/kg, 4 J/kg.**
  - ○ Give first dose of **epinephrine, 0.01 mg/kg (1:10,000), via IV/IO,** or **0.1 mg/kg (1:1000), via ET.** Give subsequent doses of **epinephrine, 0.1 mg/kg (1:1000) via IV/IO/ET. Repeat every 3 to 5 minutes.**
    NOTE: Intravenous/intraosseous doses at up to 0.2 mg/kg may be effective.
  - ○ **Defibrillate at 4 J/kg 30 to 60 seconds after the medication is given.**
  - ○ Assess pulse and rhythm: keep in mind that a change in pulse or rhythm will change the algorithm. If there has been no change in VF or VT, the patient is considered to be in refractory VF or VT. The following antifibrillatory agents should be employed in a drug-shock, drug-shock pattern. The patient should be defibrillated at 4 J/kg 30 to 60 seconds following each medication. **Lidocaine 1.0 mg/kg IV bolus. Dose may be repeated once in 3 to 5 minutes. Bretylium 5 mg/kg IV bolus. Dose may be repeated once at 10 mg/kg.**
  - ○ Should the patient's rhythm convert to a supraventricular rhythm after a defibrillation, infuse lidocaine to prevent recurrence. If no antifibrillatory agent has been given previously, lidocaine, 1.0 mg/kg, should be given, followed by the 20 to 50 μg per minute lidocaine infusion.
- **Pulseless Electrical Activity**
  - ○ Consider possible causes and therapy.
- **Hypovolemia**—volume infusion.
- **Cardiac tamponade**—transport rapidly to ED for pericardiocentesis.
- **Hypothermia**—see hypothermia algorithm.

- **Drug overdoses** such as tricyclic agents, digitalis, beta blockers, calcium channel blockers—transport to ED.
- **Hypoxia**—ensure adequate ventilations with high concentration oxygen.
- Tension pneumothorax—needle thoracentesis.
- **Hyperkalemia**—(patients in renal failure, tall peaked T waves)—consider sodium bicarbonate and transport to ED
- **Acidosis**—ensure adequate ventilations, consider sodium bicarbonate.

> Continue **CPR**.
> Secure the **airway**.
> **Hyperventilate** with 100% oxygen.
> **Establish IV or IO access** with 0.9% NaCl or RL.
> Give first dose of **epinephrine, 0.01 mg/kg (1:10,000), via IV/IO**, or **0.1 mg/kg (1:1000), via ET**. Give subsequent doses of **epinephrine 0.1 mg/kg (1:1000), via IV/IO/ET. Repeat every 3 to 5 minutes. NOTE:** IV/IO doses at up to 0.2 mg/kg may be effective.

- Asystole

> Continue **CPR**.
> Secure the **airway**.
> **Hyperventilate** with 100% oxygen.
> **Establish IV or IO access** with 0.9% NaCl or RL.
> Give first dose of **epinephrine, 0.01 mg/kg (1:10,000), via IV/IO**, or **0.1 mg/kg (1:1000), via ET**. Give subsequent doses of **epinephrine 0.1 mg/kg (1:1000) via IV/IO/ET. Repeat every 3 to 5 minutes.**

NOTE: IV/IO doses at up to 0.2 mg/kg may be effective.

- *Supraventricular Tachycardia* (SVT).

This is the most commonly occurring, clinically significant arrhythmia in infants. It occurs less commonly in older pediatric patients. Because wide-complex tachycardias are uncommon in children, any wide-complex tachycardia should be considered VT. Often children will be able to tolerate an SVT; however, when the rate is very fast, a low cardiac output state may occur. These unstable children should be treated with **high-concentration oxygen and adenosine, 0.1 mg/kg IV** (dose may be repeated at 0.2 mg/kg if ineffective; maximum single dose 12 mg). If **IV access is unavailable synchronized cardioversion, starting at 0.5 J/kg,** should be performed.

- *Ventricular Tachycardia*. VT with a pulse is best treated with **lidocaine 1 mg/kg IV/IO**, before synchronized cardioversion; however, if IV/IO access is not promptly available, **synchronized cardioversion, starting at 0.5 J/ kg**, should be performed. The lidocaine bolus should be followed by a lidocaine infusion at 20 to 50 µg per minute.
- *Hypovolemia*. It is important to restore circulating blood volume in the pediatric patient to prevent progression to refractory shock and cardiac arrest. The preferred intravenous or intraosseous solutions are crystalloids—0.9% NaCl or LR, or colloid solutions. Blood products should be reserved for severe acute blood loss. Dextrose-containing fluids should not be used in children because large amounts of dextrose will cause hyperglycemia, leading to an osmotic diuresis and possibly a poor neurologic outcome. The pediatric patient in shock should receive high-concentration oxygen, endotracheal intubation, as indicated, fluid resuscitation with **0.9% NaCl or lactated Ringer's solution at 20 ml/kg,** and expeditious transport to the appropriate ED. The fluid bolus **may be repeated** if there is inadequate response to the first bolus. Consider transfusion if 40 mL/ kg has failed to satisfactorily treat hemorrhagic shock.
- **Vasopressors** will not often be needed. Their use should be limited to the treatment of hypotension in the euvolemic patient, or in those patients who have not responded to significant fluid resuscitation. The AHA recommended vasopressors for use in pediatric patients are:

   Epinephrine 0.1 to 1.0 µg/kg per minute.
   Dopamine 2.0 to 20.0 µg/kg per minute.
   Dobutamine 2.0 to 20.0 µg/kg per minute.

Bibliography

American Academy of Pediatrics, American College of Emergency Physicians: APLS: The Pediatric Emergency Medicine Course, ed 2. 1993.

Neonatal Resuscitation. In Guidelines for Cardiopulmonary Resuscitation and Emergency Cardiac Care. JAMA 268: 2276–2282, 1992.

Pediatric Advanced Life Support. In Guidelines for Cardiopulmonary Resuscitation and Emergency Cardiac Care. JAMA 268: 2262–2276, 1992.

Notes

CHAPTER 56

Pulse Oximetry
Robert L. Kerner, RN, Jr., CEN, EMT-CC

Assessment and maintenance of a patent airway is an important skill required of every EMS provider. A thorough and accurate patient assessment is the starting point to detect your patient's airway status and oxygen requirements. After you are satisfied that the airway is open and patent and that the patient is being adequately ventilated, either spontaneously or mechanically, you must next address the patient's oxygenation status. The three most practical methods for assessing a patient's oxygen status is through physical examination, arterial blood-gas analysis, or pulse oximetry.

The pulse oximeter, or "pulse ox," is frequently seen in intensive care units and emergency departments, and has recently made its way into the prehospital setting. The devices are easy to use, noninvasive, and cost-effective when compared with arterial blood-gas analysis. Yet, despite its widespread acceptance as an important tool for EMS practitioners, many do not know how it works or how to properly apply the data that they obtain from it.

Gas Transport

To understand how a pulse oximeter works, it is necessary to comprehend the physiology of oxygen transport within the human body. Oxygen may be transported either bound to hemoglobin or dissolved in the blood. A vast majority of the oxygen, approximately 98.5%, is bound to hemoglobin molecules, while the remaining 1.5% is dissolved in the circulating blood. Carbon dioxide also competes for hemoglobin as a transport mechanism. Approximately 30% of carbon dioxide is bound to hemoglobin, while 10% is dissolved in the blood and 60% is removed as bicarbonate.

The concentration of oxygen dissolved in the blood plays a major role in determining the hemoglobin saturation. During respiration, oxygen diffuses from the alveoli and is dissolved in the blood. As the amount of oxygen dissolved in blood increases, the partial pressure of oxygen (PO_2) increases. The increase in PO_2 facilitates oxygen-hemoglobin bonding because there is now increased availability of oxygen in the blood. When PO_2 is increased, oxygen and hemoglobin bond, forming oxyhemoglobin. This is the mechanism that is present in the pulmonary capillaries. When the PO_2 is decreased, as it is in the systemic capillaries, the reaction is driven in the other direction and oxygen is released (dissociates) from hemoglobin. Therefore, a rise in PO_2 will lead to an increase in hemoglobin saturation, whereas a decrease in PO_2 will lead to desaturation of the hemoglobin molecules.

The relationship between hemoglobin saturation and PO_2 is not linear. In other words, doubling the PO_2 will not necessarily lead to twice as much hemoglobin saturation. This can be seen on the oxygen dissociation curve that follows. The S-shaped curve shows the relationship between percent hemoglobin saturation and PO_2.

Notice that between a PO_2 of 60 to 100 mm Hg the curve is

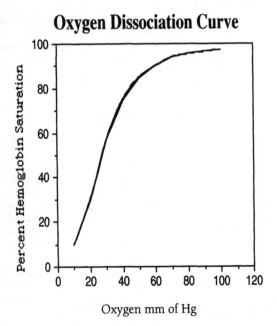

Oxygen Dissociation Curve

Oxygen mm of Hg

relatively flat. An increase in PO_2 in this range will produce only a small increase in hemoglobin saturation. At the steep portion of the curve, between PO_2 of 0 to 60 mm Hg, a small change in the PO_2 will yield a significant change in the hemoglobin saturation. The significance of this concept is that a small decrease in PO_2 can lead to a tremendous decrease in hemoglobin desaturation.

There are other factors that affect hemoglobin saturation and these factors must be taken into account when using the pulse oximeter. An increase in PCO_2 will decrease the affinity of hemoglobin for oxygen, causing an increased oxygen-hemoglobin dissociation at the tissue level, thereby shifting the curve to the right. A shift in the curve to the right means that the hemoglobin will bind less avidly to the oxygen, resulting in increased oxygen delivery to the tissues. An increase in acidity or an increase in temperature also shifts the curve to the right.

The presence of carbon monoxide will also affect hemoglobin-oxygen saturation. Carbon monoxide's affinity for hemoglobin is 240 times greater than that of oxygen, and a relatively small amount of carbon monoxide can bind with a much greater amount of hemoglobin. This phenomenon may lead to serious oxygen deprivation. The presence of carboxyhemoglobin shifts the oxygen dissociation curve to the left, resulting in oxygen that is strongly bound to hemoglobin. This means decreased oxygen delivery to the tissues.

Pulse Oximeter

The pulse oximeter is a noninvasive method of measuring the oxygen saturation of arterial blood. Although many models of pulse oximeters are now available, all work on the same basic principle. A probe is applied to the patient and a beam of light is passed through the tissues to a photodetector on the other half of the probe. The photodetector senses the amount of light absorbed by the oxyhemoglobin molecules in the arterial blood as it passes through the tissues beneath the probe. This information is transmitted to the processing unit of the oximeter, and the percentage of oxygen saturation is displayed. Most pulse oximeters also provide a readout of the patient's pulse rate as well as alarm features such as low saturation or high pulse rate. There are numerous battery-powered oximeters that allow the device to be used in the prehospital setting.

The probe-patient interface is perhaps the weakest link in the system. Probes come in many sizes, including adult, pediatric, and neonatal models. Of these, some models have multiple-use probes, such as finger clips, whereas others have single-use probes, such as a tape-type probe. In general, the probe should be applied snugly to a clean dry surface to allow an accurate reading. Common areas for probe placement include the fingers, toes, nose, and foot. In most cases, nail polish should be removed from fingers or toes before probe placement, because colored polish may interfere with the probe. The probe must then be plugged into the oximeter unit directly or to a connecting cable. Check the operation manual to see which types of probes are recommended for the particular machine being used. A probe which is not applied properly will give inaccurate information.

Clinical use of pulse oximetry is increasing. The fact that it is noninvasive means that prehospital care providers can perform an important diagnostic test with no patient discomfort involved. Even small children are able to tolerate this procedure when it is presented in a calm, nonthreatening manner. When applied properly, the results gathered from oximetry are reliable. Prehospital EMS providers can be taught to use the oximeter in a short time span, and it is perhaps one of the easiest biomedical devices to apply and use.

The pulse oximeter is not without a few drawbacks that must be taken into account each time the device is used. The device must sense a pulse in order to calculate the oxygen saturation. States of decreased cardiac output, such as low heart rate, decreased blood pressure, tachycardia, and cardiovascular collapse, will greatly limit the probe's ability to sense the pulse. Likewise, vasoconstrictive states such as shock or hypothermia will have a similar effect. A tourniquet or automated blood pressure cuff proximal to the probe will also interfere with oximetry for the same reasons. Excessive patient movement may cause artifact, and carbon monoxide poisoning has actually been shown to cause high saturation readings.

Remember that the pulse oximeter only measures arterial oxygen saturation. It does not measure the actual PO_2, nor does it measure the PCO_2 or the pH. It also does not assess ventilation. A patient with chronic obstructive pulmonary disease who has a hypoxic drive may have an excellent PO_2 when given 100% oxygen, but will soon hypoventilate and have dangerously high carbon dioxide levels while maintaining the excellent PO_2.

Troubleshooting

When the patient's chief complaint, physical examination, and pulse oximeter measurements do not correlate, you must troubleshoot the situation. Does the patient appear sicker than the pulse oximeter reading or vice versa? Always base your interventions on the total evaluation of the patient; treat the patient, not the device. Gather more data if necessary.

Check the mechanical aspects of the machine. Is it plugged in and does it have sufficient power to operate? Is the probe on properly? Is there any indication that the machine is sensing a pulse? Is the pulse being occluded by a blood pressure cuff? Is the probe placed somewhere that is not being perfused adequately? Has someone accidentally disconnected the cable?

Reassess your patient. Is the patient hypothermic, in shock, or seizing? Could the patient be compensating well for an occult problem such as a pneumonia? Could the patient be anemic? The possibility exists that if the hemoglobin level is low and if all hemoglobin molecules are bound to oxygen, then the oxygen saturation will be 100%. Yet, the patient is still hypoxic because they have a reduced oxygen-carrying capacity. Is there a possibility that the patient has carbon monoxide poisoning?

The Bottom Line for Field Use

A pulse oximeter can provide you with important information about the oxygen saturation of patients in respiratory distress. This information was not previously available to the paramedic. Oxygen saturation is only part of the picture. The assessment of the ventilatory status remains one of clinical judgment.

Room air oxygen saturation should be greater than 95%. Most pulse oximeters are accurate plus or minus 5%. This means that a patient with an oxygen saturation of 95%, as measured by a pulse oximeter, may have a true oxygen saturation of 90% to 100%. Recall that at 90%, the patient is standing at the steep downhill portion of the oxyhemoglobin dissociation curve. A small decrease in saturation will result in significant hypoxia. Watch these patients closely.

> NOTE: Never use the pulse oximeter as a tool to withhold oxygen from a patient in respiratory distress.

Bibliography

de Asla R and Smith R: Instrumentation. In Kinney M, Packa D, and Dunbar S (eds): AACN'S Clinical Reference for Critical Care Nursing. McGraw-Hill, New York, 1988, pp 60–62.

Groosbach I: Case Studies in Pulse Oximetry Monitoring. Critical Care Nurse, 13(4): 63–65, 1993.

Guyton A: Textbook of Medical Physiology. WB Saunders, Philadelphia, 1991, pp 433–443.

Tortora G and Anagnostakos N. Principles of Anatomy and Physiology. Harper & Row, New York, 1987, pp 575–578.

Notes

SECTION III

Procedures

SECTION III

Procedures

Chapter 57
Basic Life Support Summary

	Adult (8 years and older)		Child (1–8 years)	Infant (birth–1 year)
	One Rescuer	Two Rescuers	One or Two Rescuers	One Rescuer
Airway technique	Head tilt-chin lift in the nontrauma patient. Jaw thrust with cervical spine precautions in the context of trauma			
Breathing	2 breaths: 1.5–2 sec/breath initially, then 10 to 12 breaths/min		2 breaths: 1–1.5 sec/breath initially, then 20 breaths/min	
Pulse check	Carotid			Brachial or Femoral
Compression depth	1.5–2 inches		1–1.5 inches	0.5–1 inch
Compression rate	80–100/minute		100/minute	>100/minute
Ratio of compressions to ventilations	15:2		5:1	
Foreign body obstructed airway technique	Heimlich maneuver, with finger sweeps in the unconscious patient		Back blows and chest thrusts, finger sweeps only if the foreign body is visualized	

Data from Guidelines for Cardiopulmonary Resuscitation and Emergency Care. JAMA 1992 268:2184-2198, 2251-2261.

CHAPTER 58

Cardioversion and Defibrillation

Thomas J. Rahilly, MS, EMT-CC

NOTE: Use body substance isolation whenever the possibility exists of contact with blood or any body fluids. This should include gloves, eye protection, masks, and other protective barriers as necessary.

Cardioversion

INDICATIONS

Patients with supraventricular tachycardias with signs and symptoms of decompensation. Cardioversion is also indicated in patients with ventricular tachycardia who have a pulse and signs and symptoms of decompensation.

CONTRAINDICATIONS

Patients with permanent (implanted) pacemakers may suffer loss of pacemaker action from the electrical shock of a defibrillator. Advise physician before cardioverting these patients.

EQUIPMENT

A defibrillator and monitor with synchronized cardioversion capabilities, defibrillator pads or a conductive medium, sedative.

PROCEDURE

1. Confirm the order to cardiovert or proceed on standing orders.
2. Sedate the patient if indicated.
3. Turn on the defibrillator and activate the synchronizer mode.

4. Ensure that the synchronizer is marking the R wave. The R wave must be at least 1 to 3 cm high for cardioversion, depending on the unit being used. Adjust the gain as necessary.
5. Place conductive medium on the paddles (gel) or on the patient (saline pads or defibrillator pads).
6. Turn on the recorder.
7. Charge the paddles to the appropriate energy level.
8. Advise all present to stand away from the patient and to avoid contact with the patient.
9. Place paddles on the patient's chest in the proper locations and apply firm pressure.
10. Begin audible countdown to cardioversion ("I am going to shock on three; one, two, three"). During the countdown check to ensure that no one is in contact with the patient.
11. Make a final confirmation of the dysrhythmia requiring cardioversion.
12. Shout "clear" and make a visual check to ensure that there is no contact with the patient.
13. Simultaneously press both discharge buttons until the defibrillator discharges on the next R wave.
14. Check the patient's pulse and ECG.

Defibrillation

INDICATIONS

Patients with ventricular fibrillation with signs of cardiac arrest or pulseless ventricular tachycardia.

CONTRAINDICATIONS

None in the presence of a pulseless patient.

EQUIPMENT

Defibrillator and monitor, defibrillator pads or conductive medium.

PROCEDURE

1. Confirm the order to defibrillate or proceed on standing orders.

2. Turn on the defibrillator power.
3. Place conductive medium on the paddles (gel) or on the patient (saline pads or defibrillator pads).
4. Turn on the recorder.
5. Charge the paddles to the appropriate energy level.
6. Advise all present to stand away from the patient and to avoid contact with the patient.
7. Place paddles on the patient's chest in the proper locations and apply firm pressure.
8. Begin audible countdown to defibrillation ("I am going to shock on three; one, two, three"). During countdown check to ensure that no one is in contact with the patient.
9. Make a final confirmation of ventricular fibrillation.
10. Shout "clear" and make a visual check to ensure that there is no contact with the patient.
11. Simultaneously press both discharge buttons until the defibrillator discharges.
12. Check the patient's pulse and ECG.

Bibliography

Allison EJ Jr (ed): Advanced Life Support Skills. Mosby–Year Book, St. Louis, MO, 1994, pp 145–154.
Grauer K and Cavallaro D: ACLS Certification Preparation. Mosby–Year Book, St. Louis, MO, 1993, p 281.

Notes

CHAPTER 59

Central Venous Catheterization Via the Subclavian Vein

John Wilkinson, MD

NOTE: This procedure should be performed only when indicated and authorized by the local medical control physician. Use universal precautions whenever the possibility exists of contact with blood or any body fluids. This should include gloves, eye protection, masks, and other barriers as necessary.

Indications

- High-flow infusion of fluids or blood in hypovolemic shock.
- Lack of peripheral access secondary to burns; trauma; plaster casts; chemically sclerosed, thrombosed, or inadequate peripheral veins.
- Access during cardiac arrest. The supraclavicular route is recommended for access during CPR as it allows for minimal interference with compressions and airway management.
- Preparation for passage of Swan-Ganz catheter or transvenous pacemaker.

Contraindications

- Distorted local anatomy or landmarks (use the opposite side instead).
- Chest wall deformities.
- Extremes of weight.
- Suspected superior vena cava injury.
- Suspected subclavian vessel injury (use the opposite side instead).

- Pneumothorax (cannulate same side so as to avoid creation of bilateral pneumothoraces).
- Bleeding disorders or anticoagulation therapy.
- Combative patient.

Equipment

Sterile swabs or sponges, sterile drapes, introducer needle (usually 18 gauge thin walled needle), catheter or sheath introducer, IV tubing and solution, antibiotic ointment, antiseptic solution, 1% lidocaine solution, 5 ml non–Luer-lok syringe, vessel dilator, silk sutures, gauze pads, sterile gloves, 25 gauge, 1.5 inch needle with 3 ml Luer-lok syringe, guidewire, No. 11 scalpel, suture scissors, cloth tape.

The selection of the type of needle and catheter set depends on the indication for the procedure. Hypovolemic shock is an indication for high-flow infusion. Although the placement of peripheral large-bore catheters is preferred, the aforementioned indications may preclude the use of the peripheral route. In such cases, one may elect to place a large-bore (8.5 French [Fr]) catheter in the subclavian vein. In cases that do not require high-flow infusion, one may opt to place a smaller device such as a 16 gauge, 20 cm catheter.

Procedure

The infraclavicular and supraclavicular approaches to the subclavian vein will be described. Both use the Seldinger or guidewire technique. The Seldinger technique has many positive aspects. Less chance exists for significant trauma to adjacent structures due to the smaller introducer needle. It is also excellent for placement of large-bore introducers for high-volume infusion.

The infraclavicular approach is more widely used. The anatomic landmarks are consistent and are generally rapidly located. The right subclavian vein is usually chosen due to anatomic considerations, but the aforementioned indications and contraindications must be considered.

1. Explain the procedure to the awake patient during preparation.
2. Place the patient in the supine position with the head in a neutral position and with arms at the patient's side. Placing the patient in the Trendelenburg posi-

tion (10 to 15 degrees) helps to decrease risk of air embolism.

3. The area of needle entry is prepared with an appropriate antiseptic solution and should include the anterior neck, supraclavicular fossa, and the anterior chest to 3 cm across the midline and just above the nipple. Once the area is prepared, sterile gloves should be worn for the remainder of the procedure. If time permits, the area may be draped.

4. The area of needle entry should be just inferior to the junction of the middle third and medial third of the clavicle (costoclavicular junction). This area may be infiltrated with 1% lidocaine using the 3-ml syringe and the 25 gauge needle.

5. The forefinger is placed in the sternal notch, while the thumb is placed at the costoclavicular junction for points of reference.

6. The non–Luer-lok syringe with the introducer needle attached is inserted, bevel down, immediately inferior to the clavicle at the costoclavicular junction, while gently aspirating on the syringe. The needle should be kept nearly flush with the skin and directed behind the clavicle toward the sternal notch.

7. Return of blood signals penetration of the vein. If the blood is bright red, the artery has been penetrated. In such a case, the needle should be removed and, if possible, pressure applied in the area of puncture.

8. Remove the syringe and cover the end of the needle with a finger. This should be performed during exhalation of the breathing patient or during inspiration of the mechanically ventilated patient to avoid air embolism.

9. Thread the guidewire through the needle and into the vein. The wire should thread easily and should never be forced if difficulty is encountered. If the wire must be removed, the needle and wire should be removed together to prevent shearing off the wire.

10. The needle is removed while always holding the wire either above or below the needle. This is to avoid losing the wire in the central circulation.

11. Make a small incision in the skin with the scalpel at the site of the wire.

12. Advance the dilator and catheter with a twisting mo-

tion into the vein after placing the dilator and catheter assembly on the guidewire. The wire must be visible through the back of the device before entering the vein.

13. Remove the dilator and wire. Cover the catheter with a finger until the intravenous tubing can be attached.

14. If placing a smaller catheter, rather than the 8.5 Fr introducer, thread the dilator over the wire and insert into the vein. Remove the dilator and thread the catheter over the wire until the tip is approximately 2 cm below the sternal angle. This distance may be determined by placing the catheter along the chest wall before insertion.

15. Secure the catheter to the skin with the silk suture if time permits.

The supraclavicular approach is reportedly easier for the less experienced EMS provider, and it does not interfere with the performance of CPR. Also, some studies have shown that there are fewer complications with this approach as compared with the infraclavicular approach. Of the several methods described in the literature, the following was chosen for its simplicity. Just the approach to the vein will be described. The remainder of the procedure will be the same as described for the infraclavicular approach.

1. Explain the procedure to the awake patient during preparation.

2. Place the patient in the supine position with the head in a neutral position and with arms at the patient's side. Placing the patient in the Trendelenburg position (10 to 15 degrees) helps to decrease risk of air embolism.

3. The area of needle entry is prepared with an appropriate antiseptic solution and should include the anterior neck, supraclavicular fossa, and the anterior chest to 3 cm across the midline and just above the nipple. Once the area is prepared, sterile gloves should be worn for the remainder of the procedure. If time permits, the area may be draped.

4. With the patient in the neutral position, place a finger on the most anterior part of the shoulder. Draw an imaginary line medially until it intersects the clavicle. The site of needle entry is just posterior to the clavicle. This area may be infiltrated with 1% lidocaine using the 3 ml syringe and the 25 gauge needle.

5. Keeping the needle parallel to the surface of the stretcher, advance toward the ipsilateral sternoclavicular joint while gently aspirating. The bevel should be directed superiorly.

6. The non–Luer-lok syringe with the introducer needle attached is inserted, bevel down, immediately inferior to the clavicle at the costoclavicular junction, while gently aspirating on the syringe. The needle should be kept nearly flush with the skin and directed behind the clavicle toward the sternal notch.

7. Return of blood signals penetration of the vein. If the blood is bright red, the artery has been penetrated. In such a case, the needle should be removed and, if possible, pressure applied in the area of puncture.

8. Remove the syringe and cover the end of the needle with a finger. This should be performed during exhalation of the breathing patient or during inspiration of the mechanically ventilated patient to avoid air embolism.

9. Thread the guidewire through the needle and into the vein. The wire should thread easily and should never be forced if difficulty is encountered. If the wire must be removed, the needle and wire should be removed together to prevent shearing off the wire.

10. The needle is removed while always holding the wire either above or below the needle. This is to avoid losing the wire in the central circulation.

11. Make a small incision in the skin with the scalpel at the site of the wire.

12. Advance the dilator and catheter with a twisting motion into the vein after placing the dilator and catheter assembly on the guidewire. The wire must be visible through the back of the device before entering the vein.

13. Remove the dilator and wire. Cover the catheter with a finger until the intravenous tubing can be attached.

14. If placing a smaller catheter, rather than the 8.5 Fr introducer, thread the dilator over the wire and insert into the vein. Remove the dilator and thread the catheter over the wire until the tip is approximately 2 cm below the sternal angle. This distance may be determined by placing the catheter along the chest wall before insertion.

15. Secure the catheter to the skin with the silk suture if time permits.

Complications

Pneumothorax, hemothorax, hydrothorax
Hemomediastinum
Tracheal perforation
Artery puncture, arteriovenous fistula
Air embolism
Hematoma at puncture site
Infection leading to cellulitis and sepsis
Phrenic nerve and brachial plexus injury

Bibliography

Conroy JM, et al.: A Modification of the Supraclavicular Approach to the Central Circulation. South Med J 83:1178–1181, 1990.

Dronen SC: Central Venous Catheterization: Subclavian Vein Approach. In Roberts JR and Hedges JR (eds): Clinical Procedures in Emergency Medicine, ed 2. WB Saunders, Philadelphia, 1991, pp 325–340.

Iserson KV: High-Flow Infusion Techniques. In Roberts JR and Hedges JR (eds): Clinical Procedures in Emergency Medicine, ed 2. WB Saunders, Philadelphia, 1991, pp 301–307.

MacDonnell JE, et al.: Supraclavicular Subclavian Vein Catheterization: Modified Landmarks for Needle Insertion. Ann Emerg Med 21:421–424, 1992.

Samlhetti AD: Seldinger (Guidewire) Technique for Venous access. In Roberts JR and Hedges JR (eds): Clinical Procedures in Emergency Medicine, ed 2. WB Saunders, Philadelphia, 1991, pp 307–314.

Sladen A: Invasive Monitoring and Its Complications in the Intensive Care Unit. CV Mosby, St. Louis, 1990, pp 101–117.

Notes

CHAPTER 60

Cricothyrotomy: Needle and Surgical
Donall E. Kenney, EMT-P

NOTE: Use body substance isolation whenever the possibility exists of contact with blood or any body fluids. This should include gloves, eye protection, masks, and other protective barriers as necessary. When sharp instruments are used (ie, needles), a sharps container must be available for their safe disposal.

Needle Cricothyrotomy

INDICATIONS

Cricothyrotomy is indicated for relief of life-threatening upper airway obstruction when:
- There is a history suggestive of airway obstruction.
- Manual measures (head tilt methods, triple airway maneuver, and attempts at ventilation) have failed and there is severe respiratory distress or respiratory arrest as indicated by:
  - An absent or ineffective respiratory effort as indicated by a lack of air movement at the nares or absent breath sounds on both sides of chest
  - Central cyanosis
- Endotracheal intubation, for whatever reason, is not feasible or possible.

CONTRAINDICATIONS

There are no contraindications in emergency situations.

EQUIPMENT

Oxygen, tubing, and a device capable of delivering oxygen at 50 psi (demand valve), No. 12 or No. 14 gauge, 8.5 cm over-the-needle catheter attached to a 3 ml syringe, povidone-iodine (Betadine), 7.5 mm endotracheal tube, and BVM adapter.

PROCEDURE

1. Locate the cricothyroid membrane by palpating the trachea just above the sternal notch and proceeding upward until the prominence of the cricoid cartilage is identified or palpate the thyroid notch and proceed downward until the prominence of the cricoid cartilage is identified.
2. Palpate the junction of the trachea and the cricothyroid membrane, which forms a "T," to ensure proper identification of the cricothyroid membrane.
3. Stabilize the larynx with fingers of the nondominant hand.
4. Cleanse the overlying skin with povidone-iodine solution.
5. Introduce a 12 to 14 gauge over-the-needle catheter attached to a 3 ml syringe through the skin just above the cricoid cartilage at a 45 degree downward angle.
6. Advance the needle into the cricothyroid membrane and into the airway.
7. When air is aspirated, stop advancing the needle, advance the catheter over the needle into the trachea, and remove the needle.
8. Attach the barrel only of the 3 ml syringe to the over-the-needle catheter. Attach a 7.5 mm endotracheal tube adapter to the 3 ml syringe barrel.
9. Deliver oxygen at 15 liters per minute with a bag-valve-mask device or via an intermittent jet insufflation device capable of delivering oxygen at 50 psi, with a timed or manual cycle of 3 seconds "on" and 5 seconds "off" and an exhaust port.
10. Auscultate lungs for air entry.

11. Look for chest expansion, and check for egress of air.
12. Rule out the possibility of obstruction below the cricothyroid membrane.
13. After completion of the procedure, transport patient and notify the receiving hospital about the need for surgical airway intervention.
14. If the airway remains obstructed, transport patient immediately and continue basic life-support procedure for obstructed airway.

NOTE: Adequate Pao_2 can be maintained for a maximum of 30 to 45 minutes.

COMPLICATIONS

Asphyxia
Aspiration
Cellulitis
Esophageal perforation
Exsanguinating hematoma
Hematoma
Posterior tracheal wall perforation
Subcutaneous or mediastinal emphysema, or both
    types
Thyroid perforation
Inadequate ventilation leading to hypoxia and death

Surgical Cricothyrotomy

NOTE: This procedure should be performed only when indicated and authorized by the local medical control physician.

INDICATIONS

- Any life-threatening situation in which no other technique can be used to establish a patent airway.

    NOTE: This is a last resort attempt at establishing an airway.

CONTRAINDICATIONS

- Patients with an established airway.
- Patients in whom endotracheal intubation can be accomplished quickly when there are no contraindications to endotracheal intubation.
- Transection of the trachea with retraction of the distal segment into the mediastinum.
- Fractured or crushed larynx or cricoid cartilage.
- Inability to locate the cricothyroid membrane.

RELATIVE CONTRAINDICATIONS

- Patients with a bleeding disorder.
- Pediatric patients younger than 5 years of age.
- Patients with massive neck edema.

EQUIPMENT

A No. 10 scalpel, curved hemostat or Trousseau dilator, bag-valve-mask, gauze pads, 1% lidocaine with epinephrine, tracheostomy tubes or 5 and 6 mm endotracheal tubes, povidine-iodine (Betadine) solution, supplemental oxygen, protective eyewear, 10 mL syringe, stethoscope, surgical gloves. Alternatively, a cricothyrotomy kit may be used.

This procedure requires the paramedic to be proficient in its performance. A needle cricothyrotomy may be easier and safer to perform by those with little experience performing surgical cricothyrotomies.

PROCEDURE

1. Check responsiveness and confirm the need for a surgical airway
2. Place the patient in the supine position with the head in a neutral position and with arms at the patient's side. If there is no need to protect the cervical spine, the neck may be hyperextended. Consider the use of sedation and analgesia, if appropriate.
3. Prepare the site with a povidine-iodine antiseptic solution if time permits. Once the area is prepared, sterile gloves should be worn for the remainder of the pro-

cedure. If time permits, the area may be draped. Local infiltration with lidocaine and epinephrine may also be used if appropriate.

4. If possible, hyperventilate the patient with 100% oxygen before the procedure.

5. Identify the cricothyroid membrane by placing the index finger of the nondominant hand on the larynx and running it inferiorly until the soft depression of the cricothyroid membrane is palpated.

6. Stabilize the trachea, holding it between the thumb and middle finger of the nondominant hand, keeping the index finger on the cricothyroid membrane.

7. Make a skin incision using the dominant hand and the No. 10 scalpel. Experts disagree as to whether a midline incision or a horizontal incision should be made. A 3 to 4 cm midline incision, if performed, minimizes the likelihood of cutting the laryngotracheal vessels and nerves. If the incision is made too high, it can easily be extended, obviating the need for a second incision. If the midline incision is not made, a 2 cm horizontal incision should be made over the cricothyroid membrane. The midline incision minimizes the chance of cutting the vascular thyroid gland.

8. A 1 cm horizontal stabbing incision is made in the cricothyroid membrane.

9. Widen the incision by inserting the curved hemostat into the incision and spreading the incision horizontally. This is felt to be superior to simply inserting the handle of the scalpel into the wound and rotating it 90 degrees.

10. Place the curved hemostat or Trousseau dilator into the widened cricothyroid incision, with the blades oriented inferiorly.

11. Pass the tracheostomy tube (or endotracheal tube) between the spread blades of the curved hemostat or Trousseau dilator.

12. Remove the hemostat (or Trousseau dilator) and inflate the balloon of the tube.

13. Ventilate the lungs using the bag-valve-mask.

14. Confirm tube placement by auscultating breath sounds, listening over the stomach, and using end-tidal carbon dioxide detectors or pulse oximetry.
15. Secure the tube to the skin by using a circumferential tie around the neck or by suturing.

COMPLICATIONS

Bleeding
Incorrect tube placement
Unsuccessful tube placement
Pneumothorax, pneumomediastinum
Tracheal perforation
Vocal cord injury
Aspiration
Subcutaneous emphysema
Esophageal perforation
Tracheal perforation
Infection leading to cellulitis and sepsis
Phrenic nerve and brachial plexus injury

Bibliography

American College of Surgeons: Advanced Trauma Life Support: Instructor Manual. American College of Surgeons, 1993, pp 71–73.

Caroline N: Emergency Care in the Streets, ed 4. Little, Brown & Co, Boston, 1991, pp 96–97.

Ho MT and Saunders CE (eds): Current Emergency Diagnosis and Treatment. Lange Medical Publications, Norwalk, CT, 1990, pp 809–810.

Jones S, Weigel A et al. (eds): Advanced Emergency Care for Paramedic Practice. JB Lippincott, Philadelphia, 1992, pp 160–169.

Mace SE: Cricothyrotomy. In Roberts JR and Hedges JR (eds): Clinical Procedures in Emergency Medicine, ed 2. WB Saunders, Philadelphia, 1991, pp 40–59.

Notes

CHAPTER 61

Endotracheal Intubation and Extubation

Owen T. Traynor, MD

NOTE: Use body substance isolation whenever the possibility exists of contact with blood or and body fluids. This should include gloves, eye protection, masks, and other barrires as necessary. When sharp instruments are used (ie, needles), a sharp instrument container must be available for their safe disposal.

Orotracheal Intubation

INDICATIONS

Any situation when there is a need to secure the airway of a patient who has lost airway control. Patients who would benefit from the insertion of an endotracheal tube (ET) include those who have experienced cardiac or respiratory arrest, coma, or ventilatory or respiratory failure.

NOTE: Endotracheal tube intubation may be performed in the multitrauma patient if cervical-spine stabilization is maintained by a second EMS provider.

CONTRAINDICATIONS

If the endotracheal intubation procedure will compromise cervical-spine control or precipitate laryngospasm, it is contraindicated.

EQUIPMENT

Laryngoscope handle and blade, ET, 10 ml syringe, malleable stylet, water-soluble lubricant (K-Y jelly), suction device and equipment, Magill forceps, bag-valve-mask (BVM), oxygen source, tape, Kling or commercial ET tube holder.

PROCEDURE

1. Confirm the order to intubate or proceed on standing order.

2. Determine the correct size tube needed, and assemble and check the equipment, including inflation and deflation of the ET tube cuff. Lubricate tip of ET tube.
3. Hyperventilate the patient for at least 30 seconds before ET attempt.
4. If cervical spine precautions are not indicated, place the patient in the "sniffing" position, and remove the oropharyngeal airway. If cervical spine precautions are indicated, an assistant must continue to stabalize the cervical spine throughout this procedure.
5. Hold the laryngoscope in the left hand and insert into the patient's mouth without causing trauma.
6. Maneuver the laryngoscope to visualize the vocal cords (do not use the teeth or gums as a fulcrum).
7. While maintaining direct visualization of the vocal cords, insert the ET tube into the trachea.
8. Remove the laryngoscope blade from the patient's mouth and the stylet from the ET tube, taking care to manually stabilize the tube in place.
9. Ventilate the patient no later than 30 seconds from the time of the last ventilation.
10. Note the rise and fall of the chest.
11. Instruct another EMS provider to continue ventilations using a BVM.
12. Auscultate the chest and abdomen to ensure correct placement of the ET tube.
13. Check tube placement with an end-tidal carbon dioxide monitor.
14. Inflate the cuff with the minimum volume of air needed to seal the tube.
15. Auscultate the chest and abdomen to ensure correct placement of the ET tube.
16. Insert an oropharyngeal airway and secure the ET tube in place with tape or Kling or a commercial holder.

Nasotracheal Intubation

INDICATIONS

Any situation where there is a need for control of the airway and orotracheal intubation is not feasible, owing to spontaneous respirations, clenched teeth, intact gag reflex, facial trauma, and so forth.

CONTRAINDICATIONS

Patients with a known bleeding disorder, severe facial trauma, or basilar skull fracture should not be intubated by the nasotracheal method.

EQUIPMENT

Endotracheal tubes (7.0, 7.5, and 8.0 mm for adults), 10 ml syringe, water-soluble lubricant and anesthetic agent (lidocaine jelly), oxymetazoline spray (Afrin) or 0.25% phenylephrine (Neo-Synephrine), suction device and equipment, Magill forceps, bag-valve-mask (BVM), oxygen source, tape or Kling holder.

PROCEDURE

1. Confirm the order to intubate or proceed on standing order.
2. Determine the correct size tube needed and assemble and check the equipment, including inflation and deflation of the ET tube cuff. Lubricate the ET tube with viscous lidocaine.
3. Apply intranasal oxymetazoline spray or 0.25% phenylephrine to vasoconstrict vessels in nasal passages to decrease bleeding.
4. Gently insert the tip of the ET tube into the nare and push (do not jab) until the tip is at the tracheal opening (breathing sounds will be loudest). If sounds diminish, indicating entry into the esophagus, pull back slightly until sounds increase. Be prepared to suction the patient.
5. Listen at the open end of the ET tube for the sound of inspiration and gently insert the tube into the trachea.
6. Connect a BVM to the ET tube and ventilate the patient.
7. Note the rise and fall of the chest.
8. Instruct another EMS provider to continue ventilations using a BVM.
9. Auscultate the chest and abdomen to ensure correct placement of the ET tube. If the tube has entered the esophagus, withdraw to the nasopharynx and attempt to place the tube in the trachea again.
10. Check tube placement with end-tidal carbon dioxide monitor.

11. Inflate the cuff with the minimum volume of air needed to seal the tube.
12. Auscultate the chest and abdomen to ensure correct placement of the ET tube.
13. Secure the ET tube in place with tape or a cling wrap.

Extubation

INDICATIONS

Any time the patient regains control of the airway and exhibits nontolerance (ie, gagging) of the ET tube.

CONTRAINDICATIONS

None; however, vomiting may occur and you should be prepared to suction the airway.

EQUIPMENT

Suction device and equipment, bandage, and scissors.

PROCEDURE

1. Turn on and test the suction unit.
2. Turn the patient's head to the side. If patient is immobilized to a spine board, turn the entire body.
3. Remove the oral airway and the device securing the tube.
4. Deflate the distal cuff.
5. Remove ET tube on inspiration.
6. Suction as needed.
7. Reassess the airway.

Foreign Body Removal

INDICATIONS

Any situation where there is a history of airway obstruction and basic life support techniques to clear the airway have failed.

CONTRAINDICATIONS

None if the airway remains obstructed.

EQUIPMENT

Laryngoscope handle and blade, Magill forceps, suction device and equipment, bag-valve-mask, oxygen source.

PROCEDURE

1. Confirm obstruction and reattempt basic life support procedures.
2. Position the patient's head and neck in a sniffing position.
3. Insert a laryngoscope and visualize glottic opening.
4. Identify obstruction. **NOTE:** If no foreign body is visible, intubate the patient. If the patient still can not be ventilated, consider passing the ET tube distally into the right mainstem bronchus. This may potentially push the foreign body into the right bronchus, and allow ventilating the left lung after the ET tube is withdrawn to its normal location. DO NOT force the ET tube distally.
5. Insert Magill forceps and position at the obstructing object.
6. Grasp obstruction and remove, using caution not to cause trauma.
7. Remove the laryngoscope.
8. Reassess and position the airway.
9. Attempt ventilation.

Bibliography

Bledsoe BE, Porter RS, and Shade BR (eds): Paramedic Emergency Care. Prentice-Hall, Englewood Cliffs, NJ, 1991, pp 234–262.
Caroline NL: Emergency Care in the Streets. ed 4. Little, Brown & Co, Boston, 1991, pp 77–89.

Notes

CHAPTER 62

Esophageal Obturator and Esophageal Gastric Tube Airways

Patrick R. Coonan, RN, EdD,CEN, EMT-CC

NOTE: Use body substance isolation whenever the possibility exists of contact with blood or any body fluids. This should include gloves, eye protection, masks, and other protective barriers as necessary. When sharp instruments are used (ie, needles), a sharp instrument container must be available for their safe disposal.

Indications

The esophageal obturator airway (EOA) and esophageal gastric tube airway (EGTA) may be used for control of the airway when it is not feasible to insert an endotracheal tube in a comatose or cardiac or respiratory arrest patient.

Contraindications

The EOA and EGTA should not be used in persons under the age of 16 years, those shorter than 5 feet or taller than 6 feet 7 inches, those who have ingested caustic poisons, or those with a history of esophageal disease or alcoholism.

Equipment

Esophageal obturator airway or EGTA, water-soluble lubricant (ie, K-Y jelly), oxygen, bag-valve-mask.

Procedure

The procedure for inserting both the EOA and EGTA is the same except for the insertion of a Levine tube through the EGTA.

1. Ensure effective ventilations using a bag-valve-mask and an oropharyngeal airway (OPA).
2. Check and assemble the equipment, including inflation and deflation of the EOA/EGTA cuff.
3. Apply a water-soluble lubricant to the tip of the EOA or EGTA.
4. Order the ventilator to stop ventilations.
5. If cervical spine precautions are not indicated, place the patient's head in a neutral position, otherwise maintain cervical spine stabilization.
6. Remove the OPA.
7. Insert the EOA or EGTA properly following the natural curvature of the pharynx.
8. Ventilate the patient within 15 seconds of the last ventilation.
9. Note the rise and fall of the chest, indicating proper placement.
10. Instruct another provider to take over ventilations using the BVM and to continue to ventilate the patient once every 5 seconds throughout the remainder of the procedure.
11. Auscultate the chest and abdomen to ensure correct placement of the EOA or EGTA.
12. Inflate the EOA or EGTA cuff with 25 to 35 ml of air and remove the syringe immediately.
13. Auscultate the chest and abdomen to ensure correct placement of the EOA or EGTA.

The following step applies to the EGTA only:

14. Measure, lubricate, and insert the Levine tube. Place the end of the Levine tube in a suitable container to collect gastric contents.

Bibliography

Allison EJ Jr (ed): Advanced Life Support Skills. Mosby–Year Book, St. Louis, 1994, pp 145–154.

Bledsoe BE, Porter RS, and Shade BR (eds): Paramedic Emergency Care, ed 2. Englewood Cliffs, NJ, Prentice Hall, 1994, pp 235–238.

Notes

CHAPTER 63

External Cardiac Pacing
Thomas J. Rahilly, MS, EMT-CC

This technique is the initial pacing method of choice in emergency cardiac care because of the speed with which it can be instituted and because it is the least invasive pacing technique available.

Indications

EMERGENT PACING

- Hemodynamically compromising bradycardias (systolic BP less than 80 mm Hg, change in mental status, myocardial ischemia, pulmonary edema).
- Bradycardia with malignant escape rhythms (unresponsive to pharmacologic therapy).
- Overdrive pacing of refractory tachycardia (supraventricular or ventricular [currently indicated only in special situations refractory to pharmacologic therapy or cardioversion]).
- Bradyasystolic cardiac arrest. Pacing not routinely recommended in such patients. If used at all, pacing should be used as early as possible after onset of arrest.
- Asystole

STANDBY MODE

- Stable bradycardias (BP greater than 80 mm Hg, no evidence of hemodynamic compromise, or hemodynamic compromise responsive to initial drug therapy).
- Prophylactic pacing in acute myocardial infarction.
- Symptomatic sinus node dysfunction.
- Mobitz II second-degree heart block.
- Third-degree heart block.
- Newly acquired left bundle-branch block, right bundle-branch block, alternating bundle-branch block, or bifascicular block.

Contraindications

None in the presence of indicators.

Equipment

Monitor and defibrillator equipped with external pacing option, pacing cable, and electrodes.

Procedure

NOTE: Not all external pacing-equipped monitors and defibrillators operate alike. Follow the manufacturer's operating guide for the one in use by your service.

ELECTRODE PLACEMENT

- Anteroposterior (AP) is preferred.
  - Anterior electrode (negative)—left anterior chest at the level of nipple midway between xiphoid and left nipple.
  - Posterior electrode (positive)—left posterior chest beneath scapula.
- Anteroanterior is an acceptable alternate if AP placement is not possible.
  - Apical electrode (negative)—fourth intercostal space midaxillary line.
  - Sternal electrode (positive)—right anterior chest midclavicular line.

PACING FOR BRADYARRHYTHMIAS

1. Confirm the order for transcutaneous pacing.
2. Explain the procedure to the patient (if alert) and obtain the patient's consent.
3. Turn monitor and defibrillator power on.
4. Prepare the skin at electrode sites.
5. Attach monitor electrodes (lead II).
6. Connect the pacing cable.
7. Attach and apply the pacing electrodes.
8. Turn pacer on.
9. Set the desired rate, usually 60 to 80 bpm (start at 40 bpm; increase by 10-bpm increments).
10. Adjust QRS size until R wave is sensed.

11. Press start/stop.
12. Increase current until capture occurs (start at zero).
13. Verify pulse, run rhythm strip, and monitor vital signs.

PACING FOR ASYSTOLE

1. Confirm the order for transcutaneous pacing.
2. Turn monitor and defibrillator power on.
3. Prepare the skin at electrode sites.
4. Attach monitor electrodes (lead II).
5. Connect the pacing cable.
6. Attach and apply the pacing electrodes.
7. Turn pacer on.
8. Set the rate at 80 bpm.
9. Press start/stop.
10. Increase current until capture occurs or maximum current is reached.
11. Verify pulse, run rhythm strip, and monitor vital signs.

EVIDENCE OF CAPTURE

- Wide QRS complex: tall, wide T
- Palpable pulse at "set" rate
- Improved BP
- Improved level of consciousness
- Improved skin color and temperature

Side Effects

- Skeletal muscle contractions
- Chest muscle discomfort (use lowest current possible)

Bibliography

Allison EJ Jr (ed): Advanced Life Support Skills. Mosby–Year Book, St. Louis, 1994, pp 157–160.

Bledsoe BE: The Acute Abdomen. In Bledsoe BE, Porter RS, and Shade BR (eds): Paramedic Emergency Care. Prentice-Hall, Englewood Cliffs, NJ, 1991, p 721.

Caroline NL: Emergency Care in the Streets. ed 4. Little, Brown & Co, Boston, 1991, pp 539–540.

Notes

CHAPTER 64

Intraosseous Infusion
Patrick R. Coonan, RN, EdD, CEN, EMT-CC

NOTE: Use body substance isolation whenever the possibility exists of contact with blood or any body fluids. This should include gloves, eye protection, masks, and other protective barriers as necessary. When sharp instruments are used (ie, needles), a sharp instrument container must be available for their safe disposal.

Indications

Intraosseous infusion (IO) should be used with critically ill or injured children (younger than 6 years of age) when there is a need for venous access and:
- Attempts at IV access have failed.
- There is no evident peripheral venous access.

Contraindications

Intraosseous infusion should not be attempted if:
- The child is alert.
- There was a previous IO attempt in the same tibia.
- There is a fracture above the intended site.
- Infected or burned skin is evident at the insertion site.

Equipment

IV fluid, microdrip or burette solution administration set, two 15 gauge IO or bone marrow needles, povidone-iodine (Betadine) swabs, antibiotic ointment, 10 ml syringe, injectable sterile saline solution, arm board, sterile dressings (4″ × 4″), 2-inch cling tape.

Procedure

1. Assemble and prepare all necessary equipment.
2. Locate the insertion site on the flat surface of the tibia, approximately 1 to 3 cm below the tibial tuberosity.

3. Prepare the site with povidone-iodine. Keep the site aseptic throughout the procedure.
4. Insert the IO needle at a 60 degree angle from the leg and aim **away** from the knee. This will prevent accidental damage to the knee.
5. Apply firm steady pressure with a twisting motion to reduce the chances of fracturing the tibia.
6. Continue to twist and apply firm pressure until you feel a sudden decrease in resistance. This sudden "pop" means you have entered the marrow space.
7. Remove the stylet and attach the syringe. Correct position is assumed if 5 to 10 ml of fluid can be infused without resistance or subcutaneous infiltration or if bone marrow can be freely aspirated by drawing back on the syringe plunger.
8. Infuse fluids or medications as ordered.
9. Secure the IO needle. Apply antibiotic ointment around the site and stabilize the IO needle as you would any impaled object using tape, bulky dressings, and Kling. The needle should be freestanding because it is being supported by the patient's bone, but requires added stabilization to prevent accidental removal.

Complications

- Swelling of soft tissues resulting in compartment syndrome
- Injury to the growth plate
- Fracture of the tibia
- Local bleeding
- Injection into the knee joint
- Periostitis
- Embolism of clots or bone marrow
- Fat embolism (rare)
- Osteomyelitis (rare)

Bibliography

Allison EJ Jr (ed): Advanced Life Support Skills. Mosby–Year Book, St. Louis, 1994, pp 186–189.
Bledsoe BE, Porter RS, and Shade BR: Paramedic Emergency Care, ed 2. Englewood Cliffs, NJ, Prentice Hall, 1994, pp 947–949.

Notes

CHAPTER 65

Medication Administration

Thomas J. Rahilly, MS, EMT-CC

NOTE: Use body substance isolation whenever the possibility exists of contact with blood or any body fluids. This should include gloves, eye protection, masks, and other protective barriers as necessary. When sharp instruments are used (ie, needles), a sharp instrument container must be available for their safe disposal.

Intravenous Bolus Administration

INDICATIONS

Any situation when there is a need for the rapid administration of a medication.

CONTRAINDICATIONS

None if the IV is functioning properly.

EQUIPMENT

Medication, syringe with needle or prefilled syringe, alcohol-prepared pads, sharp instruments container.

PROCEDURE

1. Confirm order, including medication, dosage, and route.
2. Explain the procedure to the patient and confirm that the patient is not known to be allergic to the medication.
3. Assemble the necessary medication and equipment.
4. Select the correct medication and inspect it for expiration date, discoloration, and particulate matter.
5. Fill syringe with medication or assemble the prefilled syringe.

6. Expel air and excess medication from the syringe (only the ordered dosage should remain in the syringe).
7. Select the medication administration port closest to the cannula and cleanse the port with an alcohol preparation.
8. Pinch close the IV tubing above the medication administration port. Closing the drip rate control valve is also acceptable.
9. Insert needle into the port and inject the correct amount of medication. In cardiac arrest, medications should be followed by a 20 ml flush and the extremity elevated to speed medication delivery to the central circulation.
10. Remove the needle and syringe and dispose of it safely.
11. Flush the IV line by opening the drip rate control valve.
12. Readjust the drip rate.

Intravenous Infusion (Piggyback) Administration

INDICATIONS

Any situation where there is a need for the immediate administration of a second IV fluid or titrated infusion of a specific medication.

CONTRAINDICATIONS

None if the primary IV is functioning properly.

EQUIPMENT

Appropriate IV fluid, medication, secondary administration set, needle, syringe with needle or prefilled syringe, alcohol-prepared pads, tape, and sharp instrument container.

PROCEDURE

1. Confirm order, including medication, dosage, and route.
2. Explain the procedure to the patient and confirm that the patient has no known allergies to the medication.
3. Assemble the necessary medication and equipment including the secondary IV setup.
4. Select the correct medication and inspect it for expiration date, discoloration, and particulate matter.

5. Calculate the required amount of medication and fill the syringe or assemble the prefilled syringe.
6. Expel air and excess medication from the syringe (only the ordered dosage should remain in the syringe).
7. Cleanse the medication port of the secondary IV bag with an alcohol preparation, inject the medication into the port, and gently shake the bag to mix the medication and solution.
8. Label the IV bag with the medication, amount injected, medication concentration, the time and date, and your initials.
9. Attach a sterile needle to the administration set, cleanse the injection port closest to the patient, and insert the needle up to the hub.
10. Close the primary IV control valve and open the secondary IV control valve to the desired drip rate.
11. Secure the secondary needle to the primary set with tape.

Intramuscular Injection

INDICATIONS

Administration of medications that require a slow rate of absorption.

CONTRAINDICATIONS

Hypotensive patients.

EQUIPMENT

Medication, syringe, 21 gauge needle, alcohol prep pads.

PROCEDURE

1. Confirm order, including medication, dosage, and route.
2. Explain the procedure to the patient and confirm that the patient has no known allergies to the medication.
3. Assemble the necessary medication and equipment.
4. Select the correct medication and inspect it for discoloration, particulate matter, and expiration date.
5. Select the proper size syringe and needle.

6. Shake down the ampule and safely break the ampule.
7. Withdraw the medication aseptically and expel air and excess medication from the syringe (only the ordered dosage should remain in the syringe).
8. Locate the deltoid area and prepare the injection site with an alcohol preparation using a concentric motion.
9. Stretch the skin taut around the injection site and insert the needle at a 90 degree angle.
10. Aspirate for blood; if blood appears, withdraw the needle and select another site.
11. Inject full dosage of medication with a slow steady push of the syringe.
12. Withdraw needle at same entry angle.
13. Massage the injection site with an alcohol preparation.
14. Properly dispose of needle and syringe.

Subcutaneous Injection

INDICATIONS

Administration of medications requiring injection into the fatty subcutaneous tissue, such as those for allergic or anaphylactic reactions.

CONTRAINDICATIONS

Patients with inadequate perfusion should not receive medication by the subcutaneous route.

EQUIPMENT

Medication, 1 ml tuberculin syringe, 25 gauge 5/8-inch needle, alcohol prep pads.

PROCEDURE

1. Confirm order, including medication, dosage, and route.
2. Explain the procedure to the patient and confirm that the patient has no known allergies to the medication.
3. Assemble the necessary medication and equipment.
4. Select the correct medication and inspect it for expiration date, discoloration, and particulate matter.

5. Select the proper size syringe and needle.
6. Shake down the ampule and safely break the ampule.
7. Withdraw the medication aseptically and expel air and excess medication from the syringe (only the ordered dosage should remain in the syringe).
8. Locate the deltoid area and prepare the injection site with an alcohol prep using a concentric motion.
9. Pinch the skin away from the underlying tissue and insert the needle at 45 degree angle.
10. Aspirate for blood; if blood appears, withdraw the needle and select another site.
11. Inject the full dosage of medication with a slow steady push of the syringe.
12. Withdraw needle at same entry angle.
13. Massage the injection site with an alcohol preparation.
14. Properly dispose of needle and syringe.

Endotracheal Tube Administration

INDICATIONS

Any situation where there is a need for the rapid administration of certain medications when no IV access is available and an endotracheal tube (ET) tube is in place.

CONTRAINDICATIONS

None, although the medications administered by this route include only the "NAVEL" drugs: naloxone (Narcan), atropine, diazepam (Valium), epinephrine, and lidocaine.

EQUIPMENT

Medication, syringe without needle or prefilled syringe, injectable normal saline, sharp instrument container.

PROCEDURE

1. Confirm order, including medication, dosage, and route.
2. If possible, confirm that the patient has no known allergic reaction to the medication.
3. Assemble the necessary medication and equipment.
4. Select the correct medication and inspect it for expiration date, discoloration, and particulate matter.

5. Prepare the medication aseptically and expel air and excess medication from the syringe (only the ordered dosage should remain in the syringe). Drugs administered through the ET tube are usually 2 to 2.5 times the recommended dose. In addition, the drug should be diluted in or flushed by 10 ml of normal saline or sterile water.
6. Hyperventilate the patient.
7. Stop ventilations and remove the ventilating device from the ET tube.
8. Stop CPR (if in progress) and quickly spray the medication down the ET tube. **NOTE:** Remove the needle from the syringe before administration.
9. Reconnect the ventilating device to the ET tube and hyperventilate the patient.
10. Resume CPR after the medication has been nebulized (several brisk ventilations).
11. Properly dispose of needle and syringe.

Bibliography

Allison EJ Jr (ed): Advanced Life Support Skills. Mosby–Year Book, St. Louis, 1994, pp 105–125.

Bledsoe BE, Poreter RS, and Shade BR (eds): Paramedic Emergency Care, ed 2. Prentice-Hall, Englewood Cliffs, NJ, 1994, pp 356–364.

Caroline NL: Emergency Care in the Streets, ed 4. Little, Brown & Co, Boston, 1991, pp 211–223.

Notes

CHAPTER 66

Needle Chest Decompression

Owen T. Traynor, MD

This procedure should be performed only when indicated and authorized by local medical control.

NOTE: Use body substance isolation whenever the possibility exists of contact with blood or any body fluids. This should include gloves, eye protection, masks, and other protective barriers as necessary. When sharp instruments are used (ie, needles), a sharp instrument container must be available for their safe disposal.

Indications

Life-threatening tension pneumothorax.

Contraindications

None when used in the treatment of a tension pneumothorax.

Equipment

Povidone-iodine solution, sterile gauze sponges, 14 to 16 gauge over-the-needle IV catheters, 1 inch adhesive tape, flutter-type valve.

Procedure

1. Assess the patient's respiratory status and breath sounds.
2. Administer high-flow oxygen and ventilate as necessary.
3. Explain the procedure to the awake patient, without delaying the procedure.
4. Place the patient supine, with the head of the stretcher

elevated 30 degrees, if cervical-spine precautions are not necessary.

5. Locate the second intercostal space at the midclavicular line on the side of the tension pneumothorax.
6. Rapidly prepare the site using the povidone-iodine solution, if time permits.
7. Insert a 14 to 16 gauge over-the-needle catheter into the second intercostal space at the midclavicular line, by passing just superior to the third rib. Thus, you will avoid puncturing the neurovascular bundle found inferior to the rib.
8. Advance the needle until the parietal pleura is punctured. A rush of escaping air will occur as the chest is decompressed.
9. Advance the catheter over the needle and remove the needle. Safely dispose of the needle.
10. Attach a flutter device (Penrose drain) to the hub of the catheter.
11. Secure the catheter to the chest wall using adhesive tape.
12. Be sure to frequently reassess the patient's respiratory status and breath sounds. Maintain high-concentration oxygen therapy.

Complications

- Pneumothorax
- Hemorrhage
- Pleural infection
- Local hematoma
- Skin infection.

Bibliography

Chest Trauma Management. In American College of Surgeons (ed): Advanced Trauma Life Support Student Manual. American College of Surgeons, Chicago, 1993, pp 135–138.

Ross DS: Thoracentesis. In Roberts JR and Hedges JR (eds): Clinical Procedures in Emergency Medicine, ed 2. WB Saunders, Philadelphia, 1991, pp 112–117.

Notes

CHAPTER 67

Peripheral Intravenous Insertion

Owen T. Traynor, MD

NOTE: Use body substance isolation whenever the possibility exists of contact with blood or any body fluids. This should include gloves, eye protection, masks, and other protective barriers as necessary. When sharp instruments are used (ie, needles), a sharp instrument container must be available for their safe disposal.

Indications

An intravenous line should be placed whenever the need for the administration of intravenous fluids or medications exists or potentially exists.

Contraindications

There are no contraindications in emergency situations; however, intravenous (IV) insertion should not significantly delay the transport of a critically ill or injured patient to the ED.

Equipment

Appropriate IV fluid, administration set and catheters, alcohol or povidone iodine (Betadine) preparations, venous constricting band (VCB), blood tubes and collection equipment, sterile dressings (4″ × 4″ squares), armboard, tape, or commercial site cover.

Procedure

1. Inform the patient about the procedure and obtain the patient's consent.
2. Assemble and ready the equipment.

3. Select the proper fluid and inspect it for expiration date, contaminants, and leaks.
4. Select the appropriate administration set, unroll tubing, and position and close the drip rate control valve.
5. Remove the protective cover and insert the administration set into the fluid bag port using an aseptic technique.
6. Open the control valve, squeeze the drip chamber, and fill one half of the chamber with fluid.
7. With the fluid flowing, bleed all of the air from the IV tubing.
8. Close the control valve and inspect for air bubbles in the IV tubing.
9. Place a VCB and palpate a radial pulse.
10. Select a suitable vein.
11. Prep the IV site with Betadine and alcohol (use concentric circles).
12. Stabilize the vein distal to the IV site.
13. Aseptically puncture the skin with the catheter (bevel up), enter the vein (from the top or side), and obtain a flashback.
14. Release the VCB.
15. Remove the needle aseptically and draw blood if necessary and then connect the IV tubing to the catheter.
16. Dispose of the needle safely.
17. Open the drip control valve and note the free flow of fluid.
18. Adjust flow rate to the appropriate rate as directed by medical control physician or protocol.
19. Inspect the surrounding tissue for infiltration of fluid.
20. Secure the catheter and IV tubing using tape or commercial site cover.

Bibliography

Allison EJ Jr (ed): Advanced Life Support Skills. Mosby–Year Book, St. Louis, 1994, pp 88–91.

Bledsoe BE, Porter RS, and Shade BR (eds): Paramedic Emergency Care, ed 2. Prentice-Hall, Englewood Cliffs, NJ, 1994, pp 233–236.

Notes

SECTION IV

Medicolegal Documentation

CHAPTER 68

Oral Case Presentations

Patrick R. Coonan, RN, EdD, CEN, EMT-CC

The oral case presentation is the primary means by which clinicians convey to each other information about patients. Excellence of oral presentation reflects your basic grasp of the patient's condition and your capacity to reduce complex data to a readily understandable form. In learning to present well, you will develop skills in obtaining, organizing, and conveying clinical information.

An oral presentation, like a written case report, gives a concise, compressed account of only the most essential facts. Moreover, the content of the oral report varies markedly, depending on its purpose. This can be providing a quick overview at the scene to fellow caregivers to an in-depth review at a continuing medical education (CME) course or other event. One of the keys to good patient care is communication. The quality of the oral case presentation given to the medical control physician may influence the nature of orders granted. Your report given to the ED staff can make the difference in the patient's outcome and is a synopsis of your evaluation and intervention with the patient.

In making oral presentations, you should bear in mind the limitations of the listener, whether that be the ED physician, nurse, or colleague. The listener has only you to listen to and must register all of the important details of a case and to synthesize the information while listening. To help the listener with this task, your presentation needs to be especially clear, uncluttered, and easily grasped. The listener should be guided through a reasoning process that helps them consider a differential diagnosis. The organization of the oral presentation is similar to that used in newspaper articles: begin with headlines, follow with lead sentences, and progress to more detailed matters that are not essential to the case.

The format of the oral presentation should somewhat parallel the written report.

- A headline sentence that includes identifying data and the reason for the visit. Age, sex, and the patient's chief complaint.
- A brief history of the current event followed by a brief past history, including the patient's medication and drug allergy history.
- The primary and secondary survey findings begin with a statement about appearance and vital signs and then proceed with a head-to-toe assessment, concluding with neurologic assessment if appropriate.
- Your working or presumptive diagnosis, which can be as specific as myocardial infarction or as general as chest pain.
- Any interventions given, including the response to therapy.
- How long the call has been in progress, if applicable.
- Your assessment, which includes a brief summary, then addresses the most severe, acute, or central medical problem, and then goes on to secondary matters.

A sample presentation follows:

The patient is a 45-year-old-man, with a past medical history significant for coronary artery disease, status post three MIs, hypertension, and insulin-dependent diabetes mellitus, who presents with a chief complaint of crushing retrosternal chest pain. The pain began at rest 1 hour ago and is associated with dyspnea, nausea, and vomiting. The patient reports this pain is similar to previous MI chest pain. The patient took two sublingual NTG prior to our arrival and reports no relief of symptoms. The patient's medications include Procardia, Lasix, and insulin.

- On physical examination, the patient is a 45-year-old man who appears dyspneic.
- His vital signs are HR, 96, regular; RR, 18, shallow; BP, 156/100 mm Hg
- Skin: cool, pale, moist
- No JVD
- Lungs: clear to auscultation, except basilar inspiratory rales.
- Abdomen is soft, nontender.
- Extremities have strong distal pulses and no peripheral edema.
- ECG shows NSR without ventricular ectopy. There are ST elevations in the lateral leads.

In summary, this is a 45-year-old man with a history of previous MIs now presenting with 1 hour of chest pain similar to previous MI pain. Our presumptive diagnosis is acute MI. We have placed the patient on 100% O$_2$ and have established IV access. We would like to give an additional sublingual NTG— if there is insufficient pain relief— we would like permission to give 3 mg of morphine IV. We are prepared to transport the patient to the ED, with an ETA of 15 minutes.

The opening statement should give a broad overview of the patient. These are the headlines that orient your listener to the remainder of the presentation. Begin with the patient's age and sex. If relevant, include marital status, race, ethnicity, or occupation. If the patient has a history of major medical problems that bear strongly on the present illness, such as recent heart attack, diabetes, alcoholism, and so forth, mention them in a few words. Next give the chief complaint, the reason for this trip to the emergency department. This is just a few words that set the stage for more detailed consideration of the patient's problem. The duration of the patient's symptoms can be included here.

The body of the report focuses on one or more major problems in the history of present illness. Present the most important problem first, along with all relevant information including pertinent abnormal findings. Cover all data about one problem before going on to another. Do not be under the illusion that a good presentation involves just the recital of all the data you know about the patient. You need to select essential information and organize it into a coherent story that can be told in a limited time. The inclusion of any data should be justifiable in terms of its usefulness in figuring out the patient's problem(s). The presentation of the primary and secondary survey begins with a few broad comments about the patient's general appearance and condition. Most times only abnormal findings are presented, and all else is considered unremarkable. As a rule, include all significant abnormal findings and any normal findings that contributed to the process of figuring out the patient's problem; omit insignificant or irrelevant abnormalities and other normal findings.

The content and organization of an oral case presentation reflect your fundamental appreciation of the patient and the problem. All healthcare providers develop their own styles of presenting, and no single format is right for every case or patient. The two most common problems are excessive length and poor organization. Practice your presentations with the following points in mind:

- Paint a broad picture, and then follow with details that the listener needs to understand the patient.
- Do not simply recite facts. A presentation should give a fair and undistorted report of the data in an organized fashion.
- Make the format appropriate to the setting. If you are giving a report to colleagues in the field, a "quick and dirty" report may be appropriate. Be familiar with the interests and expectations of the listeners, their time constraints, and their goals for the case.
- Be brief and lucid. Consider whether anything can be condensed, clarified, or omitted. Try not to repeat yourself.
- Speak clearly and crisply. Give an energetic account and engage your listeners.

What makes this case special? A few well-chosen words about how this case is interesting can help you to get more attention and thus help the patient to receive better care.

An effective, organized, and concise oral report can make a difference in the care your patient receives. Practice the method presented here and use it whenever possible. It will expedite patient care and improve your relationship with the ED staff.

Bibliography

Billings AJ and Stoeckle JD: The Clinical Encounter: A Guide to the Medical Interview and Case Presentation. Yearbook Medical Publishers, Chicago, 1989, pp 259–269.

Notes

CHAPTER 69

Written Reports
Bruce M. Cohn, JD, EMT-CC

Written documentation of the prehospital encounter serves a number of essential purposes. First and foremost, it is part of the patient's medical record. The information contained in the prehospital patient care report may be used by the hospital in formulating a plan of treatment for the patient. The prehospital report is a legal document. It will become vital in the event a lawsuit ensues over any aspect of the patient's evaluation, treatment, and care within the medical system. A detailed, properly completed record may help you successfully defend allegations of wrongdoing or prevent the filing of a lawsuit in the first place. The prehospital report is also a valuable document for retrospective analysis, as a learning experience and as the basis for a quality assurance/improvement program.

A prehospital patient care report should be completed for every call, no matter how trivial. You should make every effort to generate a document that is legible and accurate and that includes as much information as possible. Although the specific information on the form varies by locality and by local protocol and needs, the following considerations apply in most situations and to all EMS provider–patient interactions:

- Ensure that date and times are accurate. Making up or estimating times may seem harmless at the time, but can be detrimental in the event of a legal problem. Times noted on the run sheet must conform with times noted on any other documents, including the electronic data stored by computer-aided dispatch systems.
- Document the "chief complaint" using the patient's own language as it was given. If the information comes from a source other than the patient, note from whom it came, this person's relationship to the patient, and the basis of this person's knowledge.
- Detail your assessment of the problem within the scope of your training and experience. Making even educated guesses about complex diagnoses that require extensive

hospital testing and evaluation by a physician create potential problems and do not serve the patient's best interest. For example, instead of guessing and making a diagnosis of acute pancreatitis, it is better to make your presumptive diagnosis abdominal pain.

- The history of the present illness and past medical history should be included to facilitate rapid diagnosis and treatment by the emergency department staff. Having been at the location where the illness first occurred or at the scene of the accident, you are in a unique position to obtain vital information that would otherwise to be lost to the attending physicians.
- Carefully note the patient's vital signs, level of consciousness, and any physical change while in your care. Vital signs should be complete with times and manner they are obtained. If a particular vital sign is omitted owing to patient comfort, refusal or any other reason, document the circumstances.
- Any medications administered should be noted on the form with dosage, route, and time of administration. Be specific; for example, when an IV is started, the catheter gauge and fluid administered is important information for both medical and legal purposes.
- Note any patient response to therapy and any problems encountered en route to the hospital. This includes the patient's reaction to medications, problems with treatment, or difficulties in communications with the medical control physician or the patient.
- Any information obtained from medical devices such as ECG, electronic blood pressure monitors, or pulse oximetry should be noted with copies of printouts attached, consistent with your local protocols and procedures.

The patient care report should not contain any gratuitous negative comments about the patient or the activity prompting the call for the ambulance. Any information obtained other than from the patient or bystanders (such as seat belt use) should indicate whether this was an observation of the crew or was obtained from some other source. On forms with check boxes or fill-in-the-blanks, take special care to ensure that the correct information is listed in the appropriate space. Check the form carefully before submitting it to ensure that all necessary items have been filled out accurately.

One of the greatest areas of potential liability for EMS providers is spinal immobilization precautions. In patients who require immobilization, note in detail the equipment and technique used. The patient's neurologic status on your arrival, after immobilization, and on transfer to the hospital must be documented.

All treatments rendered to a patient, whether inside or outside of the hospital, require the consent of the patient or the patient's healthcare representative. If a patient refuses a particular procedure or does not want to be transported to the hospital, proper documentation becomes critical. Never assume that your recollection of the events will coincide with that of the patient or your fellow crew members. Conflicts between documents written at the time in question and testimony as to someone's recollection generally favor the document. Any information given to the patient regarding the possible consequences of refusing care should be noted in detail. If the conversation was held in the presence of a family member or a police officer, indicate this on the report. The signed refusal of the patient must be obtained and witnessed properly. Police officers are generally considered to be the most appropriate witnesses. They are also required to document their official actions and are more likely to be available for corroboration at a later date.

Effective documentation of the prehospital encounter is a necessary part of the EMS process. A carefully prepared patient care report provides benefits to the patient, the provider, and the system in promoting good patient care, quality assurance, and reducing legal liability.

Bibliography

Instruction Manual for Prehospital Care Report, New York State Department of Health, Emergency Medical Services Program, Albany, NY, 1985.

Goldstein AS: Observing Record Keeping Requirements. In EMS and the Law. Robert J Brady & Co, 1983.

Valenzuela TD and Criss EA: Data Collection and Ambulance Call Report Design. In EMS Medical Director's Handbook. CV Mosby, St. Louis, 1989.

Notes

APPENDIX A

**Medications
Administered by
the Paramedic**

Activated Charcoal

Class
- Chemical-binding agent.

Mode of Action
- Activated charcoal binds to, or absorbs to, various chemical agents, limiting their absorption from the gastrointestinal tract.

Indications
- Certain overdoses and poisonings in the alert patient

Contraindications
- None.

Side Effects/Precautions
- May cause vomiting, constipation, or diarrhea.

Adult Dosage
- 25 to 50 g by mouth (PO) or via nasogastric (NG) tube.

Pediatric Dosage
- 10 to 25 g PO or via NG tube.

Adenosine (Adenocard)

Class
- Antiarrhythmic agent.

Mode of Action
- Adenosine is a naturally occurring nucleoside that slows conduction through the atrioventricular (AV) node.

Indications
- As an aid in diagnosis of narrow complex tachycardias.
- For the treatment of narrow complex tachycardias, except atrial fibrillation and atrial flutter.

Contraindications
- Avoid in patients with known adenosine hypersensitivity.
- Avoid in patients with bradycardias or second- or third-degree AV block.

Side Effects/Precautions
- May cause transient chest discomfort, palpitations, flushing, headache, nausea, and bronchoconstriction.
- May produce transient arrhythmias, such as second- or third-degree AV block, asystole, sinus bradycardia, premature atrial contractions (PACs), or premature ventricular contractions (PVCs).

Adult Dosage

- 6 mg rapid IV bolus. Drug may be repeated in 1 to 2 minutes at 12 mg rapid IV bolus. If unsuccessful, it may be repeated a second time at 12 mg IV bolus. Dosage may need to be increased if patient is using theophylline preparations. Dosage may need to be reduced in the presence of dipyridamole (Persantine).

Pediatric Dosage

- 0.1 mg/kg rapid IV bolus initially, then repeated at 0.2 mg/kg rapid IV bolus in 1 to 2 minutes. If unsuccessful, drug may be repeated a second time at 0.2 mg/kg IV bolus. Maximum single dose is 12 mg.

Albuterol (Proventil, Ventolin)

Class

- β_2 sympathetic agonist.

Mode of Action

- Albuterol dilates smooth muscle in the bronchial tree through β_2 stimulation. Also has some adrenergic effects on the heart and central nervous system (CNS) when given in high doses.

Indications

- For treatment of reversible bronchoconstriction, such as asthma, chronic bronchitis, emphysema, or other reactive airway disease.

Contraindications

- Avoid in patients with known hypersensitivity.
- Use with caution in patients with hypertension and in patients with a heart rate (HR) greater than 150 bpm.
- Do not use in the context of an MI.

Side Effects/Precautions

- May cause tachycardias, hypertension, chest pain, nervousness, tremor, headache, nausea, or vomiting.

Adult Dosage

- 2.5 mg in 3 mL normal saline (0.9% NaCl) via nebulizer. Dose may be repeated every 6 hours; however, in cases of severe bronchospasm, it may be given as frequently as back to back. More frequent dosing may result in greater incidence of side effects.

Pediatric Dosage

- Age younger than 12 years: one half of the adult dose (1.25 mg); age older than 12 years: use adult dosing. Dose may be repeated every 6 hours; however, in cases of severe bronchospasm, it may be given as frequently as back to back.

Aminophylline (Aminophyllin)

Class
- Methylxanthine bronchodilator

Mode of Action
- Aminophylline relaxes smooth muscle in the respiratory tract, resulting in bronchodilation. It has mild diuretic properties, in addition to cardiac and CNS stimulatory effects.

Indications
- Treatment of reversible bronchoconstriction, such as asthma, chronic bronchitis, emphysema, or other reactive airway disease.
- Possible contribution to the treatment of acute pulmonary edema.

Contraindications
- Patients with known hypersensitivity.
- Should be used with caution in patients with tachydysrhythmias and ectopic beats.

Side Effects/Precautions
- May cause tachycardias, atrial and ventricular arrhythmias, palpitations, chest pain, nervousness, tremor, headache, nausea, or vomiting.
- Should be used with caution in patients with liver disease or congestive heart failure (CHF).

Adult Dosage
- Loading dose: 5 to 6 mg/kg IV infusion over 20 to 30 minutes. Drug may be used in patients who are not currently using aminophylline or theophylline. For patients using a theophylline or aminophylline agent, this loading dose should be reduced by one half (2.5 to 3 mg/kg).

Pediatric Dosage
- 6 mg/kg IV infusion over 20 to 30 minutes. For patients using a theophylline or aminophylline agent, this loading dose should be reduced by one half (2.5 to 3 mg/kg).

Atropine Sulfate

Class
- Parasympathetic blocker

Mode of Action
- Atropine sulfate increases the HR by blocking the action of the parasympathetic nervous system on the sinoatrial (SA) node and the AV node.

Indications
- Symptomatic bradycardias, heart blocks, or both.
- Asystole.
- Organophosphate insecticide poisoning.

Contraindications
- None when used in emergency situations.

Side Effects/Precautions
- May cause tachycardia, palpitations, seizures, hypertension, respiratory failure, and anticholinergic symptoms (i.e., blurred vision, dilated pupils, confusion, fever, decreased GI motility).
- May worsen narrow-angle glaucoma.
- Slow administration or a low dose (less than 0.4 mg) may cause a paradoxic slowing of the HR.

Adult Dosage
- 0.5 to 1.0 mg IV for bradycardias and heart blocks. Drug may be repeated every 3 to 5 minutes up to a maximum dosage of 3 mg (0.04 mg/kg).
- 1 mg IV for asystole. Drug may be repeated every 3 to 5 minutes up to a maximum dosage of 3 mg (0.04 mg/kg).
- 2 mg IV for organophosphate poisoning. Drug may be repeated as necessary.
- Drug may be given via endotracheal tube (ET) if IV unavailable.

Pediatric Dosage
- 0.02 mg/kg IV for bradycardias, heart blocks, and asystole.

Bretylium Tosylate (Bretylol)

Class
- Antiarrhythmic agent

Mode of Action
- Bretylium raises the ventricular fibrillation (VF) threshold of ischemic heart muscle. It initially causes an adrenergic discharge followed by adrenergic blockade.

Indications
- Recurrent VF and/or VT that has remained unresponsive to lidocaine therapy or defibrillation.

Contraindications
- Avoid in patients with known hypersensitivity.
- None when used as indicated.

Side Effects/Precautions
- May cause hypotension, orthostatic hypotension, brady-cardia, nausea, and vomiting.
- May aggravate digitalis toxicity.

Adult Dosage
- VF: 5 mg/kg IV followed by defibrillation. Drug may be repeated at 10 mg/kg IV after an unsuccessful defibrillation attempt. It may be repeated every 5 minutes to a maximum total dosage of 30 to 35 mg/kg.
- 1 to 2 mg per minute infusion if bretylium therapy is successful.
- VT (stable hemodynamics): 5 to 10 mg/kg diluted and infused via IV over 8 to 10 minutes. Drug may be repeated at 5 to 10 mg/kg every 1 to 2 hours.
- 1 to 2 mg per minute infusion if bretylium therapy is successful.

Diazepam (Valium)

Class
- Benzodiazepine.

Mode of Action
- Diazepam possesses CNS depressant, antiepileptic, anxiolytic, and skeletal muscle relaxant properties.

Indications
- Prehospital indication is for the treatment of status epilepticus.

Contraindications
- Avoid in patients with known hypersensitivity.
- No prehospital contraindications when used in the case of status epilepticus.

Side Effects/Precautions
- May cause CNS depression, respiratory depression, and increased intraocular pressure in patients with narrow-angle glaucoma.

Adult Dosage
- 5 to 10 mg IV bolus (or IM). Drug may be repeated every 10 minutes to maximum total dose of 30 mg.

Pediatric Dosage
- Younger than 5 years: 0.2 to 0.5 mg IV every 2 to 5 minutes to a maximum dose of 5 mg.
- Older than 5 years: 1 mg IV every 2 to 5 minutes to a maximum dose of 10 mg.

Dextrose 50% (D⁵⁰)

Class
- Carbohydrate.

Mode of Action
- D⁵⁰ elevates blood glucose levels.

Indications
- Hypoglycemia.
- Diagnostic test for hypoglycemia in patients with an altered mental state of unknown etiology.

Contraindications
- None when used in emergency situations.

Side Effects/Precautions
- Infiltration of D⁵⁰ may cause local tissue necrosis.
- A sample of blood should be drawn before the administration of D⁵⁰ to determine premedication serum glucose levels.
- Thiamine should also be administered to patients before administration of D⁵⁰ to avoid an acute thiamine deficiency.

Adult Dosage
- 25 g D⁵⁰ (50 mL) IV.

Pediatric Dosage
- 0.5 mL/kg of D⁵⁰ IV or 1 mL/kg of dextrose 25% (D²⁵) IV.

  NOTE: It is preferable to use an infusion of dextrose 10% (D¹⁰) IV in pediatric patients whose symptoms of hypoglycemia are not serious (coma or seizures) to avoid overshoot hyperglycemia.

Diphenhydramine (Benadryl)

Class
- Antihistamine (H_1 histamine blocker).

Mode of Action
- Competitive blocker of H_1 histamine receptors, prevent-

ing histamine from causing vasodilation, hypotension, tachycardia, and increased GI secretions. Histamine plays a significant role in allergic reactions. Diphenhydramine also has anticholinergic effects.

Indications
- Severe allergic reactions, such as anaphylaxis.

Contraindications
- Avoid in patients with known hypersensitivity.
- Should be used with caution in asthmatic patients; may thicken bronchial secretions and thereby worsen mucus plugging.
- May worsen narrow-angle glaucoma.
- Use with caution in patients with hypertension.

Side Effects/Precautions
- Side effects are largely due to the anticholinergic effects and include drowsiness, dry mouth, urinary retention, hypotension, thickened bronchial secretions, wheezing, and GI symptoms.

Adult Dosage
- 10 to 50 mg slow IV bolus, or deep IM injection.

Pediatric Dosage
- 2 to 5 mg/kg IV or deep IM injection. Usual dose is 10 to 30 mg.

Dopamine

Class
- Adrenergic vasopressor.

Mode of Action
- Dopamine is an epinephrine precursor with dose-dependent dopaminergic, α-adrenergic, and β-adrenergic effects.
- 0.5 to 2 µg/kg per minute IV infusion for dopaminergic effects: vasodilation of renal and mesenteric vessels without affecting heart rate or blood pressure.
- 2 to 10 µg/kg per minute IV infusion for predominantly β-adrenergic effects: increasing HR and contractility and some vasodilation.
- Greater than 10 µg/kg per minute IV infusion for predominantly α-adrenergic effects: vasoconstriction, increasing peripheral vascular resistance and HR.

Indications
- Significant hypotension.

Contraindications
- Avoid in patients with known hypersensitivity.
- Avoid in patients with hypovolemic hypotension, unless patient has failed aggressive IV fluid resuscitation, including resuscitation with blood products.
- Contraindicated in hypotensive patients who have hypotension that is caused by a tachyarrhythmia.

Side Effects/Precautions
- May cause tachyarrhythmias, hypotension (at low doses), chest pain, palpitations, nausea, and vomiting.
- May also cause tissue necrosis if IV infiltrates (hospital treatment of site with phentolamine if this occurs).

Adult Dosage
- 2 to 5 µg/kg minute IV infusion, titrating upward until desired effect is achieved.

Pediatric Dosage
- 1 µg/kg minute IV infusion, titrating upward until desired effect is achieved.

Epinephrine

Class
- Sympathetic agonist possessing both α and β properties.

Mode of Action
- Its α effects are primarily vasoconstriction, which increases peripheral vascular resistance (PVR) and perfusion. Its β effects are increased automaticity, increased HR, increased contractility, increased cardiac output, increased myocardial oxygen demand, and bronchodilation. It also decreases the threshold for successful defibrillation.

Indications
- Cardiac arrest: asystole, electromechanical dissociation, VF, pulseless VT.
- Asthma.
- Anaphylaxis.

Contraindications
- None when used during cardiac arrest.
- Use with caution in patients who are elderly, hypertensive, pregnant, or in patients who have a cardiovascular or hyperthyroid disease.

Side Effects/Precautions
- May cause tachycardia, palpitations, hypertension, ven-

tricular irritability, increased myocardial oxygen demand, cerebrovascular accident (CVA), and MI.

Adult Dosage
- Cardiac arrest: 1 mg epinephrine (1:10,000) IV; dose may be repeated every 3 to 5 minutes. If given via ET, use 2 to 2.5 times IV dose. High-dose epinephrine may also be employed (5 mg or 0.1 mg/kg IV) if the initial low dose is ineffective.

  NOTE: Current use of high-dose epinephrine is controversial.
- Anaphylaxis: 0.3 to 0.5 mg epinephrine (1:10,000) IV if poor perfusion. 0.3 to 0.5 mg epinephrine (1:1000) SC if adequate perfusion.
- Asthma: 0.3 mg to 0.5 mg epinephrine (1:1000) SC; dose may be repeated every 20 minutes.

Pediatric Dosage
- Cardiac arrest: 0.01 to 0.1 mg/kg epinephrine (1:10,000) IV; dose may be repeated every 3 to 5 minutes. If given via ET, use 2 to 2.5 times IV dose.
- Anaphylaxis: 0.01 mg/kg epinephrine (1:10,000) IV if poor perfusion; maximum single dose: 0.3 mg. 0.01 mg/kg epinephrine (1:1000) SC if adequate perfusion; maximum single dose 0.3 mg.
- Asthma: 0.01 mg/kg epinephrine (1:1000) SC; maximum single dose: 0.3 mg. Dose may be repeated twice at 20 minute intervals.

Furosemide (Lasix)

Class
- Diuretic.

Mode of Action
- Furosemide is a potent diuretic, acting within 5 to 30 minutes. In addition to its diuretic action, it produces a vasodilatative effect.

Indications
- Acute pulmonary edema.

Contraindications
- Avoid in patients with known hypersensitivity.
- Avoid in anuric patients.
- Use with caution in patients with hepatic failure or renal failure.

Side Effects/Precautions
- May cause hypokalemia, hypovolemia, orthostatic hypotension, and ototoxicity.

Adult Dosage
- 40 mg to 80 mg furosemide IV.

Pediatric Dosage
- 1 to 3 mg/kg furosemide IV.

Glucagon

Class
- Antihypoglycemic agent.

Mode of Action
- Glucagon converts glycogen, a stored form of glucose found in the liver and muscles, into glucose. It also inhibits glycogen synthesis and elevates blood glucose levels. Glucagon is only effective if the patient has sufficient stores of glycogen in the liver. The administration of glucagon should be followed by glucose as soon as possible. The onset of action is within 5 to 20 minutes.
- In addition, glucagon enhances myocardial contractility and increases HR and AV conduction through a cellular receptor-mediated pathway distinct from the adrenergic receptor pathway. It is, therefore, able to stimulate the myocardium during β blockade.

Indications
- Hypoglycemia, especially when IV access is unavailable and D^{50} has not been given.
- Beta blocker overdose

Contraindications
- None when used in an emergency.

Side Effects/Precautions
- May cause nausea and vomiting.

Adult Dosage
- Hypoglycemia: 1 mg IM or SC; dose may be repeated twice.
- Beta blocker overdose; 3 to 10 mg IV bolus, followed by a 2 to 5 mg per hour infusion.

Pediatric Dosage
- Not recommended for prehospital use in pediatrics.

Isoproterenol (Isuprel)

Class
- Sympathetic agonist possessing 100% β effects.

Mode of Action
- Isoproterenol is a 100% β agent and its effects are increased automaticity, increased HR, increased contractility, decreased PVR, increased cardiac output, increased myocardial oxygen demand, and bronchodilation.

Indications
- Symptomatic bradycardias, heart blocks, or both that are unresponsive to atropine therapy.

Contraindications
- None when used emergently as indicated.

Side Effects/Precautions
- May cause tachydysrhythmias, ventricular ectopy; PACs, hypotension, angina pectoris, and headache.

  NOTE: Isoproterenol has been implicated in causing cellular damage to the myocardium. It also increases the myocardial workload and myocardial oxygen demand. This may extend the area of an infarction.

Adult Dosage
- 2 μg per minute to 10 μg per minute IV infusion (1 mg in 250 mL of D_5W, to a concentration of 4 μg/mL).

Infusion Amount	Drip Rate
2 μg/min	30 gtts/min
4 μg/min	60 gtts/min
6 μg/min	90 gtts/min
8 μg/min	120 gtts/min
10 μg/min	150 gtts/min

Pediatric Dosage
- 0.1 to 0.2 μg per minute IV infusion. Dose may be titrated to desired effect.

Lidocaine

Class
- Antiarrhythmic agent.

Mode of Action
- Lidocaine suppresses ventricular ectopic activity by decreasing the irritability of the heart muscle and the conduction system, and raises the fibrillatory threshold.

Indications
- Ventricular ectopy in the context of an MI.
- VT and recurrent VF.

Contraindications
- Avoid in patients with known hypersensitivity.
- Avoid in patients with bradydysrhythmias, heart blocks, and idioventricular escape rhythms.

Side Effects/Precautions
- May cause hypotension, numbness, drowsiness, confusion, respiratory depression, and seizures.

Adult Dosage
- 1 to 1.5 mg per kg IV bolus, which may be repeated at 0.5 to 0.75 mg/kg every 8 to 10 minutes until a maximum dose of 3 mg/kg or 225 mg has been administered.
- 2 to 4 mg per minute (1 g of lidocaine in 250 mL of D_5W or 2 g in 500 mL in concentration of 4 mg/mL). Lidocaine infusion should be begun if lidocaine is effective.

NOTE: Give the typical loading dose and reduce the maintenance dose by 50% in adults older than 70 years of age who have CHF, liver disease, or impaired hepatic blood flow to prevent toxicity.

Infusion Amount	Drip Rate
2 mg/min	30 gtts/min
3 mg/min	45 gtts/min
4 mg/min	60 gtts/min

Pediatric Dosage
- 1 mg/kg IV bolus (maximum dose of 50 mg), followed by an infusion of 20 to 50 µg/kg per minute.

Meperidine (Demerol)

Class
- Narcotic analgesic agent.

Mode of Action
- Meperidine binds to opiate receptors in the CNS.

Indications
- Treatment of moderate to severe pain.

Contraindications
- Avoid in patients with known hypersensitivity.
- Should be used with caution in patients with chronic obstructive pulmonary disease (COPD) because narcotics may cause respiratory depression.

- Use with caution in patients with a history of a seizure disorder because narcotics may lower the seizure threshold.

Side Effects/Precautions
- May cause CNS depression, respiratory depression, depression of the seizure threshold, hypotension, nausea, and vomiting.

Adult Dosage
- 50 to 100 mg IM every 3 to 4 hours.

Pediatric Dosage
- 1.1 to 1.8 mg/kg IM every 3 to 4 hours. Maximum single dose: 100 mg.

Magnesium Sulfate

Class
- CNS depressant, anticonvulsant, and antiarrhythmic.

Mode of Action
- Magnesium sulfate depresses the CNS.
- Improves muscle cell membrane stability.
- Relaxes smooth and cardiac muscle.

Indications
- Convulsions associated with eclampsia and pre-eclamsia.
- VT.

Contraindications
- Avoid in patients with heart block.
- Avoid in patients with a history of renal disease.

Side Effects/Precautions
- May cause respiratory distress or failure.
- May cause cardiac arrest.

Adult Dosage
- Eclampsia: 2 to 4 g slow IV over a minimum of 3 minutes.
- VT: 1 to 2 g IV over 1 minute.

Pediatric Dosage
- Not recommended for prehospital use.

Methylprednisolone (Solumedrol)

Class
- Glucocorticoid steroid.

Mode of Action
- Methylprednisolone suppresses the body's immune system and thereby decreases the severity of the inflammatory response.

Indications
- Treatment of anaphylaxis.
- Treatment of severe bronchospasm.
- Treatment of spinal cord injury.

Contraindications
- None when used in the emergent treatment of anaphylaxis.

Side Effects/Precautions
- May cause euphoria, hypertension, hyperglycemia, fluid retention, nausea, and vomiting
- Use with caution in patients with CHF, diabetes mellitus (DM), renal disease, and hypertension.

Adult Dosage
- Anaphylaxis or bronchospasm regimen: 100 to 200 mg IV bolus or IM. Drug must be reconstituted.
- Spinal cord injury regimen: 30 mg/kg IV infusion given over 15 minutes.

Pediatric Dosage
- Anaphylaxis or bronchospasm regimen: 2 mg/kg IV bolus or IM. Drug must be reconstituted.
- Spinal cord injury regimen: 30 mg/kg IV infusion given over 15 minutes.

Morphine Sulfate

Class
- Narcotic analgesic agent.

Mode of Action
- Morphine sulfate binds to opiate receptors in the CNS.

Indications
- Treatment of moderate to severe pain.
- Treatment of cardiogenic acute pulmonary edema.

Contraindications
- Avoid in patients with known hypersensitivity.
- Contraindicated for use in patients with a depressed level of consciousness or respiratory depression.
- Should be used with caution in patients with COPD, because narcotics may cause respiratory depression.

- Use with caution in patients with a history of a seizure disorder, because narcotics may lower the seizure threshold.

Side Effects/Precautions
- CNS depression, respiratory depression, depression of the seizure threshold, hypotension, nausea, and vomiting.

Adult Dosage
- 2 to 5 mg IV every 5 to 30 minutes until desired effect is achieved.

Pediatric Dosage
- Not recommended for prehospital use in pediatric patients.

Naloxone (Narcan)

Class
- Narcotic antagonist.

Mode of Action
- Naloxone reverses the effects of narcotics.

Indications
- Known or suspected narcotic overdose.
- Diagnostic test for narcotic overdose.

Contraindications
- Avoid in patients with known hypersensitivity.

Side Effects/Precautions
- May cause an acute withdrawal syndrome in the narcotic-dependent patient. The duration of naloxone is, in general, less than that of the narcotic. Therefore, patients who initially respond well to naloxone may fall back into coma as the naloxone wears off. Naloxone is not effective against nonopiates such as cocaine and marijuana.

Adult Dosage
- 0.4 mg to 2 mg IV, IM, or SC. Dose may be repeated as necessary.
- May be given as a continuous infusion (2.0 mg naloxone in 500 mL of 0.9% NaCl or D_5W in a concentration of 0.004 mg/mL), titrating the dose to clinical response. Usual dose is 0.4 mg per hour.

Pediatric Dosage
- 0.01 mg/kg IV, IM, or SC; dose may be repeated as necessary. If no response is achieved, dose may be increased to 0.1 mg/kg.

Nifedipine (Procardia)

Class
- Calcium channel blocker.

Mode of Action
- Nifedipine dilates systemic and coronary arteries by blocking the calcium channels found in the myocardium, the cardiac conduction system, and in the vascular bed, thus decreasing calcium's entry into the cells and resulting in decreased cardiac contractility, decreased conduction through the AV node, and vasodilation. Nifedipine's greatest effects are on the vascular calcium channels, thus causing predominantly vasodilation and thereby decreasing blood pressure.

Indications
- For quick lowering of blood pressure in hypertensive emergencies.
- As an antianginal agent.

Contraindications
- Avoid in patients with known hypersensitivity.
- Avoid in patients with hypotension.

Side Effects/Precautions
- Headache, CHF, cough, wheezing, ventricular arrhythmias, and hypotension.

Adult Dosage
- 10 mg by mouth or SL. Dose may be repeated in 20 to 30 minutes.

Pediatric Dosage
- Not recommended for prehospital use in pediatric patients.

Nitroglycerin

Class
- Antianginal analgesic.

Mode of Action
- Nitroglycerin dilates coronary arteries, thus increasing myocardial oxygenation. Peripheral vasculature dilates as well, promoting pooling of the blood, thereby reducing preload.

Indications
- Relief of the pain of angina pectoris, MI, or both.
- Treatment of pulmonary edema.

Contraindications
- Avoid in patients with known hypersensitivity.
- Avoid in patients with hypotension.
Side Effects/Precautions
- May cause hypotension, headache, dizziness, reflex tachycardia, syncope, and a burning sensation in the mouth.
- Be sure to remove topical nitroglycerin preparations from patients when giving additional nitroglycerin to avoid overdosing. Topical nitroglycerin preparations should be removed from the chest before defibrillation or cardioversion to avoid electrical arcing.
Adult Dosage
- Nitroglycerin comes in several forms, each with its own dosing regimen.
- 1/150 g (0.4 mg) sublingual. Dose may be repeated every 5 minutes.
- 1 to 2 metered dose sprays (0.4 mg/dose) of translingual nitroglycerin onto oral mucosa. Dose may be repeated every 5 minutes.
- 1/2 to 2 inches of 2% nitroglycerin ointment (1 inch equals 15 mg nitroglycerin). Duration is approximately 6 hours.
- 0.2 to 0.4 mg per hour transdermal nitroglycerin (patches in 0.1 to 0.6 mg per hour dosing). Duration is approximately 12 to 24 hours.

Nitrous Oxide-Oxygen 50:50 Mixture (Nitronox)

Class
- Medicinal gas.
Mode of Action
- Nitrous oxide produces rapid onset and readily reversible analgesia and CNS depression when inhaled.
Indications
- Relief of moderate to severe pain.
Contraindications
- Avoid in patients with known hypersensitivity.
- Contraindicated under the following conditions:
  - Decreased level of consciousness
  - Patient unable to follow simple commands

- Concurrent use of CNS depressants
- Pregnancy
- Abdominal distension or trauma (nitrous oxide may accumulate in gas-filled spaces, worsening abdominal obstruction)
- Chest trauma (nitrous oxide may accumulate in gas-filled spaces, worsening chest injuries)
- Respiratory compromise
- Hypoxia

Side Effects/Precautions
- May cause lightheadedness, respiratory depression, nausea, and vomiting.
- Patient must be monitored during administration. Use of a pulse oximeter is helpful.

Adult Dosage
- Patient self-administers the drug until pain is relieved or patient is unable to self-administer.

Pediatric Dosage
- Patient self-administers the drug until pain is relieved or patient is unable to self-administer.

Oxygen

Class
- Medicinal gas.

Mode of Action
- Oxygen diffuses across membranes to act as a necessary agent for aerobic metabolism. Hypoxia, anoxia, or both leads inevitably to death.

Indications
- Suspected hypoxia or anoxia, be it local, as in patients with ischemia, or systemic, as in patients with cardiac arrest.

Contraindications
- None when used emergently.

Side Effects/Precautions
- May cause respiratory depression in patients with a hypoxic drive.
- Although oxygen toxicity may occur after prolonged ventilatory support with a high-oxygen concentration, even 100% oxygen is not hazardous to the patient's lungs during the time frame that prehospital care is rendered. Oxygen should never be withheld from anyone who needs it.

Adult Dosage/Pediatric Dosage
- 85% to 100% via non-rebreather mask.
- 24% to 40% via Venturi mask.
- 24% to 40% via nasal cannula.
- Bag-valve-mask (BVM) devices fitted with reservoirs and liter flow of 15 liters per minute supply approximately 85% to 100% oxygen. Use of a BVM allows continuous assessment of pulmonary compliance. Pop-off valves are not recommended for use in pediatric patients.
- Intermittent positive-pressure devices supply approximately 100% oxygen.

Oxytocin (Pitocin, Syntocinon)

Class
- Hormone.

Mode of Action
- Oxytocin causes the uterus to contract after delivery of a fetus, thereby decreasing uterine bleeding.

Indications
- Control of postpartum bleeding after delivery of the placenta.

Contraindications
- None when used emergently; however, ensure that there is no undelivered fetus.

Side Effects/Precautions
- May cause nausea and vomiting.
- May cause cardiac dysrhythmias.

Adult Dosage
- 10 U (1 mL) in 1000 mL of 0.9% NaCL IV, titrated to patient's response (1 to 2 mL per minute initially).

Pediatric Dosage
- Not recommended for prehospital use in pediatric patients.

Procainamide (Procan, Pronestyl)

Class
- Antiarrhythmic agent.

Mode of Action
- Procainamide increases the refractory period of the atria and to a lesser extent the AV node, bundle of His, and

the Purkinje system. It slows conduction velocity throughout the conduction system. Its actions on the AV node are variable—a direct slowing action coexists with a mild vagolytic effect (slightly increasing AV conduction). It also decreases automaticity. The net effects make this drug effective for the treatment of both atrial and ventricular arrhythmias.

Indications
- Treatment of PVCs and recurrent VT when lidocaine is contraindicated or fails to control ventricular ectopy.
- Treatment of wide-complex tachycardias that cannot be distinguished from VT.

Contraindications
- Avoid in patients with known hypersensitivity.
- Do not use in the presence of prolonged QT interval or torsades de pointes.

Side Effects/Precautions
- May cause hypotension, nausea, vomiting, and ventricular arrhythmias such as torsades de pointes, AV block, and asystole.
- May depress cardiac contractility; therefore, use with caution in the context of an acute MI.

Adult Dosage
- 20 mg per minute IV infusion until arrhythmia is suppressed, patient becomes hypotensive, QRS complex widens by 50%, or a maximum dose of 17 mg/kg has been given. If the patient is unstable, procainamide may be given at a rate of 30 mg per minute. Maintenance infusion rate of 1 to 4 mg per minute.

Pediatric Dosage
- Not recommended for prehospital use in pediatric patients.

Sodium Bicarbonate

Class
- Alkalinizing agent.

Mode of Action
- Sodium bicarbonate reacts with hydrogen to form water and cabon dioxide to buffer metabolic acidosis. Sodium bicarbonate's high carbon dioxide content readily diffuses into cells, causing a paradoxical worsening of intracellu-

lar hypercarbia and acidosis. Bicarbonate diffuses into cells more slowly.

Indications

- During cardiac arrest resuscitation (if at all), only after the use of more definitive and better substantiated interventions, such as prompt defibrillation, effective CPR, ET intubation, hyperventilation with 100% oxygen, and the use of drugs such as epinephrine and lidocaine. The administration of sodium bicarbonate has not been demonstrated to improve ventricular defibrillation or survival in cardiac arrest.

Contraindications

- Pulmonary edema.

Side Effects/Precautions

- The performance of the ischemic heart is depressed by the high levels of carbon dioxide that result from the administration of sodium bicarbonate. Sodium bicarbonate administration may inhibit hemoglobin release of oxygen to the tissues. Sodium bicarbonate forms a precipitate when mixed with calcium chloride and deactivates epinephrine.

Adult Dosage/Pediatric Dosage

- 1 mEq/kg IV initial dose.
- Drug may be repeated at 0.5 mEq/kg, which should not be given more frequently than every 10 minutes.

Streptokinase

Class

- Thrombolytic agent.

Mode of Action

- Streptokinase is an enzyme that activates the conversion of plasminogen into plasmin, helping to dissolve thrombi.

Indications

- Thrombolytic therapy is indicated in all MI patients with ST-segment elevations who present within 6 hours of the onset of symptoms, if there are no contraindications. There is some evidence that patients who are up to 24 hours out may also benefit from the use of thrombolytics. The most benefit has been seen with patients who are having an anterior wall MI, but some benefit has been seen in inferior wall MIs as well. The benefit of thrombolytics decreases with time: therefore, they should be administered as soon as possible.

Contraindications

- The following are absolute contraindications to thrombolytic therapy:
  - GI bleeding
  - Intracranial neoplasm
  - Pregnancy
  - Prolonged (greater than 1 minute) or traumatic CPR
  - Arteriovenous malformation or aneurysm
  - Recent (less than 2 months) intracranial or intraspinal surgery or trauma
  - History of a previous hemorrhagic CVA
- The relative contraindications are:
  - Recent (less than 10 days) trauma or surgery
  - Previous CVA
  - Any hemorrhagic retinopathy
  - Poorly controlled severe hypertension
  - Known bleeding disorder
  - If streptokinase or anisoylated plasminogen streptokinase activator complex (APSAC) is to be used, a prior exposure to streptokinase or APSAC (absolute contraindication if there was a previous allergic reaction)
  - Active peptic ulcer disease
  - Hepatic insufficiency

Side Effects/Precautions

- Streptokinase therapy is associated with the following adverse effects: intracranial bleeding, reperfusion arrhythmias, bronchospasm, anaphylaxis, GI bleeding, and bleeding from IV sites.

Adult Dosage

- 1.5 million-IU IV infusion over 60 minutes.

Pediatric Dosage

- Not recommended for prehospital use in pediatric patients.

Syrup of Ipecac

Class

- Emetic agent.

Mode of Action
- Syrup of ipecac stimulates the chemotactic (emetic) area of the brain and irritates the GI mucosa to stimulate vomiting.

Indications
- To induce vomiting in the alert patient with a suspected or known poisoning or overdose.

Contraindications
- Avoid patients with known hypersensitivity.
- Contraindicated in patients with a decreased level of consciousness, without an intact gag reflex, or who have ingested caustic or petroleum-based products.

Side Effects/Precautions
- May cause CNS depression, arrhythmias, hypotension, and diarrhea.
- Take care to use only syrup of ipecac and not ipecac extract which is several-fold more concentrated.

Adult Dosage
- 15 to 30 mL by mouth, followed by several glasses of warm water. Dose may be repeated once in 20 minutes.

Pediatric Dosage
- 6 months to 1 year: 5 to 10 mL by mouth followed by warm water.
- Older than 1 year: 15 to 25 mL by mouth followed by warm water.

Thiamine (Vitamin B1)

Class
- Vitamin.

Mode of Action
- Thiamine is a necessary co-enzyme in the metabolism of glucose. Thiamine deficiency may cause Wernicke's syndrome. Sign and symptoms of Wernicke's syndrome include an altered mental state, involuntary muscular contractions, and ophthalmoplegia (most commonly bilateral nystagmus).

Indications
- Known or suspected thiamine deficiency.
- Altered mental state of unknown etiology, especially if alcohol abuse or malnourishment is suspected.
- The administration of D^{50} may precipitate Wernicke's syn-

drome in the thiamine-deficient patient, and therefore
thiamine is often administered whenever D⁵⁰ is administered.

Contraindications
- None when used emergently.

Side Effects/Precautions
- IV Thiamine has been associated with anaphylaxis; administer slowly IV.

Adult Dosage
- 100 mg (1 mL) IM or IV.

Pediatric Dosage
- Thiamine is rarely used for pediatric patients.

Tissue Plasminogen Activator
(Alteplase, Activase)

Class
- Thrombolytic agent.

Mode of Action
- Tissue plasminogen activator (tPA) is an enzyme that activates the conversion of plasminogen into plasmin, helping to dissolve thrombi.

Indications
- Thrombolytic therapy is indicated in all MI patients with
  ST segment elevations who present within 6 hours of the
  onset of symptoms, if there are no contraindications.
  There is some evidence that patients who are up to 24
  hours out may also benefit from the use of thrombolytics.
  The most benefit has been seen with patients who are
  having an anterior wall MI, but some benefit has been
  seen in inferior wall MIs as well. The benefit of
  thrombolytics decreases with time; therefore, they should
  be administered as soon as possible.

Contraindications
- The following are absolute contraindications to
  thrombolytic therapy:
  - GI bleeding
  - Intracranial neoplasm
  - Pregnancy
  - Prolonged (greater than 1 minute) or traumatic CPR
  - Arteriovenous malformation or aneurysm

Recent (less than 2 months) intracranial or intraspinal surgery or trauma

History of a previous hemorrhagic CVA

- The relative contraindications are:

Recent (less than 10 days) trauma or surgery

Previous CVA

Any hemorrhagic retinopathy

Poorly controlled severe hypertension

Known bleeding disorder

If streptokinase or APSAC is to be used, a prior exposure to streptokinase or APSAC (absolute contraindication if there was a previous allergic reaction)

Active peptic ulcer disease

Hepatic insufficiency

Side Effects/Precautions

- Thrombolytic therapy is associated with the following adverse effects: intracranial bleeding, reperfusion arrhythmias, hypotension, GI bleeding, nausea, vomiting, and bleeding from IV sites.

Adult Dosage

- 15 mg IV bolus, followed by 0.75 mg/kg up to 50 mg IV infusion over 30 minutes, then 0.5 mg/kg up to 35 mg IV infusion over 60 minutes. Total dose is not to exceed 100 mg over 3 hours.

Pediatric Dosage

- Not recommended for prehospital use in pediatric patients.

Verapamil (Calan, Isoptin)

Class

- Calcium channel blocker.

Mode of Action

- Verapamil blocks the calcium channel found in the myocardium, in the cardiac conduction system, and in the vascular bed, decreasing calcium's entry into the cells, resulting in decreased cardiac contractility, decreased conduction through the AV node, and vasodilation.

Indications

- Symptomatic supraventricular tachycardias, including rapid atrial fibrillation and rapid atrial flutter.

Contraindications
- Verapamil is contraindicated under the following circumstances: bradycardias, second- and third-degree AV block, and Wolf-Parkinson-White syndrome with rapid atrial fibrillation or atrial flutter, severe CHF.

Side Effects/Precautions
- The most significant side effects are hypotension, bradycardias, development of AV blocks, asystole, and CHF.

Adult Dosage
- 2.5 to 5 mg IV bolus over 1 minute: drug may be repeated at 5 to 10 mg IV bolus in 15 to 30 minutes.

Pediatric Dosage
- Younger than 1 year: 0.1 to 0.2 mg/kg IV bolus over 2 minutes. Typical dose: 0.75 to 2 mg.
- 1 year to 15 years: 0.1 to 0.3 mg/kg IV bolus over 2 minutes. Typical dose: 2 to 5 mg.

Bibliography

Beck R: Pharmacology for Prehospital Emergency Care. FA Davis, Philadelphia, 1992.

Deglin JH and Hazard AH: Davis' Drug Guide for Nurses, ed 4. FA Davis, Philadelphia, 1994.

Appendix B
Commonly Used Medications

DRUG NAME	DRUG TYPE
Accupril	See QUINIPRIL
Accutane	See ISOTRETINOIN
Accutrim	See PHENYLPROPANOLAMINE
ACEBUTOLOL	Cardioselective β adrenergic blocker
ACETAMINOPHEN	Nonopioid analgesic, antipyretic
ACETAZOLAMIDE	Carbonic anhydrase—glaucoma,CHF
ACETOPHENAZINE	Phenothiazine—antipsychotic
ACETYLCYSTEINE	Mucolytic agent
ACETYLSALICYLIC ACID	See ASPIRIN
Actifed	Combination decongestant, antihistamine
ACYCLOVIR	Antiviral agent
Adalat	See NIFEDIPINE
Adapin	See DOXEPIN
Advil	See IBUPROFEN
Aerobid	See FLUNISOLIDE
Aerolate	See THEOPHYLLINE
Afrin	See OXYMETAZOLINE
Akineton	See BIPERIDEN
ALBUTEROL	β_2 agonist bronchodilator
Aldactazide	See HYDROCHLOROTHIAZIDE–SPIRONOLACTONE
Aldactone	See SPIRONOLACTONE
Aldoclor–150, –250	See CHLOROTHIAZIDE–METHYLDOPA
Aldomet	See METHYLDOPA
Aldoril 15, 25, D30, D50	See HYDROCHLOROTHIAZIDE–METHYLDOPA
Allerest	Combination antihistamine, sympathomimetic
ALLOPURINOL	Xanthine oxidase inhibitor for gout
ALPRAZOLAM	Benzodiazepine—anxiolytic
Altace	ACE inhibitor—HTN
Alternagel	See ALUMINUM HYDROXIDE
ALUMINUM CARBONATE	Antacid
ALUMINUM HYDROXIDE	Antacid
ALUMINUM PHOSPHATE	Antacid
Alupent	See METAPROTERENOL
AMANTADINE	Antiparkinson agent
AMIKACIN	Antibiotic
AMILORIDE	K⁺ sparing diuretic
AMINOPHYLLINE	Methylxanthine bronchodilator
AMIODARONE	Antiarrhythmic
AMITRIPTYLINE	Tricyclic antidepressant

Generic names are in capital letters; trade names are in lower case.

DRUG NAME	DRUG TYPE
AMLODOPINE	Ca^{2+} channel blocker
AMOBARBITAL	Barbiturate—anxiolytic, hypnotic
AMOXAPINE	Tricyclic antidepressant
AMOXICILLIN	Antibiotic
AMOXICILLIN CLAVULANATE	Antibiotic
Amoxil	See AMOXICILLIN
Amphojel	See ALUMINUM HYDROXIDE
AMPHOTERICIN B	Antifungal antibiotic
AMPICILLIN	Antibiotic
AMPICILLIN SULBACTAM	Antibiotic
AMRINONE	Inotrope with vasodilator effects—CHF
Amytal	See AMOBARBITAL
Anafranil	See CLOMIPRAMINE
Anaprox	See NAPROXEN
Ancef	See CEFAZOLIN
Anhydron	See CYCLOTHIAZIDE
Antabuse	See DISULFIRAM
Antivert	See MECLIZINE
Anusol	Anti hemorrhoid
Apresazide	Combination HYDRALAZINE–HYDROCHLOROTHIAZIDE
Apresoline	See HYDRALAZINE
Aquatensen	See METHYCLOTHIAZIDE
Artane	See TRIHEXYPHENIDYL
Asendin	See AMOXAPINE
ASPIRIN	Analgesic, antipyretic, antiplatelet
ASPIRIN–BUTALBITAL	Combination antimigraine
ASPIRIN–MEPROBAMATE	Combination antimigraine
ASTEMIZOLE	Long–acting antihistamine
Atarax	See HYDROXYZINE
ATENOLOL	Cardioselective β adrenergic blocker
Ativan	See LORAZEPAM
Atromid–S	See CLOFIBRATE
Atrovent	See IPRATROPIUM
Augmentin	See AMOXICILLIN CLAVULANATE
Aventyl	See NORTRIPTYLLINE
Axid	See NIZATIDINE
Axotal	See ASPIRIN–BUTALBITAL
Axsain	See CAPSAICIN
Azactam	See AZTREONAM
AZATHIOPRINE	Immunosuppressive agent
AZITHROMYCIN	Antibiotic
Azmacort	Inhaled TRIAMCINOLONE

Generic names are in capital letters; trade names are in lower case.

DRUG NAME	DRUG TYPE
AZT	See ZIDOVUDINE
AZTREONAM	Antibiotic
Azulfidine	See SULFASALINE
BACITRACIN	Topical Antibiotic
Bacitrin	See BACITRACIN
BACLOFEN	Centrally acting antispastic agent
Bactrim	Antibiotic
Basaljel	See ALUMINUM CARBONATE
BECLOMETHASONE	Inhaled corticosteroid for bronchospasm
Beclovent	See BECLOMETHASONE
Beconase	Inhaled BECLOMETHASONE for sinusitis
Bellergal–S	Combination antimigraine
Benadryl	See DIPHENHYDRAMINE
BENAZEPRIL	ACE inhibitor—antihypertensive
BENDROFLUMETHIAZIDE	Thiazide diuretic
BENTHIAZIDE	Thiazide diuretic
Benzamycin	Topical antibacterial—acne vulgaris
BENZONATATE	Cough suppressant
BENZTROPINE	Antiparkinson agent
BEPRIDIL	Ca^{2+} channel blocker—refractory angina
Betagan	See LEVOBUNOLOL
BETAMETHASONE	Steroid—antiinflammatory agent
BETAMETHASONE cream	Topical steroid—dermatologic disorders
BETAXOLOL	Topical β blocker—glaucoma
BETHANECHOL	Parasympathomimetic–urinary retention
Betoptic	Cardioselective β adrenergic blocker–glaucoma
Biaxin	See CLARITHROMYCIN
BIPERIDEN	Antiparkinson agent
BISACODYL	Laxative
BITOLTEROL MESYLATE	Adrenergic bronchodilator
Blenoxane	See BLEOMYCIN
BLEOMYCIN	Anticancer agent
Blocadren	See TIMOLOL
Bonine	See MECLIZINE
Brethaire	See TERBUTALINE
Brethine	See TERBUTALINE
Brevibloc	See ESMOLOL
Bricanyl	See TERBUTALINE

Generic names are in capital letters; trade names are in lower case.

DRUG NAME	DRUG TYPE
BROMOCRIPTINE	Antiparkinson agent
Bronkodyl SR	Sustained action THEOPHYLLINE
Bronkometer	See ISOETHARINE
Bronkosol	See ISOETHARINE
Bucladin–S	See BUCLIZINE
BUCLIZINE	Antihistamine—antivertigo, anti-motion sickness
BUMETANIDE	Loop diuretic
Bumex	See BUMETANIDE
BUPROPION	Atypical antidepressant
Buspar	See BUSPIRONE
BUSPIRONE	Anxiolytic
BUSULFAN	Anticancer agent
Cafergot P–B	Combination antimigraine
Calan SR	Sustained release VERAPAMIL
CALCIUM CARBONATE	Antacid
Capoten	See CAPTOPRIL
Capozide	Combination CAPTOPRIL–HYDROCHLOROTHIAZIDE
CAPSAICIN cream	Topical analgesic—neuralgias, arthritis
CAPTOPRIL	ACE inhibitor
Carafate	See SUCRALFATE
CARBACHOL eye drops	Glaucoma
CARBAMAZEPINE	Anticonvulsant
CARBOPLATIN	Anticancer agent
Cardene	See NICARDIPINE
Cardilate	See ERYTHRITYL TETRANITRATE
Cardioquin	See QUINIDINE
Cardizem SR	Sustained release DILTIAZEM
Cardura	See DOXAZOSIN
CARISOPRODOL	Muscle relaxant
CARTEOLOL	β adrenergic blocker
Cartrol	See CARTEOLOL
Catapres	See CLONIDINE
Ceclor	See CEFACLOR
CEFACLOR	Antibiotic
CEFADROXIL	Antibiotic
CEFAZOLIN	Antibiotic
CEFIXIME	Antibiotic
Cefizox	See CEFTZOXIME
Cefobid	See CEFOPERAZONE
CEFOPERAZONE	Antibiotic
Cefotan	See CEFOTETAN

Generic names are in capital letters; trade names are in lower case.

DRUG NAME	DRUG TYPE
CEFOTAXIME	Antibiotic
CEFOTETAN	Antibiotic
CEFOXITIN	Antibiotic
CEFPROZIL	Antibiotic
CEFTAZIDIME	Antibiotic
Ceftin	See CEFUROXIME
CEFTRIAXONE	Antibiotic
CEFTZOXIME	Antibiotic
CEFUROXIME	Antibiotic
Cefzil	See CEFPROZIL
Celontin	See METHSUXIMIDE
Centrax	See PRAZEPAM
CEPHALEXIN	Antibiotic
Chlor–Trimeton	See CHLORPHENIRAMINE
CHLORAL HYDRATE	Hypnotic
CHLORAMBUCIL	Anticancer agent
CHLORAMPHENICOL	Antibiotic
CHLORAZEPATE	Antiepileptic
CHLORDIAZEPOXIDE	Benzodiazepine—anxiolytic
Chloromycetin	See CHLORAMPHENICOL
CHLOROTHIAZIDE	Thiazide diuretic
CHLORPROMAZINE	Phenothiazine—antipsychotic, antiemetic
CHLORPROPAMIDE	Hypoglycemic agent, antidiuretic therapy for diabetes insipidus
CHLORPROTHIXENE	Antipsychotic
CHLORTHALIDONE	Thiazide–related diuretic
CHLOZOXAZONE	Relief of local muscle spasm
Choledyl	See OXTRIPHYLLINE
CHOLESTYRAMINE	Antihypercholesterolemic agent
CHOLINE MAGNESIUM TRISALICYLATE	Nonopioid analgesic, antipyretic
Cholybar	See CHOLESTYRAMINE
CHORPHENIRAMINE	Antihistamine
CIMETIDINE	H_2 blocker—peptic ulcer disease
Cipro	See CIPROFLOXACIN
CIPROFLOXACIN	Antibiotic
CISAPRIDE	Gastric motility agent—treatment of esophageal reflux
CISPLATIN	Anticancer agent
Claforan	See CEFOTAXIME
CLARITHROMYCIN	Antibiotic
Cleocin	See CLINDAMYCIN
CLINDAMYCIN	Antibiotic

Generic names are in capital letters; trade names are in lower case.

DRUG NAME	DRUG TYPE
Clinoril	See SULINDAC
CLOFIBRATE	Hypoglycemic agent, antidiuretic therapy for diabetes insipidus
CLOMIPRAMINE	Tricyclic antidepressant
CLONAZEPAM	Benzodiazepine—anxiolytic, antiepileptic
CLONIDINE	Centrally acting α agent
CLORAZEPATE	Benzodiazepine—anxiolytic, hypnotic
CLOTRIMAZOLE	Topical antifungal
CLOZAPINE	Antipsychotic
Clozaril	See CLOZAPINE
COBALAMIN	Vitamin B12
CODEINE	Opioid analgesic, antitussive
Cogentin	See BENZTROPINE
Colace	See DOCUSATE SODIUM
COLCHICINE	Antiinflammatory agent—gout
Colestid	See COLESTIPOL
COLESTIPOL	Anti hypercholesterol agent
Combipres	Combination CHLORTHALIDONE–CLONIDINE
Compazine	See PROCHLOROPERAZINE
Constant–T	See THEOPHYLLINE
Cordarone	See AMIODARONE
Corgard	See NADOLOL
CORTISONE	Steroid
Corzide	Combination NADOLOL–BENDROFLUMETHIAZIDE
Coumadin	See WARFARIN
CROMOLYN SODIUM	Inhaled mast cell stabilizer for bronchospasm
CYANOCOBALAMIN	Vitamin B12
CYCLIZINE	Antihistamine—antivertigo, antiemetic
CYCLOBENZAPRINE	Skeletal muscle relaxant
CYCLOPHOSPHAMIDE	Anticancer agent
CYCLOSPORIN A	See CYCLOSPORINE
CYCLOSPORINE	Immunosuppressant—transplants
CYCLOTHIAZIDE	Thiazide diuretic
Cylert	See PEMOLINE
CYPROHEPTADINE	Antihistamine
Cytotec	See MISOPROSTOL
Cytoxan	See CYCLOPHOSPHAMIDE
Dalmane	See FLURAZEPAM

Generic names are in capital letters; trade names are in lower case.

DRUG NAME	DRUG TYPE
Dantrium	See DANTROLENE
DANTROLENE	Peripherally acting antispasm agent
DAPSONE	Antibiotic
Darvocet–N 50, 100	Combination PROPOXYPHENE–ACETAMINOPHEN
Darvon Compound–65	Combination PROPOXYPHENE–CAFFEINE–ASPIRIN
Darvon–N	See PROPOXYPHENE
DDAVP	See DESMOPRESSIN
Decabid	See INDECAINIDE
Delaxin	See METHOCARBAMOL
Delta–Cortef	See PREDNISOLONE
Demerol APAP	Combination MEPERIDINE–ACETAMINOPHEN
Depakote	See DIVALPROEX SODIUM
Depo–Medrol	Long acting METHYLPREDNISO–LONE
Deponit	See NITROGLYCERIN
Deprenyl	See SELEGILINE
DESERPIDINE	Antihypertensive
DESIPRAMINE	Tricyclic antidepressant
DESMOPRESSIN ACETATE	Antidiuretic therapy for diabetes insipidus
Desyrel	See TRAZODONE
Dexedrine	See DEXTROAMPHETAMINE
DEXTROAMPHETAMINE	Amphetamine—attention defifit hyperactivity disorder
DEXTROMETHORPHAN	Antitussive
D. H. E. 45	See DIHYDOERGOTAMINE
Diabeta	See GLYBURIDE
Diabinese	See CHLORPROPAMIDE
Diamox	See ACETAZOLAMIDE
Diapid	See LYPRESSIN
DIAZEPAM	Benzodiazepine—anxiolytic, hypnotic, antispastic
Dibenzyline	See PHENOXYBENZAMINE
DICLOXACILLIN	Antibiotic
DICUMAROL	Anticoagulant
Diflucan	See FLUCONAZOLE
DIFLUNISAL	NSAID—analgesic, antipyretic
DIGITALIS	Cardiac glycoside—antiarrhythmic, CHF
DIGITOXIN	Cardiac glycoside—antiarrhythmic, CHF

Generic names are in capital letters; trade names are in lower case.

DRUG NAME	DRUG TYPE
DIGOXIN	Cardiac glycoside—antiarrhythmic, CHF
DIHYDROERGOTAMINE	Antimigraine
Dilantin	See PHENYTOIN
Dilatrate–SR	Sustained release ISOSORBIDE DINITRATE
Dilaudid	See HYDROMORPHONE
Dilor	See DYPHYLLINE
DILTIAZEM	Ca^{2+} channel blocker
DIMENHYDRINATE	Anti–motion sickness
Dipentum	See OLSALAZINE SULFATE
DIPHENHYDRAMINE	Antihistamine
DIPYRIDAMOLE	Antiplatelet agent
Disalcid	See SALSALATE
DISOPYRAMIDE	Antiarrhythmic
DISULFIRAM	Alcohol–sensitizing drug
Ditropan	See OXYBUTININ
Diucardin	See HYDOFLUMETHAZINE
Diulo	See METOLAZONE
Diuril	See CHLOROTHIAZIDE
DIVALPROEX SODIUM	Anticonvulsant
DOCUSATE SODIUM	Stool softener
Dolene AP–65	Combination PROPOXYPHENE–ACETAMINOPHEN
Dolobid	See DIFLUNISOL
Dolophine	See METHADONE
Dopar	See LEVODOPA
Doral	See QUAZEPAM
Doriden	See GLUTETHIMIDE
Doxaphene	Opioid analgesic
DOXAZOSIN	α^1 blocker—antihypertensive agent
DOXEPIN	Tricyclic antidepressant
DOXYCYCLINE	Antibiotic
Dramamine	See DIMENHYDRATE
DROPERIDOL	Antivertigo, antiemetic
Dulcolax	See BISACODYL
Duragesic	See FENTANYL
Duraquin	See QUINIDINE
Duricef	See CEFADROXIL
Dyazide	Combination HYDROCHLOROTHIAZIDE–TRIAMTERENE
DynaCirc	See ISRADIPINE
DYPHYLLINE	Methylxanthine bronchodilator

Generic names are in capital letters; trade names are in lower case.

DRUG NAME	**DRUG TYPE**
Dyrenium	See TRIAMTERENE
E–mycin	See ERYTHROMYCIN
Ecotrin	See ASPIRIN
Edecrin	See ETHACRYNIC ACID
EDROPHONIUM	Anticholinesterase agent— Myasthenia gravis
Elavil	See AMITRIPTYLINE
Eldepryl	See SELEGILINE
Elixophyllin SR	Sustained release THEOPHYLLINE
ENALAPRIL	ACE inhibitor
ENALAPRILAT	ACE inhibitor
ENCAINIDE	Antiarrhythmic
Endep	See AMITRIPTYLINE
Enduron	See METHYCLOTHIAZIDE
Enduronyl	Combination METHYCLOTHIAZIDE– DESERPIDINE
Enkaid	See ENCAINIDE
EPHEDRINE	Adrenergic agent—nasal deconges– tant
EPINEPHRINE	Adrenergic bronchodilator
Equanil	See MEPROBAMATE
Ergostat	See ERGOTAMINE TARTRATE
ERGOTAMINE TARTRATE	Antimigraine
Ery–tab	See ERYTHROMYCIN
ERYTHRITYL TETRANITRATE	Nitrate—antianginal
ERYTHROMYCIN	Antibiotic
Esgic	Combination antimigraine
Esidrix	See HYDROCHLOROTHIAZIDE
ESMOLOL	Cardioselective β adrenergic blocker
ETHACRYNIC ACID	Loop diuretic
ETHAMBUTOL	Antibiotic—tuberculosis
ETHCHLORVYNOL	Hypnotic
ETHINAMATE	Hypnotic
Ethmozine	See MORICIZINE
ETHOPROPAZINE	Antiparkinson agent
ETHOSUXIMIDE	Antiepileptic
ETHOTOIN	Antiepileptic
ETODOLAC	NSAID—analgesic, antipyretic
Exna	See BENTHIAZIDE
FAMOTIDINE	H_2 blocker—peptic ulcer disease
Feldene	See PIROXICAM
FELODIPINE	Ca^{2+} channel blocker
FENOPROFEN CALCIUM	Nonopioid analgesic, antipyretic

Generic names are in capital letters; trade names are in lower case.

DRUG NAME	DRUG TYPE
FENTANYL	Narcotic analgesic
FINSATERIDE	Treatment of benign prostatic hypertrophy
Fioricet	Narcotic–containing analgesic, antipyretic
Fiorinal	Combination antimigraine
Flagyl	See METRONIDAZOLE
FLECAINIDE	Antiarrhythmic
Flexeril	See CYCLOBENZAPRINE
Florinef	See FLUDOCORTISONE
Floxin	See OFLOXACIN
FLUCONAZOLE	Antifungal antibiotic
FLUDROCORTISONE	Steroid
FLUMAZENIL	Benzodiazepine antagonist
FLUNISOLIDE	Inhaled corticosteroid for bronchospasm
FLUOXETINE	Selective serotonin reuptake inhibitor—antidepressant
FLUPHENAZINE	Phenothiazine—antipsychotic, long acting
FLUPHENAZINE DECANOATE	Phenothiazine—antipsychotic, long acting
FLUPHENAZINE ENANTHATE	Phenothiazine—antipsychotic, long acting
FLURAZEPAM	Benzodiazepine—anxiolytic, hypnotic, sedative
Fortaz	See CEFTAZIDIME
FOSINOPRIL	ACE inhibitor—antihypertensive
Fulvicin	See GRISEOFULVIN
FUROSEMIDE	Loop diuretic
Garamycin	See GENTAMICIN
GEMFIBROZIL	Cholesterol and triglyceride–lowering agent
GENTAMICIN	Antibiotic
GLIPIZIDE	Oral hypoglycemic agent
Glucotrol	See GLIPIZIDE
GLUTETHIMIDE	Hypnotic
GLYBURIDE	Oral hypoglycemic agent
Grifulvin V	See GRISEOFULVIN
Grisactin	See GRISEOFULVIN
GRISEOFULVIN	Antifungal antibiotic
GUANABENZ	Centrally acting α agent, antihypertensive
GUANETHIDINE	Antihypertensive

Generic names are in capital letters; trade names are in lower case.

DRUG NAME	DRUG TYPE
GUANFACINE	Centrally acting α agent
HALAZEPAM	Benzodiazepine—anxiolytic, hypnotic
Halcion	See TRIAZOLAM
Haldol Decanoate	See HALOPERIDOL DECANOATE
HALOPERIDOL DECANOATE	Antipsychotic, long acting
Harmonyl	See DESERPIDINE
HCTZ	See HYDROCHLOROTHIAZIDE
Hismanal	See ASTEMIZOLE
HYDRALAZINE	Arterial vasodilator—antihypertensive
HYDROCHLOROTHIAZIDE	Thiazide diuretic
HYDROFLUMETHIAZIDE	Thiazide diuretic
HYDROMORPHONE HYDROCHLORIDE	Opioid analgesic
Hydromox	See QUINETHAZONE
Hydropres-25, -50	Combination HYDROCHLOROTHIAZIDE-RESERPINE
HYDROXYZINE	Antihistamine, antiemetic, anxiolytic
Hygroton	See CHLORTHALIDONE
Hytrin	See TERAZOSIN
IBUPROFEN	NSAID—analgesic, antipyretic
IMIPRAMINE	tricyclic antidepressant, anxiolytic
Imodium	See LOPERAMIDE
Imuran	See AZATHIOPRINE
Inapsine	See DROPERIDOL
INDAPAMIDE	Thiazide-related diuretic
INDECAINIDE	Antiarrhythmic agent
Inderal LA	Long-acting PROPRANOLOL
Inderide LA	Long-acting combination PROPRANOLOL-HYDROCHLOROTHIAZIDE
Indocin	See INDOMETHACIN
INDOMETHACIN	NSAID—analgesic, antipyretic
INH	See ISONIAZID
Inocor	See AMRINONE
Intal	See CHROMOLYN SODIUM
IODINATED GLYCEROL	Expectorant
IPRATROPIUM	Inhaled anticholinergic bronchodilator
Ismelin	See GUANETHIDINE
Ismo	See ISOSORBIDE MONONITRATE
Iso-Bid	See ISOSORBIDE DINITRATE
ISOCARBOXAZID	MAO inhibitor—antidepressant

Generic names are in capital letters; trade names are in lower case.

DRUG NAME	DRUG TYPE
ISOETHARINE	β_2 agonist bronchodilator
ISONIAZID	Antibiotic—tuberculosis
ISOPROTERENOL	β adrenergic bronchodilator
Isoptin SR	Sustained release VERAPAMIL
Isopto Carpine	See PILOCARPINE
Isordil	See ISOSORBIDE DINITRATE
ISOSORBIDE DINITRATE	Nitrate—antianginal
ISOSORBIDE MONONITRATE	Nitrate—antianginal
ISOTRETINOIN	Treats cystic acne
ISRADIPINE	Ca^{2+} channel blocker
Isuprel	See ISOPROTERENOL
Janimine	See IMIPRAMINE
Keflex	See CEPHALEXIN
Keftab	See CEPHALEXIN
Kefurox	See CEFUROXIME
Kefzol	See CEFAZOLIN
Kemadrin	See PROCYCLIDINE
Kenalog	Topical TRIAMCINOLONE
Kerlone	See BETAXOLOL
KETOCONAZOLE	Antifungal agent
KETOROLAC	NSAID—analgesic, antipyretic
Klonopin	See CLONAZEPAM
Kwell	See LINDANE
L–THYROXINE	Thyroid hormone—hypothyroidism
LABETALOL	α, β adrenergic blocker
LACTULOSE	Laxative and treatment of hepatic encephalopathy
Lanoxicaps	See DIGOXIN
Lanoxin	See DIGOXIN
Larodopa	See LEVODOPA
Lasix	See FUROSEMIDE
Leukeran	See CHLORAMBUCIL
Levatol	See PHENOBUTOLOL
LEVOBUNOLOL	β blocker—glaucoma
LEVODOPA–CARBIDOPA	Combination antiparkinson agent
LEVORPHANOL	Opioid analgesic
LEVOTHYROXINE	Thyroid hormone—hypothyroidism
Libritabs	See CHLORDIAZPOXIDE
Librium	See CHLORDIAZPOXIDE
LINDANE	Treatment of lice and scabies
Lioresal	See BACLOFEN
Lipo–Nicin	Decreases LDL, triglycerides, increases HDL
LISINOPRIL	ACE inhibitor

Generic names are in capital letters; trade names are in lower case.

DRUG NAME	DRUG TYPE
LITHIUM CARBONATE	Treatment of manic episodes in bipolar disorder
Lodine	See ETODOLAC
Lomotil	Narcotic–like antidiarrheal agent
Loniten	See MINOXIDIL
LOPERAMIDE	Antidiarrheal agent
Lopid	See GEMFIBROZIL
Lopressor HCT	Combination METOPROLOL–HYDROCHLOROTHIAZIDE
LORAZEPAM	Benzodiazepine—anxiolytic, hypnotic
Lorcet	Combination HYDROCODONE–ACETAMINOPHEN
Lorelco	See PROBUCOL
Lortab	Combination HYDROCODONE–ACETAMINOPHEN
Lotensin	See BENZAPRIL
Lotrimin	See CLOTRIMAZOLE
LOVASTATIN	Treatment of hypercholesterolemia
LOXAPINE	Antipsychotic
Loxitane	See LOXAPINE
Lozol	See INDAPAMIDE
Ludiomil	See MAPROTILINE
Lufyllin	See DYPHYLLINE
LYPRESSIN	Antidiuretic therapy for diabetes insipidus
Maalox	Antacid
Macrodantin	See NITROFURANTIN
Mandol	See CEFAMANDOLE
MAPROTILINE	Tricyclic antidepressant
Marezine	See CYCLIZINE
Marplan	See ISOCARBOXAZID
Maxair	See PIRBUTEROL
Maxzide	Combination HYDROCHLOROTHIAZIDE–TRIAMTERENE
MECLIZINE	Antihistamine—antivertigo, anti–motion sickness
Medihaler Ergotamine	See ERGOTAMINE
Medipren	See IBUPROFEN
Medrol	See METHYLPREDNISOLONE
MEDROXYPROGESTERONE	Treatment of amenorrhea, uterine bleeding
MEFENAMIC ACID	Non–opioid analgesic, antipyretic

Generic names are in capital letters; trade names are in lower case.

DRUG NAME	DRUG TYPE
Mefoxin	See CEFOXITIN
Mellaril	See THIORIDAZINE
MEPERIDINE	Opioid analgesic
MEPHENYTOIN	Antiepileptic
MEPHOBARBITAL	Barbiturate—antiepileptic
MEPROBAMATE	Anxiolytic
Meprospan	See MEPROBAMATE
Mesantoin	See MEPHENYTOIN
MESORIDAZINE	Phenothiazine—antipsychotic
Mestinon	See PYRIDOSTIGMINE BROMIDE
Metahyrin	See TRICHLOROMETHIAZIDE
Metaprel	See METAPROTERENOL
METAPROTERENOL	β agonist bronchodilator
Metatensin #2, #4	Combination TRICHLOROMETHIAZIDE–RESERPINE
METHADONE	Opioid analgesic
METHAZOLAMIDE	Treatment of glaucoma
METHIMAZOLE	Treatment of hyperthyroidism
METHOCARBAMOL	Relief of local muscle spasm
METHSUXIMIDE	Antiepileptic
METHYCLOTHIAZIDE	Thiazide diuretic
METHYLDOPA	Centrally acting α agent, antihypertensive
METHYLPHENIDATE	CNS stimulant—attention deficit hyperactivity disorder
METHYLPREDNISOLONE	Steroid—inflammatory and allergic conditions
METHYPRYLON	Hypnotic
METHYSERGIDE MALEATE	Antimigraine
METOCLOPRAMIDE	Treatment of esophageal reflux, diabetic gastroparesis
METOLAZONE	Thiazide–related diuretic
METOPROLOL	β^1 blocker—angina, hypertension
METRONIDAZOLE	Antibiotic
Mevacor	See LOVASTATIN
MEXILITINE	Antiarrhythmic agent
Mexitil	See MEXILITINE
Mezlin	See MEZLOCILLIN
MEZLOCILLIN	Antibiotic
MICONAZOLE	Antifungal antibiotic
Micrainin	Combination antimigraine
Micronase	See GLYBURIDE
Midamor	See AMILORIDE

Generic names are in capital letters; trade names are in lower case.

DRUG NAME	DRUG TYPE
MIDAZOLAM	Benzodiazepine
Midol 200	See IBUPROFEN
Midrin	Combination antimigraine
Milontin	See PHENSUXIMIDE
Miltown	See MEPROBAMATE
Minipress	See PRAZOSIN
Minitran	See NITROGLYCERIN
MINOXIDIL	Arterial vasodilator—antihypertensive
Minzide 1, 2, 5	Combination PRAZOSIN–POLYTHIAZIDE
MISOPROSTOL	Prevention of gastric ulcers
Moban	See MOLIDONE
Moderil	See RESCINNAMINE
Moduretic	Combination AMILORIDE–HYDROCHLOROTHIAZIDE
MOLIDONE	Antipsychotic
Monistat	See MICONAZOLE
Monopril	See FOSINOPRIL
MORICIZINE	Antiarrhythmic
MORPHINE SULFATE	Opioid analgesic
Motrin	See IBUPROFEN
MS Contin	Long–acting MORPHINE
Mucomyst	See ACETYLCYSTEINE
MYAMBUTAL	See ETHAMBUTAL
Mycelex	See CLOTRIMAZOLE
Mycostatin	See NYSTATIN
Mykrox	See METOLAZONE
Mylanta	Antacid
Myleran	See BUSULFAN
Mysoline	See PRIMIDONE
N–ACETYLCYSTEINE	Mucolytic
NABUMETONE	NSAID—analgesic, antipyretic
NADOLOL	β blocker–angina, hypertension
Nalfon	See FENOPROFEN
Naprosyn	See NAPROXEN
NAPROXEN	NSAID—analgesic, antipyretic
Nardil	See PHENELZINE
Nasacort	Inhaled TRIAMCINOLONE—allergic rhinitis
Nasalcrom	See CROMOLYN SODIUM
Naturetin	See BENDROFLUMETHIAZIDE
Navane	See THIOTHIXENE
NebuPent	See PENTAMIDINE

Generic names are in capital letters; trade names are in lower case.

DRUG NAME	DRUG TYPE
Nembutal	See PENTOBARBITAL
Neo–Synephrine	See PHENYLEPHRINE
NEOSTIGMINE	Anticholinesterase agent— Myasthenia gravis
Neptazane	See METHAZOLAMIDE
NIACIN	Decreases LDL and triglycerides, increases HDL
NICARDIPINE	Ca^{2+} channel blocker
Nicobid	Decreases LDL and triglycerides, increases HDL
Nicorette gum	See NICOTINE POLACRILEX
NICOTINE POLACRILEX	Adjunct to smoking cessation
NICOTINIC ACID	See NIACIN
NIFEDIPINE	Ca^{2+} channel blocker
NIMODIPINE	Ca^{2+} channel blocker
Nimotop	See NIMODIPINE
Nitro–Bid	See NITROGLYCERIN
Nitro–Dur	See NITROGLYCERIN
Nitrocine	See NITROGLYCERIN
Nitrodisc	See NITROGLYCERIN
NITROFURANTOIN	Antibiotic
Nitrogard	See NITROGLYCERIN
NITROGLYCERIN	Nitrate—antianginal
Nitrol	See NITROGLYCERIN
Nitrolingual	See NITROGLYCERIN
Nitrong	See NITROGLYCERIN
Nitropaste	See NITROGLYCERIN
Nitrospan	See NITROGLYCERIN
Nitrostat	See NITROGLYCERIN
NIZATIDINE	H_2 blocker—peptic ulcer disease
Nizoral	See KETOCONAZOLE
Noctec	See CHLORAL HYDRATE
Norflex	See ORPHENADRINE CITRATE
NORFLOXACIN	Antibiotic
Normodyne	See LABETOLOL
Noroxin	See NORFLOXACIN
Norpace CR	See DISOPYRAMIDE
Norpramin	See DESIPRAMINE
NORTRIPTYLINE	Tricyclic antidepressant
Norvasc	See AMLODIPINE
Numorphan	See OXYMORPHONE
Nuprin	See IBUPROFEN
NYSTATIN	Antifungal
OFLOXACIN	Antibiotic

Generic names are in capital letters; trade names are in lower case.

DRUG NAME	DRUG TYPE
OLSALAZINE SODIUM	Treatment of ulcerative colitis
OMEPRAZOLE	Treatment of peptic ulcer disease, esophageal reflux
Orap	See PRIMOZIDE
Oretic	See HYDROCHLOROTHIAZIDE
Organidin	See IODINATED GLYCEROL
Orinase	See TOLBUTAMIDE
ORPHENADRINE CITRATE	Relief of local muscle spasm
Os–cal	Antacid
OXACILLIN	Antibiotic
OXAZEPAM	Benzodiazepine—anxiolytic, hypnotic
OXTRIPHYLLINE	Methylxanthine bronchodilator
OXYBUTYNIN	Urinary antispasmodic
OXYCODONE	Opioid analgesic
OXYMETAZOLINE	Nasal decongestant
OXYMORPHONE	Opioid analgesic
Pamelor	See NORTRIPTYLINE
Pancrease	See PANCRELIPASE
PANCRELIPASE	Digestive enzymes—treatment of pancreatic disease
Panwarfin	See WARFARIN
Paradione	See PARAMETHADIONE
Paraflex	See CHLORZOXAZONE
Parafon Forte DSC	See CHLORZOXAZONE
PARAMETHADIONE	Antiepileptic
Paraplatin	See CARBOPLATIN
Parlodel	See BROMOCRIPTINE
Parnate	See TRANCYPROMINE
PAROXETINE	Selective serotonin reuptake inhibitor—antidepressant
Parsidol	See ETHOPROPAZINE
Paxil	See PAROXETINE
Paxipam	See HALAZEPAM
Peganone	See ETHOTOIN
PEMOLINE	CNS Stimulant—attention deficit hyperactivity disorder
Pen–Vee K	See PENICILLIN
PENBUTOLOL	β adrenergic blocker
PENICILLIN	Antibiotic
PENTAERYTHRITOL	Nitrate—antianginal
Pentam	See PENTAMIDINE
PENTAMIDINE	Treatment of pneumocystis carinii pneumonia

Generic names are in capital letters; trade names are in lower case.

DRUG NAME	DRUG TYPE
PENTAZOCINE	Opioid analgesic
PENTOBARBITAL	Barbiturate—anxiolytic, hypnotic
PENTOXIFYLLINE	Treatment of peripheral vascular disease
Pepcid	See FAMOTIDINE
Percocet	Combination OXYCODONE–ACETOMINAPHEN
Percodan	Combination OXYCODONE–ASPIRIN
PERGOLIDE	Antiparkinson agent
Pericolace	Stool softener
Perilactin	See CYPROHEPTADINE
Peritrate	See PENTAERYTHRITOL
Permax	See PERGOLIDE
Permitil	See FLUPHENAZINE
PERPHENAZINE	Phenothiazine—antipsychotic, antiemetic
Persantine	See DIPYRIDAMOLE
Pertofrane	See DESIPRAMINE
PHELELZINE	MAO inhibitor—antidepressant, anxiolytic
PHENACAMIDE	Antiepileptic
PHENAZOPYRIDINE	Urinary tract analgesia
Phenergan	See PROMETHAZINE
PHENOBARBITAL	Barbiturate—anticonvulsant, sedative
PHENOXYBENZAMINE	α adrenergic blocker—antihypertensive
PHENSUXIMIDE	Antiepileptic
PHENTOLAMINE	α adrenergic blocker—antihypertensive
Phenurone	See PHENACCEMIDE
PHENYLEPHRINE	α agonist—decongestant
PHENYLPROPANOLAMINE	α agonist—appetite suppressant, stress incontinence
PHENYTOIN	Anticonvulsant, antiarrhythmic
Phosphajel	See ALUMINUM PHOSPHATE
Phrenilin	Combination antimigraine
Phyllocontin	See AMINOPHYLLINE
PILOCARPINE	Treatment of glaucoma
PINDOLOL	β adrenergic blocker
PIPERACILLIN	Antibiotic
PIRBUTEROL	Adrenergic bronchodilator
PIROXICAM	NSAID—analgesic, antipyretic

Generic names are in capital letters; trade names are in lower case.

DRUG NAME	DRUG TYPE
Pitressin	See VASOPRESSIN
Placidyl	See ETHYLCHLORVYNOL
Platinol	See CISPLATIN
Plendil	See FELODIPINE
POLYTHIAZIDE	Thiazide diuretic
Ponstel	See MEFANAMIC ACID
Pravachol	See PRAVASTATIN
PRAVASTATIN	Treats hyperlipidemia
PRAZEPAM	Benzodiazepine—anxiolytic, hypnotic
PRAZOSIN	α_1 adrenergic blocker—antihypertensive
PREDNISOLONE	Steroid—inflammation and allergic conditions
PREDNISONE	Steroid—inflammation and allergic conditions
Premarin	Estrogen supplement
Prilosec	See OMEPRAZOLE
Primaxin	See IMIPENEM
PRIMIDONE	Anticonvulsant
PRIMOZIDE	Antipsychotic—Tourette's disorder
Prinivil	ACE inhibitor
Prinzide	Combination LISINOPRIL–HYDROCHLOROTHIAZIDE
PROBUCOL	Treatment of hypercholesterolemia
PROCAINAMIDE	Antiarrhythmic
Procan SR	Long–acting PROCAINAMIDE
Procardia SR	Long–acting NIFEDIPINE
PROCHLOROPERAZINE	Phenothiazine—antiemetic
PROCYCLIDINE	Antiparkinson agent
Prolixin Decanoate	Long–acting FLUPHENAZINE
Prolixin Enenthate	See FLUPHENAZINE
PROMETHAZINE	Antihistaminic—antivertigo, antiemetic
Pronestyl	See PROCAINAMIDE
Propacet 100	Combination PROPOXYPHENE–ACETOMINAPHEN
PROPAFENONE	Antiarrhythmic
PROPOXYPHENE	Narcotic analgesic
PROPRANOLOL	β adrenergic blocker
Propulsid	See CISAPRIDE
PROPYLTHIOURACIL	Treatment of hyperthyroidism
Proscar	See FINASTERIDE
Prostigmin	See NEOSTIGMINE BROMIDE

Generic names are in capital letters; trade names are in lower case.

DRUG NAME	DRUG TYPE
PROTRIPTYLINE	Tricyclic antidepressant
Proventil	See ALBUTEROL
Provera	See MEDROXYPROGESTERONE
Prozac	See FLUOXETINE
PSEUDOEPHEDRINE	Adrenergic agent—nasal decongestant
PTU	See PROPYLTHIOURACIL
PYRAZINAMIDE	Antibiotic—tuberculosis
Pyridium	See PHENAZOPYRIDINE
PYRIDOSTIGMINE BROMIDE	Anticholinesterase agent—Myasthenia gravis
QUAZEPAM	Benzodiazepine—anxiolytic, hypnotic
Questran	See CHOLESTYRAMINE
Quibron–T	See THEOPHYLLINE
Quibron–T/SR	Sustained release THEOPHYLLINE
Quinaglute	See QUINIDINE
Quinaglute	See QUINIDINE
Quinamm	See QUININE SULFATE
QUINAPRIL	ACE inhibitor—hypertension
Quinatime	See QUINIDINE
QUINETHAZONE	Thiazide–related diuretic
Quinidex	See QUINIDINE
QUINIDINE	Antiarrhythmic
QUININE SULFATE	Relief of local muscle spasm
RAMIPRIL	ACE inhibitor
RANITIDINE	H^2 blocker—peptic ulcer disease
Raudixin	See RAUWOLFIA SERPENTINA
Rauverid	See RAUWOLFIA SERPENTINA
RAUWOLFIA SERPENTINA	Antihypertensive
Regitine	See PHENTOLAMINE
Reglan	See METOCLOPRAMIDE
Regonol	See PYRIDOSTIGMINE BROMIDE
Rela	See CARISOPRODOL
Relafen	See NABUMETONE
Renese	See POLYTHIAZIDE
RESERPINE	Antihypertensive
Respbid	See THEOPHYLLINE
Restoril	See TEMAZEPAM
Retin–A	See TRETINOIN
Retrovir	See ZIDOVUDINE
Rifadin	See RIFAMPIN
RIFAMPIN	Antibiotic—tuberculosis, meningococcal meningitis

Generic names are in capital letters; trade names are in lower case.

DRUG NAME	DRUG TYPE
Rimactane	See RIFAMPIN
Ritalin	See METHYLPHENIDATE
Robaxin	See METHOCARBAMOL
Rocephin	See CEFTRIAXONE
Romazecon	See FLUMAZENIL
Roxanol SR	Long–acting MORPHINE
Roxicodone	See OXYCODONE
Rufen	See IBUPROFEN
Rythmol	See PROPAFENONE
SALSALATE	NSAID—analgesic, antipyretic
Saluron	See HYDROFLUMETHIAZIDE
Salutensin	Combination RESERPINE—HYDROFLUMETHIAZIDE
Sansert	See METHYSERGIDE MALEATE
SCOPOLAMINE	Anticholinergic—antivertigo, antiemetic
SECOBARBITAL	Barbiturate—anxiolytic, hypnotic
Seconal	See SECOBARBITAL
Sectral	See ACEBUTOL
Seldane	See TERFENADINE
SELEGILINE	MAO inhibitor—antiparkinson agent
Septra	See TRIMETHAPRIM-SULFAMETHOXAZOLE
Ser–Ap–Es	Combination HYDROCHLOROTHIAZIDE-RESERPINE–HYDRALAZINE
Serax	See OXAZEPAM
Serentil	See MESORIDAZINE
Serpasil	See RESERPINE
SERTRALINE	Selective serotonin reuptake inhibitor—antidepressant
SIMVASTATIN	Lipid–lowering agent
Sinemet	Combination LEVODOPA–CARBIDOPA
Sinequan	See DOXEPIN
Slo–Bid	Long–acting THEOPHYLLINE
Slo–Niacin	See NIACIN
Slo–Phyllin	See THEOPHYLLINE
Solu–Medrol	See METHYLPREDNISOLONE
Soma	See CARISOPRODOL
Sorbitrate	See ISOSORBIDE DINITRATE
SPIRONOLACTONE	K$^+$ sparing diuretic
Stelazine	See TRIFLUOPERAZINE
STREPTOMYCIN	Antibiotic—tuberculosis

Generic names are in capital letters; trade names are in lower case.

DRUG NAME	DRUG TYPE
SUCRALFATE	Local therapy for peptic ulcers
Sudafed	See PSEUDOEPHEDRINE
SULFASALAZINE	Anti–inflammatory agent—treatment of ulcerative colitis
SULINDAC	NSAID—analgesic, antipyretic
Sumatrex	See SUMATRIPTAN
SUMATRIPTAN	Seratonin agonist—migraine headaches
Suprax	See CEFIXIME
Surmontil	See TRIMIPRAMINE
Sustaire	See THEOPHYLLINE
Symmetrel	See AMANTADINE
Synthroid	See LEVOTHYROXINE
Tagamet	See CIMETIDINE
Talacen	Combination PENTAZOCINE–ACETOMINAPHEN
Talwin Compound	Combination PENTAZOCINE–ASPIRIN
Talwin NX	Combination PENTAZOCINE–NALOXONE
Tambocor	See FLECAINAIDE
TAMOXIFEN	Antiestrogen properties—breast cancer
Tapazole	See METHIMAZOLE
Taractan	See CHLORPROTHIXENE
Tazicef	See CEFTAZIDIME
Tazidime	See CEFTAZIDIME
Tegretol	See CARBAMAZEPINE
TEMAZEPAM	Benzodiazepine—insomnia
Tenex	See GUANFACINE
Tenoretic	Combination ATENOLOL–CHLORTHALIDONE
Tenormin	See ATENOLOL
Tensilon	See EDROPHONIUM
TERAZOSIN	α^1 adrenergic blocker—antihypertensive
TERBUTALINE	β agonist brochodilator
TERFENADINE	Antihistamine
Tessalon	See BENZONATATE
TETRACYCLINE	Antibiotic
Thalitone	See CHLORTHALIDONE
Theo–24	See THEOPHYLLINE
Theo–Dur	Sustained release THEOPHYLLINE
Theobid	See THEOPHYLLINE

Generic names are in capital letters; trade names are in lower case.

DRUG NAME	DRUG TYPE
Theochron	See THEOPHYLLINE
Theoclear 80	See THEOPHYLLINE
Theoclear LA	See THEOPHYLLINE
Theolair	See THEOPHYLLINE
Theolair–SR	Sustained release THEOPHYLLINE
THEOPHYLLINE	Methylxanthine bronchodilator
Theostat 80	See THEOPHYLLINE
Theovent	See THEOPHYLLINE
THIETHYLPERAZINE	Phenothiazine—antiemetic
THIORIDAZINE	Phenothiazine—antipsychotic
THIOTHIXENE	Antipsychotic
Thorazine	See CHLORPROMAZINE
Ticar	See TICARCILLIN
TICARCILLIN	Antibiotic
TICARCILLIN CLAVULANATE	Antibiotic
Ticlid	See TICLOPIDINE
TICLOPIDINE	Antiplatelet agent—TIAs, thrombotic CVAs
Tigan	See TRIMETHOBENZAMIDE
Timentin	See TICARCILLIN–CLAVULANATE
Timolide	Combination TIMOLOL–HYDROCHLOROTHIAZIDE
TIMOLOL	β adrenergic blocker
Timoptic	TIMOLOL eyedrops—glaucoma
Tindal	See ACETOPHENAZINE
TOBRAMYCIN	Antibiotic
TOCAINIDE	Antiarrhythmic
Tofranil	See IMIPRAMINE
TOLAZAMIDE	Oral hypoglycemic
TOLBUTAMIDE	Oral hypoglycemic
Tolinase	See TOLAZAMIDE
Tonocard	See TOCAINIDE
Toprol	See Metoprolol
Toradol	See KETOROLAC
Torecan	See THIETHYPERAZINE
Tornalate	See BITOLTEROL MESYLATE
Trandate	See LABETOLOL
Transderm Scop	See SCOPOLAMINE
Transderm–Nitro	See NITROGLYCERIN
Tranxene	See CHLORAZEPATE
TRANYLCYPROMINE	MAO inhibitor—antidepressant
TRAZODONE	Atypical antidepressant
Trental	See PENTOXIFYLLINE

Generic names are in capital letters; trade names are in lower case.

DRUG NAME	DRUG TYPE
TRETINOIN	Topical therapy for acne vulgaris
TRIAMCINOLONE	Steroid—asthma, sinusitis
TRIAMCINOLONE CREAM	Topical steroid
TRIAMTERENE	K$^+$ sparing diuretic
TRIAZOLAM	Benzodiazepine—anxiolytic, insomnia
TRICHLOROMETHIAZIDE	Thiazide diuretic
Tridione	See TRIMETHADIONE
TRIFLUOPERAZINE	Phenothiazine—antipsychotic
TRIFLUPROMAZINE	Phenothiazine—antiemetic
TRIHEXYPHENIDYL	Antiparkinson agent
Trilafon	See PERPHENAZINE
Trilisate	Salicylate combination—analgesic
TRIMETHADIONE	Antiepileptic
TRIMETHAPRIM–SULFAMETHOXAZOLE	Antibiotic
TRIMETHOBENZAMIDE	Anticholinergic agent—antiemetic
TRIMIPRAMINE	Tricyclic antidepressant
Tylenol	See ACETOMINAPHEN
Tylox	Combination OXYCODONE–ACETOMINAPHEN
Unasyn	See AMPICILLIN SULBACTAM
Uniphyl	Long–acting THEOPHYLLINE
Urecholine	See BETHANECOL
Valium	See DIAZEPAM
Valmid	See ETHINAMATE
VALPROIC ACID	Antiepileptic
Valrelease	See DIAZEPAM
Vancenase	Inhaled BECLOMETHASONE—sinusitis
Vanceril	Inhaled BECLOMETHASONE—bronchospasm
Vascor	See BEPRIDIL
Vaseretic	Combination ENALAPRIL–HYDROCHLOROTHIAZIDE
VASOPRESSIN	Antidiuretic therapy for diabetes insipidus
Vasotec	See ENALAPRIL
Ventolin	See ALBUTEROL
VERAPAMIL	Ca^{2+} channel blocker
Verelan	See VERAPAMIL
Versed	See MIDAZOLAM
Vesprin	See TRIFLUOPROMAZINE
Viokase	See PANCRELIPASE

Generic names are in capital letters; trade names are in lower case.

DRUG NAME	DRUG TYPE
Visken	See PINDOLOL
Vistaril	See HYDROXYZINE
Vivactil	See PROTRIPTYLINE
WARFARIN	Anticoagulant
Wellbutrin	See BUPROPION
Wigraine	Combination ERGOTAMINE–CAFFEINE
Wygesic	Combination PROPOXYPHENE–ACETOMINAPHEN
Wytensin	See GUANABENZ
Xanax	See ALPRAZOLAM
Zantac	See RANITIDINE
Zarontin	See ETHOSUXIMIDE
Zaroxolyn	See METOLAZONE
Zestoretic	Combination LISINOPRIL–HYDROCHLOROTHIAZIDE
Zestril	See LISINOPRIL
ZIDOVUDINE	Antiretroviral agent—HIV infection
Zinacef	See CEFUROXIME
Zithromax	See AZITHROMYCIN
Zocor	See SIMVOSTATIN
Zoloft	See SERTRALINE
Zorprin	See ASPIRIN
Zostrix	See CAPSAICIN
Zovirax	See ACYCLOVIR
Zyloprim	See ALLOPURINOL

References

Deglin JH and Vallerand AH: Davis's Drug Guide for Nurses, 4 ed. F. A. Davis, Philadelphia, PA, 1994.

Generic names are in capital letters; trade names are in lower case.

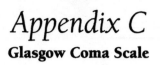

Appendix C
Glasgow Coma Scale

Glasgow Coma Scale

(GCS)

Eye	Spontaneous	4
Opening	To Voice	3
	To Pain	2
	None	1
Verbal	Oriented	5
Response	Confused	4
(Patient's Best	Inappropriate Words	3
Verbal Response)	Incomprehensible Sounds	2
	None	1
Motor	Obeys Command	6
Response	Localizes Pain	5
(Patient's Best	Withdraw (pain)	4
Motor Response)	Flexion (pain)	3
	Extension (pain)	2
	None	1

Total GCS Score   (3 to 15)

Appendix D
Trauma Score

Trauma Score

	Value	Points
Respiratory rate	10–24 bpm	4
	25–35 bpm	3
	>35 bpm	2
	<10 bpm	1
	0 bpm	0
Respiratory effort	Normal	1
	Shallow or Retractive	0
Systolic blood pressure	>90 mm Hg	4
	70–90 mm Hg	3
	50–69 mm Hg	2
	<50 mm Hg	1
	0 mm Hg	0
Capillary refill	Normal	2
	Delayed	1
	None	0

Total of the above scoring plus total GCS score (3 to 15) equals trauma score.

Appendix E
Pediatric Resuscitation Dosages

Cardiac Arrest

Age	Weight (kg)	Low-dose Epinephrine (mg) 1:10,000 IV/IO [0.01 mg/kg]	Defibrillation (J) [2J/kg, initially/ 4J/kg]	Atropine (mg) [0.02 mg/kg] Max. dose: Child, 0.5 mg; Teen, 1.0 mg	Sodium Bicarbonate (mEq) [1 mEq/kg]	Lidocaine (mg) [1 mg/kg]
Premature	1.0	0.01	2/4	0.1	1.0	1.0
	2.0	0.02	4/8	0.1	2.0	2.0
Neonate	3.0	0.03	6/12	0.1	3.0	3.0
	4.0	0.04	8/16	0.1	4.0	4.0
	5.0	0.05	10/20	0.1	5.0	5.0
	6.0	0.06	12/24	0.12	6.0	6.0
6 months	7.0	0.07	14/28	0.14	7.0	7.0
	8.0	0.08	16/32	0.16	8.0	8.0
	9.0	0.09	18/36	0.18	9.0	9.0
1 year	10.0	0.10	20/40	0.20	10.0	10.0
	11.0	0.11	22/44	0.22	11.0	11.0
2 years	12.0	0.12	24/48	0.24	12.0	12.0
	13.0	0.13	26/52	0.26	13.0	13.0
3-4 years	14.0	0.14	28/56	0.28	14.0	14.0
	15.0	0.15	30/60	0.30	15.0	15.0
	16.0	0.16	32/64	0.32	16.0	16.0

Age	Weight	Low-dose Epinephrine (mg) 1:10,000 IV/IO [0.01 mg/kg]	Defibrillation (J/J) [2J/kg, initially/ 4J/kg]	Atropine (mg) [0.02 mg/kg] Max. dose: Child, 0.5 mg; Teen, 1.0 mg	Sodium Bicarbonate (mEq) [1 mEq/kg]	Lidocaine (mg) [1 mg/kg]
	17.0	0.17	34/68	0.34	17.0	17.0
5-6 years	18.0	0.18	36/72	0.36	18.0	18.0
	19.0	0.19	38/76	0.38	19.0	19.0
	20.0	0.20	40/80	0.40	20.0	20.0
7-8 years	22.5	0.23	45/90	0.45	22.5	22.5
	25.0	0.25	50/100	0.50	25.0	25.0
9-10 years	27.5	0.28	55/110	0.55	27.5	27.5
	30.0	0.30	60/120	0.60	30.0	30.0
	32.5	0.33	65/130	0.65	32.5	32.5
	35.0	0.35	70/140	0.70	35.0	35.0
	37.5	0.38	75/150	0.75	37.5	37.5
11-12 years	40.0	0.40	80/160	0.80	40.0	40.0
	42.5	0.43	85/170	0.85	42.5	42.5
12-13 years	45.0	0.45	90/180	0.90	45.0	45.0
	47.5	0.48	95/190	0.95	47.5	47.5
14-15 years	50.0	0.50	100/200	1.0	50.0	50.0

Age	Weight (kg)	Lidocaine Infusion (mg) [20–50 µg/min] Run at 2 mL/hr for 20 µg/min	Dobutamine or Dopamine Infusion (mg) [2–20 µg/kg/min] Run at 2 mL/kg/hr for 2 µg/kg/min	Epinephrine Infusion (mg) [0.1–1.0 µg/kg/min] Run at 1 mL/hr for 0.1 µg/kg/min
Premature	1.0	60.0	6.0	0.6
Neonate	2.0	120.0	12.0	1.2
	3.0	180.0	18.0	1.8
	4.0	240.0	24.0	2.4
	5.0	300.0	30.0	3.0
6 months	6.0	360.0	36.0	3.6
	7.0	420.0	42.0	4.2
	8.0	480.0	48.0	4.8
	9.0	540.0	54.0	5.4
1 year	10.0	600.0	60.0	6.0
	11.0	660.0	66.0	6.6
2 years	12.0	720.0	72.0	7.2
	13.0	780.0	78.0	7.8
3–4 years	14.0	840.0	84.0	8.4
	15.0	900.0	90.0	9.0
	16.0	960.0	96.0	9.6

Note: Each column lists the amount of the drug that must be added to diluent to make a 100 mL solution. Add 60 × body weight (kg) for lidocaine, 6 × body weight (kg) for dopamine or dobutamine, and 0.6 × body weight (kg) for epinephrine.

Age	Weight (kg)	Lidocaine Infusion (mg) [20–50 μg/kg/min] Run at 2 mL/hr for 20 μg/kg/min	Dobutamine or Dopamine Infusion (mg) [2 –20 μg/kg/min] Run at 2 mL/hr for 2 μg/kg/min	Epinephrine Infusion (mg) [0.1–1.0 μg/kg/min] Run at 1 mL/hr for 0.1 μg/kg/min
	17.0	1020.0	102.0	10.2
	18.0	1080.0	108.0	10.8
5-6 years	19.0	1140.0	114.0	11.4
	20.0	1200.0	120.0	12.0
	22.5	1350.0	135.0	13.5
7-8 years	25.0	1500.0	150.0	15.0
	27.5	1650.0	165.0	16.5
9-10 years	30.0	1800.0	180.0	18.0
	32.5	1950.0	195.0	19.5
	35.0	2100.0	210.0	21.0
	37.5	2250.0	225.0	22.5
	40.0	2400.0	240.0	24.0
11-12 years	42.5	2550.0	255.0	25.5
	45.0	2700.0	270.0	27.0
12-13 years	47.5	2850.0	285.0	28.5
14-15 years	50.0	3000.0	300.0	30.0

Note: Each column lists the amount of the drug that must be added to diluent to make a 100 mL solution. Add 60 × body weight (kg) for lidocaine, 6 × body weight (kg) for dopamine or dobutamine, and 0.6 × body weight (kg) for epinephrine.

Age	Weight (kg)	Adenosine (mg/mg) [0.1 mg/kg initially, then 0.2 mg/kg]	Bretylium (mg/mg) [5mg/kg / 10mg/kg]	Cardioversion (J) [0.5 J/kg, increasing to 2 J/kg]	Epinephrine (mg) 1:1000 SC [Asthma]	Diazepam (mg) [0.1–0.3 mg/kg]
Premature	1.0	0.1/0.2	5/10	0.5	0.01	0.1
	2.0	0.2/0.4	10/20	1.0	0.02	0.2
Neonate	3.0	0.3/0.6	15/30	1.5	0.03	0.3
	4.0	0.4/0.8	20/40	2.0	0.04	0.4
	5.0	0.5/1.0	25/50	2.5	0.05	0.5
	6.0	0.6/1.2	30/60	3.0	0.06	0.6
6 months	7.0	0.7/1.4	35/70	3.5	0.07	0.7
	8.0	0.8/1.6	40/80	4.0	0.08	0.8
	9.0	0.9/1.8	45/90	4.5	0.09	0.9
1 year	10.0	1.0/2.0	50/100	5.0	0.10	1.0
	11.0	1.1/2.2	55/110	5.5	0.11	1.1
2 years	12.0	1.2/2.4	60/120	6.0	0.12	1.2
	13.0	1.3/2.6	65/130	6.5	0.13	1.3
3-4 years	14.0	1.4/2.8	70/140	7.0	0.14	1.4
	15.0	1.5/3.0	75/150	7.5	0.15	1.5
	16.0	1.6/3.2	80/160	8.0	0.16	1.6

Please note the following maximum single doses: adenosine—12 mg, epinephrine (1:1000)—0.3 mg.

Age	Weight	Adenosine (mg/mg) [0.1 mg/kg initially, then 0.2 mg/kg]	Bretylium (mg/mg) [5mg/kg / 10mg/kg]	Cardioversion (J) [0.5 J/kg, increasing to 2 J/kg]	Epinephrine (mg) 1:1000 SC [Asthma]	Diazepam (mg) [0.1–0.3 mg/kg]
	17.0	1.7/3.4	85/170	8.5	0.17	1.7
5-6 years	18.0	1.8/3.6	90/180	9.0	0.18	1.8
	19.0	1.9/3.8	95/190	9.5	0.19	1.9
	20.0	2.0/4.0	100/200	10.0	0.20	2.0
	22.5	2.3/4.6	112.5/225	11.0	0.23	2.3
7-8 years	25.0	2.5/5.0	125/250	12.5	0.25	2.5
	27.5	2.8/5.6	137.5/275	14.0	0.28	2.8
9-10 years	30.0	3.0/6.0	150/300	15.0	0.30	3.0
	32.5	3.3/6.6	162.5/325	16.0	0.30	3.3
	35.0	3.5/7.0	175/350	17.5	0.30	3.5
	37.5	3.8/7.6	187.5/375	18.5	0.30	3.8
11-12 years	40.0	4.0/8.0	200/400	20.0	0.30	4.0
	42.5	4.3/8.6	212.5/425	21.0	0.30	4.3
12-13 years	45.0	4.5/9.0	225/450	22.5	0.30	4.5
	47.5	4.8/9.6	237.5/475	23.5	0.30	4.8
14-15 years	50.0	5.0/10.0	250/500	25.0	0.30	5.0

Please note the following maximum single doses: adenosine—12 mg, epinephrine (1:1000)—0.3 mg.

Appendix F
Pediatric Vital Signs
Advanced Airway Adjunct Sizes

Age	Heart Rate (bpm)	Respiratory Rate (bpm)	Systolic Blood Pressure (mm Hg)	Laryngoscope (Straight Blade Size)	Endotracheal Tube Size (Uncuffed Tube*)
Premature	100–190	40–60		0	2.0–2.5*
Neonate	90–190	30–60	50–70	0–1	3.0*
6 months	80–180	25–40	60–110	1	3.5–4.0*
1 year	80–150	20–40	70–110	2	4.0–4.5*
2 years				2	5.0*
3–4 years	80–140	20–30	80–115	2	5.0–5.5*
5–6 years	70–120	20–25	80–115	3	5.5–6.0*
7–8 years	70–110	20–25	85–120	3	6.0–6.5
9–10 years				3	6.5
10–11 years				3	6.5
11–12 years	60–110	15–20	95–135	3	6.5–7.0
12–13 years				3	7.0
14–15 years	55–100	12–20	110–140	3	7.0–7.5

American Academy of Pediatrics, American College of Emergency Physicians: APLS: The Pediatric Emergency Medicine Course, ed 2. 1993.

Guidelines for Cardiopulmonary Resuscitation and Emergency Cardiac Care. JAMA 268:2184–2198, 2251–2261, 1992.

Luten R: Pediatric Cardiopulmonary Resuscitation. In Tintinalli JE, Krome LR, and Ruiz E (eds): Emergency Medicine: A Comprehensive Study Guide, ed 3. McGraw-Hill, New York, 1992, 177–182.

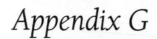

Appendix G

Intravenous Infusion Dosages for Hypoglycemia and Shock

Age	Weight (kg)	Lorazepam (mg) [0.05 mg/kg]	Naloxone Hydrochloride (mg) [0.1 mg/kg] Max. dose: 2 mg	Dextrose 25% (mL) [2 mL/kg]	Fluid Resuscitation Bolus (mL) [20 mL/kg]
Premature	1.0	0.05	0.1	2	10
	2.0	0.10	0.2	4	20
Neonate	3.0	0.15	0.3	6	30
	4.0	0.20	0.4	8	80
	5.0	0.25	0.5	10	100
	6.0	0.30	0.6	12	120
6 months	7.0	0.35	0.7	14	140
	8.0	0.40	0.8	16	160
	9.0	0.45	0.9	18	180
1 year	10.0	0.50	1.0	20	200
	11.0	0.55	1.1	22	220
2 years	12.0	0.60	1.2	24	240
	13.0	0.65	1.3	26	260
3-4 years	14.0	0.70	1.4	28	280
	15.0	0.75	1.5	30	300
	16.0	0.80	1.6	32	320

Age	Weight (kg)	Lorazepam (mg) [0.05 mg/kg]	Naloxone Hydrochloride (mg) [0.1 mg/kg] Max. dose: 2 mg	Dextrose 25% (mL) [2 mL/kg]	Fluid Resuscitation Bolus (mL) [20 mL/kg]
	17.0	0.85	1.7	34	340
5-6 years	18.0	0.90	1.8	36	360
	19.0	0.95	1.9	38	380
	20.0	1.00	2.0	40	400
7-8 years	22.5	1.12	2.0	45	450
	25.0	1.25	2.0	50	500
9-10 years	27.5	1.38	2.0	55	550
	30.0	1.50	2.0	60	600
	32.5	1.62	2.0	65	650
	35.0	1.75	2.0	70	700
	37.5	1.88	2.0	75	750
11-12 years	40.0	2.00	2.0	80	800
	42.5	2.12	2.0	85	850
12-13 years	45.0	2.25	2.0	90	900
	47.5	2.38	2.0	95	950
14-15 years	50.0	2.50	2.0	100	1000

Please note that the fluid resuscitation bolus is 10 mL/kg in premature infants and neonates.

Appendix H
**Lund and Browder
Rule of Nines Charts**

"Rule of Nines"
Burn Chart
Adult Body Surface Area

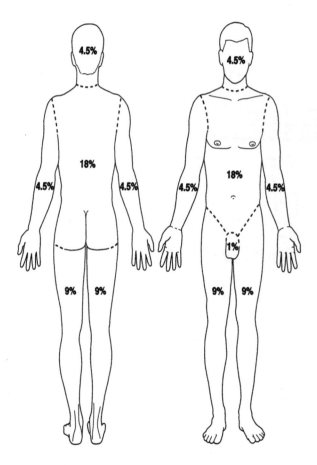

"Rule of Nines"
Burn Chart
Child Body Surface Area

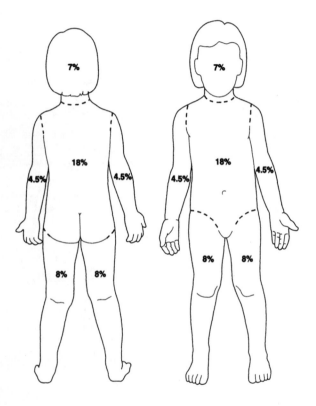

"Rule of Nines"
Burn Chart
Infant Body Surface Area

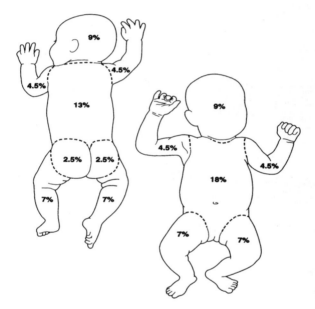

Index

Numbers followed by an *f* indicate figures; numbers followed by a *t* indicate tabular material.